Dr. Airola's
HANDBOOK OF NATURAL HEALING

HOW TO GET WELL

Other books by Dr. Paavo Airola

ARE YOU CONFUSED?

THERE IS A CURE FOR ARTHRITIS

HOW TO KEEP SLIM, HEALTHY AND YOUNG WITH JUICE FASTING

CANCER: CAUSES, PREVENTION AND TREATMENT —
    THE TOTAL APPROACH

STOP HAIR LOSS

SWEDISH BEAUTY SECRETS

WORLDWIDE SECRETS OF STAYING YOUNG

HYPOGLYCEMIA: A BETTER APPROACH

THE MIRACLE OF GARLIC

EVERYWOMAN'S BOOK

THE AIROLA DIET AND COOKBOOK

Published by
HEALTH PLUS, Publishers
P.O. Box 1027, Sherwood, Oregon 97140

Dr. Airola's

HANDBOOK OF NATURAL HEALING

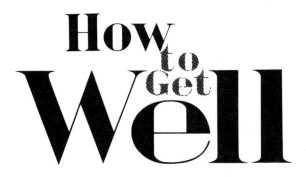

How to Get Well

Therapeutic uses of foods, vitamins, food supplements, juices, herbs, fasting, baths, and other ancient and modern nutritional and biological modalities in treatment of common ailments.

by PAAVO AIROLA, N.D.,Ph.D

With a Foreword by H. RUDOLPH ALSLEBEN, M.D.

MEDICAL EDITORS:

H. Rudolph Alsleben, M.D.
Barnet G. Meltzer, M.D.
Alan H. Nittler, M.D.

HEALTH PLUS, Publishers, Sherwood, Oregon

How To Get Well
Copyright © 1974 by
Paavo O. Airola, N.D., Ph.D.

1st printing, January, 1974
2nd printing, February, 1974
3rd printing, revised and updated edition, May, 1974
4th printing, November, 1974
5th printing, January, 1975
6th printing, completely revised edition, July, 1975
7th printing, revised edition, January, 1976
8th printing, revised edition, May, 1976
9th printing, August, 1976
10th printing, April, 1977
11th printing, August, 1977
12th printing, March, 1978
13th printing, October, 1978
14th printing, June, 1979
15th printing, September, 1979
16th printing, revised and updated edition, June 1980
17th printing, March, 1981
18th printing, May, 1982
19th printing, June, 1983
20th printing, March, 1985
21st printing, November, 1986
22nd printing, September, 1987
23rd printing, May, 1989

ISBN #0-932090-03-6
Printed in the United States of America

DEDICATED

to the multitudes who suffer and die needlessly — uninformed and unaware that simple, safe and effective means of correcting their ills and restoring health are available;

and to the small but growing number of brave, openminded and dedicated healers — a new breed of doctors — who with unprejudiced and inquiring minds search for the truth and, when and wherever they find it, have the courage to use it for the benefit of their patients — even if the truth happens to be contrary to the prevailing orthodox thinking and practices.

ACKNOWLEDGEMENTS

I wish to express my sincere thanks and indebtedness to the following doctors for their unselfish contribution and assistance in proofreading and editing the manuscript before publication, and for their most valuable expert advice regarding the various therapies presented herein:

H. Rudolph Alsleben, M.D.

Barnet G. Meltzer, M.D.

Alan H. Nittler, M.D.

My special thanks to my dear daughters, Anni Airola, B.S., R.D., and Karen and Paula Airola, whose love, cooperation, and personal sacrifices have helped make this book possible.

I also wish to thank my secretary, Karen Jensen, for her linguistic assistance in preparation of this work, — help as much appreciated as it was needed.

Last, but not least, I wish to publicly express my sincerest thanks and declare my eternal indebtedness to the Divine Creative Power, which inspired and helped me to conceive and create this book — my lifework — and endowed me with the knowledge, the courage, the strength, and the wisdom to execute it for the benefit and blessing of all those who suffer and seek help and comfort.

FOREWORD

by H. Rudolph Alsleben, M.D.

Dr. H. Rudolph Alsleben, M.D., is a founder of the Alsleben-Shute Foundation for Nutritional Research, a busy and respected director of his large clinic in Anaheim, California, and one of the leading pioneers of preventive medicine in the United States. He is also a dynamic speaker and a prolific writer, and the Editor and Publisher of the prestigious medical magazine for professionals and laymen — "THE ANSWER — Preventive Medicine". Dr. Alsleben is a co-author of a monumental book, "HOW TO SURVIVE THE NEW HEALTH CATASTROPHES", which is regarded as an important milestone in the treatment of degenerative diseases and particularly the health problems caused by heavy metal poisoning. Dr. H. Rudolph Alsleben is one of the pioneers in diagnostic uses of thermograph and the therapeutic uses of chelation — truly a giant among the growing number of medical doctors who have the courage to break away from the medical prejudice and the straightjacket of officially endorsed, conventional practices and let the welfare of their patients be their only consideration.

The Publishers thought that the following communication from Dr. Alsleben to Dr. Airola would make a fitting Foreword for the book.

Dear Paavo:

I have read your manuscript with great interest and considerable pride, because what you have accomplished fills a critical need in our society in these perilous times.

Your book is sensational! Any effort on my part to make revisions would only detract from the unique creativity that you possess. You will find a few minor corrections and suggestions on the margins of the manuscript.

This book is the beginning of a Science of Self-help, with which the public can sustain itself and more adequately select its medical purveyors.

I am so impressed with your exciting book, with the way in which you conceived and constructed it, with your fabulous and expert presentation of the philosophy of biological medicine, and with the common and academic sense that it makes, that I have changed my office sign in Anaheim, California, to read

H. Rudolph Alsleben, M.D.
Biological Medicine

Having been a practitioner in the area of Preventive Medicine for more than a decade, I, just as you have, see the need for people to help themselves in matters of health; and for those members of the medical community who are interested in nutritional and biological approaches to health and disease, the need for the authoritative guidance in the proper administration of the alternatives to the orthodox procedures, which your book so expertly provides.

Paavo, I remember one instance early in my professional career that bent my directions into a dedicated service to mankind.

Toward the end of my first year of practice, I received a telephone call in the early hours of the morning. The wife of one of my patients said, worriedly, that her husband was very ill and on his way to the hospital. Because his complaint was in the chest, I notified the intensive care personnel at the hospital and the attending heart specialist. When I arrived at the critical wing, the patient was under an oxygen tent. Intravenous fluids were running into his arms. Oscilloscopes and monitors were flashing and beeping. The cardiologist came away from the patient, and, as he passed me, he casually muttered, an unlighted cigar dangling from his lips:

"Sub-endocardial MI (myocardial infarction, heart attack), continue orders. I'll see him in the morning. Only 31 years old. Too bad . . " .

I walked to the bedside. Zipping open the flap of the oxygen tent, I leaned closely to the opening and said, with an air of surprised arrogance;

"Well, John, you've had a heart attack."

"How come, Doc? I've been coming to you for over a year now", said John with an obvious struggle and a puzzled look on his face.

We were all standing there watching our fallen comrade . . . me with embarrassment . . . his wife with panic . . . the nurses with the boredom of work . . . and the machines and monitors . . . My eyes were fixed on the heart monitor, watching for the patterns. I suddenly realized that my mind was impersonally playing with his life, I was looking for bad patterns, not good ones. I was expecting the worst, not the best. I could not stand it any longer.

I left, and as I walked down the long, tunnel-like, white corridor of the intensive care unit, I thought to myself:

— This man had hardening of the arteries. He was dying of a corruption of his blood vessels. It was growing in his body for 30 years. For all of his life, there was nothing done to avert this tragedy. No one advised him. No one warned or treated him. They merely waited until it was so bad that the patient told us of his problem by his collapse. He received no preventive care whatsoever. Now he had an "intensive care" — rather, an intensive watching. We, the doctors, the nurses, the family, and the machines, were simply watching him die.

This man's life could have been saved if the changes in his blood vessels had been diagnosed in advance. The critical developments could have been prevented by changes in his living and eating patterns and by other safe biological means.

Your book, Paavo, is a giant step in that direction.

I would be inclined to divide medical practice in this country into three parts. On the one hand we have acute and traumatic medicine: broken bones, gunshot wounds, acute illnesses such as flu and pneumonia — medicine is well-equipped to handle these problems. On the other hand, we have terminal, catastrophic diseases, such as cancers, sclerotic heart diseases, arthritis — medicine is well-equipped to handle these also . . . *Not* by helping them, but by writing death certificates.

In the middle, between these two extremes of acute and terminal illness, lies a gigantic no man's land where supposedly healthy people live, without "apparent" disease. And, according to that incredible philosophy of orthodox medicine, "you do not qualify for a *treatment* until you have a *disease*." These people must first become acutely ill or terminally sick before they can expect to find help from their medical purveyors. Medicine has *abandoned* these people and left them to their own devices to maintain health. But what devices do our people have?

None! Medicine has not equipped them with the useful knowledge to be able to maintain health and prevent disease — mainly because of medical ignorance in these vital areas. Much of the available so-called health literature is filled with faddist notions, contradictions, and unreliable "old wives tales", leaving the sincere health seeker in confusion and bewilderment.

There are but few informed and courageous leaders concerned with the well-being of the public; leaders who have not only dedicated their lives to helping their fellow men, but who have the sufficient knowledge and qualifications to accomplish this.

I am proud to tell you that I feel you to be one of those few, Paavo. By writing this book, you rendered a great service to a disease-ridden mankind. Well done.

I remain in sincerest gratitude,

H. Rudolph Alsleben, M.D.

PUBLISHER'S PREFACE

Health Plus Publishers is proud to present to the members of the healing professions, nutritionists, researchers, and students of these and allied fields, this comprehensive reference work on therapeutic uses of foods, vitamins, food supplements, juices, herbs, juice fasting, baths, heat therapies and other nutritional and biological modalities in the treatment of most common diseases. Both ancient methods of treatment, used effectively in folk medicine, as well as by ancient doctors, and modern drugless approaches based on recent scientific discoveries, are combined to form what is becoming known as *biological medicine.*

Biological medicine is a new, fast-growing branch of the healing science based on harmless nutritional and naturopathic methods of correcting disease and restoring health. A growing number of progressive medical doctors, particularly in Europe, are moving from the Pasteurian concept of disease and symptomatic drug-therapy approach towards a new concept of medicine — the total approach of treating the whole man. Biological medicine is a healing science based on the philosophy that most, if not all, diseases are of man's own making and are the end result of a long-time abuse in the form of wrong living habits, faulty nutritional patterns and other health-destroying environmental factors. New medical thinking is directed towards a concept of man as a whole entity with his physical and emotional aspects inseparably unified in one living soul. It sees man as an organic part of the biological and cosmic universe and subject to the unchangeable and irrevocable laws of nature. Man's disregard of these laws in respect to his ecological environment, nutritional, physical and emotional needs leads to disharmony with the life-giving and health-sustaining biological and spiritual universe. *Disease is a consequent result of this disharmony.*

Biological medicine is based on the principle of intelligent support of the natural healing and health-restorative powers inherent in the living organism. Although drugs have their place in medical practice, they never eliminate the basic causes of disease — at best they only suppress or alleviate the symptoms. Lasting results can be obtained only when a wise doctor assists and supports the body's own healing forces which institute the health-restoring processes and accomplish the actual cure.

Nutritional and biological therapies, as presented in this work, are directed at correcting the underlying causes of disease, strengthening the patient's resistance to disease and creating the most favorable conditions for the body's own healing processes to take place.

Biological medicine is not opposed to *any* of the healing systems, including the allopathic (medical). The nutritional and biological treatments presented in this work are not intended to *replace* the other conventional approaches to healing — medical, chiropractic, homeopathic, spiritual, etc. — but are to be used as a vital adjunct to other forms and methods of healing, *as supportive programs aimed at improving the patient's biological milieu and supporting and speeding up the body's own healing processes.*

Paavo O. Airola, N.D., Ph.D., the author of this monumental work, is the leading exponent of biological and nutritional medicine in the United States. He first introduced the concept of Biological Medicine into the United States in 1968 with his award-winning book, "There *IS* a Cure for Arthritis", followed by many other books on various aspects of health and disease. Dr. Airola is an internationally heralded nutritionist, naturopathic physician and an acknowledged authority on natural healing. He is a member of the *International Society For Research on Diseases of Civilization, Nutrition and Environment,* the most respected nutrition research organization in the world, which was founded by Dr. Albert Schweitzer. He is also a member of the British Society of Drugless Practitioners and of the International Naturopathic Association.

The priceless information in this publication is based on Dr. Airola's lifelong research of available data from various research centers and biological clinics, and the ancient and modern medical, naturopathic, nutritional and herbal literature. It is also based in part on his own clinical work and experience as a nutritional consultant and director of naturopathic and nutritional therapies in various biological clinics.

Never before has such an incredible amount of vital, authoritative and useful information on all aspects of nutritional and drugless approach to health and disease been assembled in one volume. It is truly an *ABZ of natural healing;* a comprehensive *reference work* on biological and nutritional approaches to disease; a *modern encyclopedia* in a nutshell on such vital areas of healing science as vitaminology, medicinal foods, juices, herbs, hydrotherapy, fasting, etc. It is *the first* practical and useful manual and reference book for doctors, researchers, nutritionists, teachers, nutrition consultants, and other related professions.

We are confident that even a quick glance through this volume will convince the reader — as it did us — that this is, without comparison, *the most important manual on all aspects of natural healing ever published.* Because of the wealth of authoritative and reliable information, and also because of its easy-to-read quick-reference format, this book is destined to become the most useful and treasured reference work not only for the members of the healing profession, but for all sincere students of health, nutrition, and natural healing.

Health Plus Publishers

TABLE OF CONTENTS

Introduction

HOW TO USE THIS BOOK

PART ONE of this book lists alphabetically most common diseases and disorders and shows how each condition can be treated with special nutritional considerations, diets, fasting, special vitamins and supplements, herbs, juices, therapeutic baths, and other harmless biological methods. This unique compilation is the result of several decades of research and study, and was originally made for my own private and exclusive use in my practice. However, so many doctors, nutritionists, and students expressed their desire to have an access to these records, that I decided to publish them. I was assured by all those who have seen the records that making them public would not only greatly contribute to the better public health and the renaissance of natural healing, but would be of immeasurable help to doctors and other health-oriented professions, researchers, and students. I sincerely hope that this work will meet their expectations.

FOOTNOTE numbers in *PART ONE* refer to *Directions* in *PART THREE* of the book, where description and complete, detailed instructions regarding nutritional, herbal and other therapies recommended in *PART ONE*, are given.

PART TWO of the book contains effective protective measures against common poisons in food, water, air, and environment, which are so vital in this age of universal pollution.

PART FOUR contains recipes for special foods and dietary supplements recommended in this book.

Finally, *PART FIVE* contains vitamins and mineral charts, an acid-alkaline food chart, Official Recommended Daily Allowances for vitamins and minerals, tables of Food Composition and other useful charts.

It is obvious that *PART ONE* — The Therapeutic Uses of Foods, Vitamins, Food Supplements, Juices, Herbs and Other Biological Modalities — will be the most read, studied and used section of this book, the other material being accessory and complementary.

Please understand that this is a *condensed* encyclopedia-like manual, which, for the lack of space, cannot be considered a complete treatise on each disease. Each condition would require a complete book in itself in order to give a proper evaluation of all its aspects and to outline a complete detailed program of treatment. To assist doctors, researchers and students, the additional relevant referential reading material is suggested for every condition.

The readers and users of this manual should keep in mind the following important points:

1. The New Biological Concept of Health and Disease

The rapid development of the chemical and physical sciences in the last two centuries has had a most negative influence upon medical thinking, and slowed down the progress of healing arts. In spite of all the bravura and ballyhoo about *our great medical progress*, when, in the enlightened future, the true medical history will be written, the twentieth century will be known as *the dark ages of the healing art*. Unbelievable as it may seem, the twentieth century concept of disease is not much different from the primitive voodoo concept. The only difference is that the "evil spirits" have been replaced with "evil germs", bacteria or virus, which attack the unfortunate and undeserving man. We believe that disease "strikes" the unsuspecting and totally innocent bodies. We talk about diseases as being "caught". We speak of evil creatures — the germs — as "going around", attacking every man in their way. The job of the modern medicine-man is to kill or drive out the evil intruders, the germ or virus, with the magic medical power from his medicine bottle or injection needle, and, thus, save the innocent victim from the vicious attack.

The new Biological Medicine takes an exception from such a Pasteurian concept of disease and the symptomatic drug-therapy approach to the treatment of disease. The biological concept of medicine is based on the irrefutable physiological fact that the primary cause of disease is not the bacteria or virus, but the *weakened resistance* brought about by man's health-destroying living habits and physical and emotional stresses. *The bacteria enter the picture only in its final stage*, as THE UNDERTAKER of the natural order, to complete and fulfill the natural law of "returning to dust" again the organism that was made unfit to live.

Bacteria are always present in our environment, as well as in a latent state in every cell of all living organisms. They are completely harmless if the organism maintains its natural health and natural resistance – but ever-ready to step in and destroy the host organism as soon as its life- force, vitality and resistance are lowered.

2. The Basic Cause of Disease

The basic premise of Biological Medicine is that most diseases have the same basic underlying causes. These are: the systemic derangement and biochemical and metabolic disorder brought about by prolonged physical and mental stresses to which the patient has been subjected – such as faulty nutritional patterns, constant overeating, overindulgence in proteins and the body's inability to properly digest them, nutritional deficiencies, sluggish metabolism and consequent retention of toxic metabolic wastes, exogenous poisons from polluted food, water, air and environment, toxic drugs, tobacco and alcohol, lack of sufficient exercise, rest and relaxation, severe emotional and physical stresses, etc. These health-destroying environmental factors bring about derangement in all vital body functions with consequent biochemical imbalance in the tissues, autotoxemia, chronic undersupply of oxygen to the cells, poor digestion and ineffective assimilation of nutrients ... *and gradually lowered resistance to disease.* Thus the Biological Medicine considers not the bacteria but the *weakened organism or the lowered resistance* as the primary cause of disease. Bacteria is more often than not, the *result* of disease, not its *cause.*

Therefore, the only effective way to cure the disease is to *eliminate the causes of disease.* All these underlying causes of ill health, mentioned above, must be corrected and eliminated before health can be restored. When, with proper assistance and support of optimum nutrition, special dietary factors, cleansing programs, specific vitamins and supplements, juices, herbs and other harmless therapies, the underlying causes of ill health are removed, the symptoms (diseases) will disappear. *Not because we cured them, but because there would be no more reason for their existence.* The health has been restored.

3. Disease – Our Misunderstood Friend

Our body is equipped with the most extensive and intricate defensive and healing system. When we violate the elementary laws of health or subject our body to severe stresses or other adverse environmental factors, our body reacts with *self-defense.* With various defensive acute symptoms, such as pain, fever, diarrhea, fatigue or loss of appetite, the body will signal that it has taken the defensive action aimed at restoring the condition of health. But in our ignorance, we totally misunderstand these warning and healing symptoms, calling them "diseases". Instead of letting the fever, the proper rest and temporary abstinence from food accomplish the health-restoring goal for which the body had initiated these symptoms, we suppress the fever with medicines, we eliminate the pain with drugs and we try to feed the sick with as much "nourishing food" as possible to get him well soon. Thus, we counteract and break down the body's own defensive and healing efforts and cause it serious damage. Now the condition may have changed from the acute into chronic. As we continue to interfere with the body's own healing activity, the more serious chronic condition, such as elevated blood pressure, inflammations, immobility of joints, hardening of the arteries, skin eruptions, even tumors, may develop. Even these conditions, however, are not "diseases" as we understand them — the negative conditions that must be suppressed or eliminated — but are our body's own, often desperate, but nevertheless positive and beneficial attempts to cope with increasingly adverse conditions and protect the organism from the total destruction.

4. Disease — Nature's Way to Get You Well

Thus disease, as we know it, is a self-defensive effort of the body to restore the impaired health. Disease is not a negative condition which should be combatted and suppressed ("cured") with all available means, but a *positive, constructive process* initiated by the body's healing forces and aimed at restoring health. Unbelievable as it may sound, we actually need disease to get well! When the body becomes ill, only the disease (which more correctly should be called health-restoring activity) can bring it back to health again. Thus we do not cure a disease, but cure a sick body, and restore health — *often with the help of disease!* — which is nothing but nature's own way of getting you well!

5. The Basic Treatment of Disease

Since most conditions of ill health are systemic in their origin and have the same underlying causes, the basic treatment of all disease is likewise the same.

First, all the underlying causes of disease must be eliminated — health-destroying causes that produced ill health, such as nutritional, physical and emotional stresses and abuses. After that, the patient should undergo a short cleansing juice fast (see *Directions: 3*) to assist the body in throwing off all the accumulated toxins and wastes. Then the patient should be put on a special supportive health-restoring and vitality-building program with emphasis on optimum nutrition (see *Directions: 1*), specific vitamins, supplements, herbs and juices and other supportive biological treatments such as hydrotherapy, massage, manipulative treatments (if needed), exercises, etc., which will help the body's own healing forces to accomplish the restoration of health. In every case, the biological doctor must outline the therapeutic program individually; it must be adjusted to the specific individual needs and the condition of the patient.

6. Relaxation and Peace of Mind — Prime Consideration

There are many factors that interfere with successful application of nutritional and biological therapies, such as: toxic environment; ineffective digestive and assimilative system; emotional stresses; anxiety, worries, fears, etc. If the patient is under a severe stress of acute anxiety, his ability to absorb and utilize nutritional and medicinal factors will be seriously impaired, and the expected healing will not manifest as long as the emotional disturbance continues to act.

Therefore, the prime consideration should be given to help the patient to free himself from all emotional stresses and worries and acquire a state of total relaxation and peace of mind. This is absolutely imperative in order to make nutritional and biological therapies effective.

Also, the patient should have a thorough understanding of the basic philosophy of biological medicine and of the purpose of various nutritional and other therapies, and have a complete confidence and faith in the prescribed methods of treatment. Thus, educating the patient in regard to the basic laws of health and disease and how he can stay well and prevent disease, should be a most important work of a future biological doctor.

7. The Total Approach

Since the basic goal of Biological Medicine is to help and support the body's own healing activity, we advocate the *total approach* when the therapeutic program is considered. Not just this or that specific vitamin, herb or treatment, but a total combined attack on all fronts, from all directions, *at the same time.* After the thorough study of patient's background and his living and eating habits is made, and possible underlying causes of his health condition are determined, the patient's own healing and health-restoring mechanism should be assisted with all the available effective and harmless means, simultaneously: optimum diet, specific herbs and nutritive supplements, juices, vitamins, minerals, etc., which are known to be effective for his specific condition. In my experience, such *TOTAL APPROACH* brings about the fastest recovery.

8. Vitamins and Supplements

The suggested vitamins and food supplements are listed *in order of importance*, beginning with the most important for each condition — although in many (perhaps most) cases this may be considered superfluous as several vitamins or supplements can be of equal importance.

In most cases, the usual therapeutic dosage is given for each supplement. (The dosage specified is for adults and children over 12 years of age. Younger children should receive less at the doctor's discretion.) It should be kept in mind, however, that this is only a *usual* dosage, based on records of what most nutritionally-oriented doctors or nutritionists prescribe to their patients. Practitioners should never forget that there is a great difference in every patient's response to vitamins and other nutrients, depending on his condition, age, nutritional stature, his special personal needs, his ability to assimilate nutrients, the mineral content of the water he drinks, the degree of toxicity in his environment, his emotional health, etc. The doctor, upon careful examination and nutritional and metabolic evaluation of the patients condition, must determine the exact dosage and the duration of vitamin therapy.

(For more details on Vitamin Therapy, see *Directions: 2.* For commonly used therapeutic doses of vitamins and minerals see also the Vitamin and Mineral Guides in Part Five: *Charts and Tables.*)

9. "Specific" Vitamins

Please keep in mind that although only a few vitamins and food supplements are named as *specific* for any one condition, virtually in every condition of ill health the Optimum Diet should be supplemented with *all* the known vitamins and minerals, but particularly with the adequate amounts of vitamin C, A, B-complex and E. Also, kelp, brewer's yeast, lecithin, mineral supplement, as well as a moderate amount of raw fruit and vegetable juices, should be a part of virtually every effective nutritional therapeutic program (see *Directions: 2*).

10. Natural Vitamins and Supplements Preferable

If possible, only the natural vitamins (vitamin complexes), made from the natural sources, should be used, and not synthetic products. This is especially important in regard to various isolated B-vitamins.

Exception: when massive doses of some vitamins are required, particularly of vitamin C and B, synthetic vitamins can be used, but always in combination with a certain amount of natural vitamins or vitamin-rich supplements. Example: synthetic B-vitamins combined with brewer's yeast; or ascorbic acid combined with rose hips or fruit juices.

11. The Length of Vitamin Therapy

For some conditions, vitamins in massive doses are suggested. Such treatments should not exceed 1 or 2 months. If needed, the vitamin treatment may be repeated after 1 or 2 month interval. This warning is given only in regard to massive doses of vitamins A, D, and synthetic isolated vitamins of B-complex.

For other important instructions on how to use and administer vitamins therapeutically, see *Directions: 2.*

12. Specifics

Under *specifics* are listed those foods, vitamins, herbs, juices and other treatments which have been found in ancient and modern practice to be of specific value and benefit for the listed condition.

13. Herbs

Specific herbs are listed for most conditions. These herbs have been found by ancient and modern practice to possess specific health-restorative medicinal properties for the condition mentioned. In compiling this information I have used dozens of reliable herbal books from around the world. I have also had my own lifelong personal experience of collecting and using medicinal herbs therapeutically.

The most common way to use herbs is a form of tea, or what is known professionally as *infusions.*

(For detailed instructions on how to make herb teas, and on other ways to use herbs therapeutically, see *Directions: 6.*)

Most herbs mentioned are available from regular health food stores in dry and packaged form ready to use. They are also available from herb houses.

14. Notes

At the end of each section on disease or condition, a blank space is left marked *NOTES:.* Doctors, researchers and students can use this space to list additional remedies, facts and latest discoveries related to this condition which they come across.

Also, the author will appreciate it if readers and researchers will send him, in c/o the Publishers, the proven nutritional and other biological treatments they know of that are not mentioned in this book, since this work will be periodically revised and updated.

15. Healing Crisis

It has been the general observation of biological doctors, as well as my own experience, that nutritional and biological therapies, as described in this manual, almost always result in a rapid and striking improvement in the condition of the patient. However, it is not uncommon that a fasting and cleansing diet will sometimes (in fact, quite often!) result in an *apparent change for the worse.* This is particularly true in chronic conditions characterized by massive accumulation of toxic wastes in the tissues. In such case, the patient will get *temporarily* worse, before getting better. The reason for this is that a juice fasting and a cleansing diet of raw vegetables and fruits will dissolve huge amounts of accumulated toxins and debris and throw them into the blood stream for elimination. The eliminative organs — kidneys, liver, lungs, and skin — will be overloaded with work. This may result in so-called "healing crises", manifested by some temporary worsening of the condition and such unpleasant symptoms of excessive elimination as headaches, bad breath, skin eruptions, catarrhal discharge, fever, etc. In arthritis, such rapid cleansing may activate biochemical changes in the joints so fast that increased pain and a noticeable worsening of the condition can be observed.

These healing crises are, fortunately, only temporary. Eventually, the patient will experience a definite improvement as the body will cleanse itself of the accumulated poisons and become strong enough to initiate an effective healing activity. In cases of extreme toxic condition, especially in cases of severe arthritis and gout, repeated short fasts of 3 to 4 days are advised instead of longer fasts. This will prevent the "healing crisis" caused by a too rapid elimination.

16. No "Cures" Offered

The nutritional and biological modalities — diets, vitamins, juices, herbs, etc. — reported in this book, are not offered as *cures* for disease, but only as supportive means of helping the body's own inherent healing forces and assisting its own healing activity. I wish to stress the fact that no food, no vitamin, no herb — and, for that matter, no drug! — can ever cure disease. Disease can be cured only by the body's own healing and health-restoring power. *The suggested programs are aimed at helping the body's healing mechanism by eliminating the causes of disease and creating the most favorable conditions for the body's own healing forces to bring about the actual cure.*

17. Biological Medicine — the Healing Art of the Future

This brings to mind a "Definition of a Doctor: A man who entertains a patient with stories while Nature performs the cure". Actually the true doctor must do more than that. He must teach the patient how to increase his resistance against disease and prevent future illness by improved ways of eating and living. He must be an expert in not only treatment of *disease*, but in instructing his patient how to build a vigorous and glowing *health* of body and mind. This is a definition of a new breed of doctor, the doctor of the future, the *Doctor of Biological Medicine.*

Therefore, it behooves all practitioners of healing arts, be it allopathic, naturopathic, osteopathic, homeopathic, or chiropractic, to familiarize themselves with the therapeutic uses of foods, vitamins, minerals, herbs and juices, and to use this new knowledge in the management of their patients. Both doctors and patients should keep in mind that:

*"If doctors of today will not become the nutritionists
of tomorrow —
The nutritionists of today will become the doctors
of tomorrow".*

For too long the official medicine has ignored nutrition as the valid factor in causation and treatment of disease. But the truth cannot be ignored indefinitely — it will invariably come out into the open. And the indisputable truth, which is coming forth more convincingly with each passing year, is that *nutrition is singularly the most important factor affecting health and disease.*

This fact is now being universally recognized by all responsible and open-minded scientists, as well as by laymen. This is so self-evident that it is incomprehensible how our modern medical "science" can continue to insist that "what you eat has nothing to do with your health". Nutrients are what the human body has to work with in building and maintaining healthy cells, tissues, glands and organs. Nutrients are used in the operation of all bodily functions. There is not an action in the body, be it enzymatic, metabolic, hormonal, mental, nervous, physical or chemical that does not require specific nutrients for its performance. The healing mechanism is an elaborate system within the body, and it can perform healing miracles — but only if it is abundantly supplied with all the special nutritional factors it needs. *There simply could be no healing without proper nutrition*! Nutrition is, unquestionably, the most important factor in building and maintaining health and correcting disease. All the other modalities, be it drugs, surgery, manipulations, acupuncture, hydro-electro-magneto-therapy — you name it! — can be useful and have their place in the arsenal of treatments, but they will fail in most cases *unless the corrective and supportive nutritional therapy is given priority.*

It is my sincere hope that this work will contribute to the advancement of nutritional and biological medicine and the art of natural healing in this disease-ridden world. I hope that many can benefit from it; that it will become a useful reference book for the practitioners of various healing professions, helping them in the management of their patients; and that it will be a blessing to all — both professionals and sincere students of health — who are earnestly seeking the information leading to better health . . . the *natural, drugless way.*

Paavo Airola

PART ONE

HOW TO GET WELL

THERAPEUTIC USES OF FOODS, VITAMINS, FOOD SUPPLEMENTS, JUICES, HERBS, FASTING, BATHS AND OTHER ANCIENT AND MODERN NUTRITIONAL AND BIOLOGICAL MODALITIES IN TREATMENT OF COMMON DISEASES.

IMPORTANT NOTES

1.   The information in this section is intended for use by nutritionally and biologically oriented physicians, naturopaths, and members of other healing professions, as well as for researchers and students engaged in scientific research in the field of nutrition and biological medicine.

In recommending certain diets and vitamins in large doses, food supplements, juices, herbs, etc., we do not diagnose or prescribe, but offer this information purely for educational and experimental purposes. The following information must be viewed as an objective compilation of existing data and research, without the author's or publisher's endorsement. Patients who suffer from serious illnesses, should use the information in this publication in cooperation with their doctor (preferably a nutritionally-oriented doctor), and abide by his decision regarding the advisability of using the suggested therapies for their specific condition. In the event the reader of this volume uses the information without the approval of his doctor, he is prescribing for himself, and assuming the responsibility for it, which is his constitutional right to do; but the author and the publishers assume no responsibility. Likewise, the members of the healing professions, who will use the information in this book in treatment of their patients, must assume the full responsibility for the results — the author and the publisher are only supplying the printed material for educational and experimental purposes, and assume no responsibility in regard to effectiveness, or possible harm incurred through correct or incorrect application of described therapies.

2.   Nutritional, herbal, naturopathic and other biological therapies described in this section are not offered as an *alternative* to orthodox medical, osteopathic, homeopathic, or chiropractic approach to treat disease, but rather as an *adjunct* to the conventional treatments — a supportive program that can be used in combination or addition to other therapies, if desired. Biological medicine does not oppose or contradict the orthodox forms of healing — it rather complements them.

3. Neither the author nor the publishers of this book are in any way connected with the health food manufacturing or retailing industry, actively or inactively; *they do not sell vitamins or other supplements which are recommended or mentioned in this book*, and they do not own or operate any health food stores.

4. This book, or any part thereof, must not be used by anyone to advertise, promote or sell products, foods, vitamins or supplements mentioned or recommended in this book.

5. This publication in its totality, including the content, the information, the specific format and the unique idea of presentation is copyrighted with the United States and World Copyright Offices. All rights are strictly reserved. No part of this publication, and particularly no part of this section on therapeutic uses of foods, vitamins, herbs, food supplements and other biological modalities, may be reproduced or transmitted in any form or by any means, electronic or mechanical, including photocopy, recording, or any other information storage and retrival system without permission in writing from the publishers.

6. To our knowledge, all of the vitamins, supplements and herbs mentioned by the author are available in most health food stores — if not, health food stores should be able to advise as to where they can be obtained. Doctors may obtain all the mentioned vitamins and other supplements from their usual professional supply sources.

7. There is a growing demand for nutritionally-oriented doctors among the rapidly growing nutrition-conscious public. There is also a growing number of doctors and clinics who specialize in nutritional and biological therapies similar to those described in this book. To help both readers and practitioners, the author is compiling a list of biologically-oriented doctors and clinics in the U.S., Canada, Mexico and Europe, and will send it on request. Please address your inquiries to the author in care of the publisher, enclosing a self-addressed, stamped envelope.

8. Again, the nutritional and biological approach to the treatment of disease — diets, vitamins, juices, herbs, etc. — as reported in the following pages, are not offered as *cures* for

disease, but only as *supportive* means of helping the body's own inherent healing forces and *assisting* the body's own healing activity, by eliminating the underlying causes of disease and creating the most favorable conditions for the body's own healing power to bring about the actual cure. In other words, the reported natural therapies are aimed at *helping the body to heal itself.*

And, since every individual's reponse to vitamins, special foods and other nutritional therapies is greatly different, depending on his specific condition, individual requirements and needs, age, health stature, his ability to assimilate nutrients, his emotional health, etc., etc., *we again stress the importance of using the information in this book in cooperation with a nutritionally-oriented doctor and abiding by his decision regarding the advisability of using the suggested therapies for any specific condition. The information contained in this book is presented for general education purposes only. It is not intended to be a substitute for specific medical advice, which the reader can obtain only from a qualified and reliable doctor.*

Neither the author nor the publisher assume responsibility or liability for any consequences of the failure of the reader to obtain such specific medical advice from a qualified doctor, nor for any consequences of the reader attempting to treat his own health problems using any or all of the information contained in this book.

ACNE

DIETARY CONSIDERATIONS

Emphasis should be on raw foods, especially fresh fruits and vegetables and sprouted seeds, such as alfalfa seeds and soy beans, and whole grain cereals, especially millet and brown rice. Avoid animal proteins, including milk. Avoid excess fat in the diet, especially animal fats. Eliminate all sweets, even chocolate, and all refined and processed foods. Avoid all soft drinks, candies, ice cream and everything made with sugar and white flour.

BIOLOGICAL TREATMENTS

1. Begin with a detoxifying and cleansing juice fast for one week (see *Directions: 3*).
2. Expose the face to the sun and fresh air as often as possible.
3. Wash face with mild soap (castile, Ivory) morning and evening.
4. Do not use commercial shampoos; mild soaps are also excellent for hair.
5. Before going to bed, massage *Formula F Plus* into face (see *Directions: 8*).
6. If constipated, follow the anti-constipation program (see section on *Constipation*).
7. Get plenty of rest and sleep.
8. Avoid most commercial cosmetics, lotions, creams, etc. *Acne Cosmetica*, acne caused by cosmetic preparations, is a well known clinical fact.
9. Use vitamin A acid preparation, applied topically (see *Notes*).
10. Since acne is always worsened by emotional stress and imbalance, the total relaxation and peace of mind are essential.

VITAMINS & SUPPLEMENTS (Daily)

A — 50,000 to 150,000 units daily for one month (doses over 50,000 units under doctor's supervision only)

E — 200 to 400 IU

Zinc gluconate — 30 mg.

Niacin — 300 mg.; 100 mg. three times daily, with meals

B-complex, natural, high potency

C — 1,000 mg.

Dolomite — 2 tablets. Bone meal — 2 tablets.

Chlorophyl — 3 tablets

F — essential fatty acids (unrefined vegetable oils) — 1 tbsp. of cold-pressed soy bean oil, sesame oil or flaxseed oil

Natural multi-vitamin-mineral formula

JUICES

Any available fresh fruit and vegetable juices, except citrus juices. Juices must be freshly made, not canned.

HERBS

Dandelion, burdock, red clover, golden seal, chaparral.

SPECIFICS

Niacin, vitamins A and E, chlorophyl tablets, vitamin A acid, sugar- and fat-free diet.

REFERENTIAL READING

Lubowe, Irwin I., *"The Modern Guide to Skin Care and Beauty"*, E. P. Dutton & Co., Inc., N.Y. 1973.

Lubowe, Irwin I., *New Hope for Your Skin.*

Rodale, J. I., *The Encyclopedia of Healthful Living*, Rodale Books, Inc., Emmaus, Penna.

Editors of Prevention, *The Natural Way to A Healthy Skin*, Rodale Books, Inc., Emmaus, Penna.

British Medical Journal, Dec. 16, 1967.

Bicknell and Prescott, *Vitamins in Medicine*, Grune And Stratton, 1953.

Alsleben, H. Rudolph, "Help for Teenage Acne", *The Answer, Preventive Medicine*, Vol. 1, No. 7, 1973.

Plewig, G., et al., *Archives of Dermatology*, March, 1970.

Prevention, March, 1973.

NOTES:

1. Two vitamins have been used successfully to treat acne: *number one, niacin*, 100 mg. three times daily (*niacin*, which produces facial flush, has been found to be more effective than *niacinamide* for this purpose), and, *number two, vitamin A* in large doses up to 150,000 units per day. The length of the treatment for both vitamins should not exceed one month.

2. The following healing packs or masks, used externally, have been reported to be effective: a) grated cucumbers; b) oatmeal cooked in milk; c) a mixture of sulphur and black molasses; d) cooked, creamed carrots. Masks are left on for one-half hour, then washed off with cold water.

3. Washing the affected area with lemon juice has been shown to be helpful.

4. Lotion containing the female hormone, estrogen, is used by some doctors with reported success. Treatment should continue several months.

5. Vitamin A acid (0.1 percent concentration) has been used successfully by doctors of the University of Pennsylvania Acne Clinic in a several-years long study. Vitamin A acid, applied topically, has been shown to be equally effective in curing and preventing acne. It is marketed under the name Retin-A and available only by prescription. (Results of this study were presented at the 1968 annual AMA convention in San Francisco.) Several doctors reported to me that they have found Retin-A to be effective.

ALCOHOLISM

High prevalence of alcoholism in western countries is characterized mainly by malnutrition and nutritional deficiencies due to overprocessed and refined nutritionless foods. Nutritional deficiencies lead to such alcoholism-predisposing conditions as hypoglycemia, adrenal insufficiency, chronic fatigue, craving for a "lift" — sweets, snacks, drinks, etc. Excessive drinking creates a vicious cycle by further depleting the body of vitamins and leading to severe deficiencies in B-complex vitamins, especially in B_1 and B_6. Alcohol depletes body of zinc and magnesium.

The most effective way to cure alcoholism is by building the body's nutritional integrity to a state where the need for a "lift" will be eliminated.

DIETARY CONSIDERATIONS

The Airola Diet, the optimum diet of vital nutrition (see *Directions: 1*), with special supplements, is imperative. Emphasis is on whole grains, raw nuts and seeds, fresh fruits and vegetables. Avoid meat and all refined and processed foods, especially white sugar and white flour. Eat several small meals a day in preference to two or three large meals.

BIOLOGICAL TREATMENTS

1. First, it would be advisable to put the patient on a 10-14 day cleansing juice fast (see *Directions: 3*). Since during fasting there is usually no craving for alcohol even for severe alcoholics, this gives a good 2-week start toward breaking the drinking habit, thus helping remove not only the physical dependence, but also the psychogenic factors.

   After the initial fast, the Airola Diet is used, as above.

   It is advisable that in the beginning of the treatment, the patient is given a suitable substitute to relieve the craving if and when such craving occurs. The best substitute drink for the alcoholic is 1 glass of fresh fruit juice, sweetened with honey if needed. If this is inconvenient, eating wholesome candy, such as halva or others that can be bought in health food stores (and easily carried in the pocket) can be recommended. The patient should always have easily available juices, candy or other snacks to take between meals if he feels a craving for a lift.

2. Plenty of indoor and outdoor exercises. This will improve circulation, the general health, and normalize the activity of the hypothalamus, the appetite center of the brain.

3. Plenty of rest.

VITAMINS & SUPPLEMENTS (Daily)

Glutamine — 2-3 grams

B-complex, high potency, natural

B_3 — in form of niacinamide, 100 mg.

B_6 — 100 mg.

Brewer's yeast — 2-3 tbsp.

C — up to 3,000 mg., or more

A — 25,000 units

D — 1,000 units

E — up to 1,200 IU

Zinc — 60 mg.

Magnesium supplement — up to 1,000 mg.

Multi-vitamin-mineral-enzyme formula

Betaine hydrochloride, 1 or 2 tablets, after large meals

JUICES

Any fresh fruit and vegetable juices, in season.

SPECIFICS

B-complex, B_6, B_3, magnesium, glutamine, brewer's yeast. Juice fasting. Optimum nutrition.

REFERENTIAL READING

Williams, Roger J., *Nutrition Against Disease*, Pitman Publishers, Corp., N.Y., 1972.

Williams, Roger J., *Alcoholism, Nutritional Approach*, University of Texas Press, 1959.

Lovell, Harold W., *Hope and Help for the Alcoholic*, Doubleday, N.Y.

Abrahamson, E. M., and Pezet, A. W., *Body Mind and Sugar*, Holt, Rinehart and Winston, 1951.

Trulson, M. F., et al., "Vitamin Medication in Alcoholism", *The Journal of the American Medical Association*, 155:114, 1954.

Alsleben, H. Rudolph and Shute, Wilfred E., *How to Survive the New Health Catastrophes*, Survival Publications, Inc., Anaheim, Ca. 1973.

Heaton, F. W., et al., "Hypomagnesemia in Chronic Alcoholism", *Lancet*, 2:802, 1962.

In my opinion, most allergies are the result of feeding babies such foods as cereals, meat, whole cow's milk, etc., before they reach the age of 10-12 months. Before that age, babies lack proper enzymes needed for the digestion of these foods, which causes allergic reactions. Babies raised on mother's milk alone (provided mother is healthy) until the age of at least 8 months, most likely will not develop allergies later in life, unless subjected to severe malnutrition or an extremely toxic environment.

Another common cause of allergies is today's processed foods loaded with thousands of chemical additives, many of which are powerful causes of allergy. Those who have allergic sensitivities should avoid all foods that might possibly contain chemical additives or residues, and eat only organically produced foods free from man-made chemicals.

DIETARY CONSIDERATIONS

The Airola Diet (see *Directions: 1*) with emphasis on whole grains, seeds and nuts and raw fruits and vegetables, all organically grown. Avoid milk (or ice-cream) and wheat, if patient is allergic to them. Yogurt and other soured milks are usually well tolerated. Goat's milk is also well tolerated. Those suffering from allergies are usually deficient in manganese. The diet should include an abundance of manganese-rich foods: buckwheat, nuts, beans, peas, blueberries.

The most common allergens (according to Dr. Coca) are: eggs, wheat, white potato, milk, and oranges, in this order of frequency. To determine foods to which the patient is allergic, we advise using Dr. Coca's "Pulse Test" (see: *Referential Reading*).

BIOLOGICAL TREATMENTS

Fasting is an excellent way to remedy allergies. Repeated short juice fasts (see *Directions: 3*) will eventually result in better tolerance of previous allergens.

After the juice fasting, the patient can try a mono diet: only one food — vegetable or fruit — such as watermelon, carrots, grapes, or apples, should be consumed for one week. After that, one more food is added to the diet. One week later, the third food is added, and so on. After four weeks, the protein foods can be introduced, one at a time. As soon as the patient notices an allergic reaction to a newly-added food, it should be discontinued and a new food tried. This way all real allergens can be eventually eliminated from the diet.

Note: If the patient is using antihistamine drugs regularly, they should not be withdrawn abruptly, even during fasting, but discontinued gradually, replacing them with vitamin C in large doses (which acts as a natural antihistamine), up to 3,000 mg. daily.

C — massive doses up to 5,000 mg. a day (vitamin C in large doses should always be taken if patient consumes foods or drugs that he is allergic to)

Manganese supplement — 5 mg. twice a week for 10 weeks

A — 10,000-25,000 units

D — 1,000 units

E — up to 800 IU

Calcium — up to 1,000 mg.

Pantothenic acid — 100 to 200 mg. Higher doses under doctor's directions (see *NOTES*)

Betaine Hydrochloride with digestive enzymes: pepsin, pancreatin, papain, bromelain — after each meal

B-complex with B_{12}

Pollen tablets — Cernitin or other pollen preparations. If not available, raw, crude pollen, 1-2 tsp. a day

Honey — raw, crude, unfiltered

SPECIFICS

Vitamins C and E, manganese, digestive enzymes, fasting, allergen-free diet, mono-diet.

REFERENTIAL READING

Rappaport. H. G., and Linde, S. M., *The Complete Allergy Guide*, Simon and Schuster, N.Y.

Bircher, Ruth, *Eating Your Way to Health*, Faber & Faber, London, 1961.

Lee, Royal, "Introduction to Protomorphology", Lee Foundation for Nutritional Research, Milwaukee, Wisc.

Rowe, Albert H., *Food Allergy, its Manifestations and Control*, Charles C. Thomas, 1973.

Coca, Arthur F., *The Pulse Test*, Lyle Stuart, N.Y., N.Y., 1959.

Hirschfeld, M., *The Whole Truth About Allergy*, Arco Publishing Co. Inc., N.Y., N.Y.

Feingold, B. F., *Annals of Allergy*, June, 1968.

Kamimura, Mitzuo, *Journal of Vitaminology*, 8, 1972, 204-209.

Knight, Granville F., "Nutritional Approach to Allergy and Infections", *Journal of Applied Nutrition*, Vol. 10, No. 3, 1957.

NOTES:

1.   Some researchers believe that alkalosis is a major cause of allergies. It is important to bring the pH of saliva to as near as possible the neutral (pH 7.0 to 7.5). This can be done by stressing acid-forming foods, such as whole grains, nuts and seeds. Also helpful is the regular use of apple cider vinegar with honey during meals, and one tablet of Betain HCl after each meal.

2. Allergic persons should take large doses of vitamin C (1,000 mg. or more) before exposure to known or suspect allergens. Vitamin C acts as an antihistamine and detoxifying agent.
3. Vitamin E possesses effective anti-allergic and antihistamine properties, according to some animal and human studies.
4. Under doctor's supervision, high doses of pantothenic acid, 1,000-1,500 mg. four or more times daily, have been used to alleviate many allergies. Dosage should be reduced when condition is controlled.

ANEMIA

(Iron Deficiency Anemia)

DIETARY CONSIDERATIONS

The diet should be predominantly alkaline. Emphasis should be on raw fruits and vegetables which are rich in iron, particularly dark green leafy vegetables, such as spinach, alfalfa, watercress, green onions, kale, broccoli, chard, okra, squash, carrots, radishes, beets, yams, tomatoes, potatoes (with jackets). Iron-rich fruits are bananas, apples, dark grapes, apricots, plums, raisins, strawberries. Bananas are particularly beneficial as they contain, in addition to easily assimilable iron, also folic acid and vitamin B_{12}, both extremely important in treatment of anemia. Other iron-rich foods are: sunflower seeds, crude blackstrap molasses, black beans, sesame seeds (Tahini), peas, egg yokes and honey. Honey is also rich in copper which helps in iron assimilation. Sunflower seeds contain almost as much iron as liver. Liver, usually prescribed in iron deficiency anemia, would be an acceptable remedy *if healthy non-toxic liver was available*; but *it is not*, at present. Perhaps, if and when the reindeer liver from Alaska will be available again, it can be recommended. In the polluted age, the best diet for anemia would be iron-rich, organically grown vegetables, fruits and other foods named above.

The diet should also include modified amounts of whole grains, such as whole wheat, whole rice, buckwheat, beans, soybeans and millet.

Avoid tea and coffee — caffein in tea and coffee interferes with iron absorption in the body.

VITAMINS & SUPPLEMENTS (Daily)

Organic iron supplement — 10 mg. (only on doctor's recommendation)

B_{12} — 25 mcg. to 50 mcg.

B_6 — 50 mg. to 100 mg.

Pantothenic acid — up to 100 mg.

B-complex, high potency, natural

Folic acid — 0.5-1 mg.

Dessicated liver — only if guaranteed not to contain toxic residues

Beet juice or beet juice powder

PABA — up to 50 mg.

E — up to 1,000 IU

Crude Blackstrap Molasses — 2 tbsp.

Bonemeal — 3 tablets

Sesame seeds (vitamin T factor), beneficial in anemia

Betaine Hydrochloride (promotes assimilation of iron and B_{12}) —
1 tablet after each meal
C — 500 mg. (promotes iron absorption)
Kelp

JUICES

Green vegetable juice made freshly in the juicer or blender from any available greens, such as spinach, kale, alfalfa, watercress, wheat grass, parsley, etc. It can be mixed with carrot and red beet juice. Drink at least 2 glasses each day. Beneficial fruit juices: red grape, blueberry, black currant, prune and apricot.

HERBS

Comfrey, dandelion, black currant, fenugreek, raspberry leaves, kelp.

SPECIFICS

Supplementary iron, B_{12}, B_6, C, folic acid, liver, beet juice (see remarks in: *Dietary Considerations*) B-complex, blackstrap molasses, HCl, iron-rich foods.

PERNICIOUS ANEMIA

Diets, juices and herbs as above.

Specifics: B_{12}, B-complex, folic acid, HCl, liver and other B_{12}-rich foods.

Note: In pernicious anemia, B_{12} must often be administered by injection as it is not well assimilated. If B_{12} is administered orally, added HCl and calcium will promote it's assimilation.

POLYCYTHEMIA

Two or three weeks of juice fasting (see *Directions: 3*) with emphasis on fruit juices, such as red grape and black currant juice, and red beet juice.

REFERENTIAL READING

McCurdy, P. R., *Journal of The American Geriatrics Society*, Vol. 21, p. 88, February, 1973.

Deaton, John G., "How to Keep Ahead of Iron Deficiency", *Prevention*, July, 1972.

Encyclopedia of Common Diseases, Rodale Books, Inc. Emmaus, Penna.

Bothwel, T. H., and Finch, E., *Iron Metabolism*, Little, Brown & Company, N.Y.

Kervran, Louis C., *"Biological Transmutations"*, Swan House Publishing Co., Binghampton, N.Y., 1972.

The American Journal of Clinical Nutrition, April, 1968.

Vilter, Richard W., *Modern Nutrition in Health and Disease*, Lea & Febinger, 1964.

Wilson, P., "Iron-deficiency Anemia", *American Journal of Nursing*, Vol. 72, March, 1972.

NOTES:

1.   According to Louis Kervran, the most effective way to get iron into the system (in iron-deficiency anemia) is not by taking an *iron*

supplement, but a *manganese* supplement, or manganese-rich foods, such as whole grains, especially buckwheat, wheat, rice, beans, etc. By biological transmutation, manganese changes in the body into iron — the form of iron that is easily assimilated and used by the body.

2.   A sufficient amount of gastric enzymes, especially of hydrochloric acid, is needed for proper assimilation of iron. Older people are often anemic in spite of plentiful iron in the diet, because they lack sufficient hydrochloric acid in their stomachs. For these reasons, a diet for anemia in older people should always be supplemented with hydrochloric acid taken at every meal.

3.   Several studies show that vitamin C enhances the effects of iron absorption: 500 mg. of vitamin C in the diet nearly doubled the absorption of supplementary iron.

4.   Hypochromic anemia has been successfully treated with therapeutic doses of pantothenic acid (see *Ref. Reading*: McCurdy).

5.   In severe conditions, where vitamin B_{12} deficiency is involved, it may be advisable to administer B_{12} subcutaneously, as it is often poorly assimilated if administered orally.

6.   Since there are many forms of anemia, it is important to distinguish between iron deficiency, folic acid deficiency and B_{12} deficiency. One of the most common causes of iron deficiency is bleeding in gastro-intestinal system. It is, therefore, essential that the correct cause of anemia is established by doctor.

DIETARY CONSIDERATIONS

A low-sodium, high-potassium, low-calorie vegetarian diet, with emphasis on fruits and vegetables. Garlic is of specific value. Moderate amounts of whole grain products, sprouted and cooked. Millet, rice, buckwheat, barley, sesame seeds, pumpkin seeds, flax seeds. Limit dairy products to a minimum. Low-fat soured milks are best.

No salt; no meat, fish or fowl; no refined or processed foods; no sugar or white flour products; no coffee, tobacco or alcohol.

Avoid overeating.

BIOLOGICAL TREATMENTS

1. Repeated short juice fasts (see *Directions: 3*) one week to ten days. *Important Note*: Continue with vitamin E during fast!
2. A program of gradually increasing exercises, such as walking and jogging. Start with short distances and increase gradually to walk-jog at least 1-2 hours a day, more if possible. *Note*: Exercise only in pure, non-smoggy air.
3. Avoid emotional stresses and anxiety.

VITAMINS & SUPPLEMENTS (Daily)

E — up to 1,600 IU. If not taken before, start with 200 IU and increase gradually

B_{15} — 100 mg. (50 mg. morning and 50 mg. evening)

Lecithin — 2 tbsp. of granules

C — 1,500 to 3,000 mg.

A — 25,000 units

Potassium

B-complex, high potency, natural

B_{12} — 25 mcg.

Kelp

JUICES

Any available vegetable juices with added garlic juice. Fruit juices: lemon, grapefruit, orange.

HERBS

Walnut tea, prepared from the interior dividing walls of the walnut; hawthorn berries, lobelia, sarsaparilla, night-blooming cereus.

SPECIFICS

Vitamin E, vitamin B_{15}, lecithin, hawthorn, walnut tea, garlic. Avoid salt, sugar, alcohol, coffee, meat and refined foods. Avoid overeating. Avoid emotional stresses.

REFERENTIAL READING

Shute, Wilfred E., *Vitamin E for Ailing and Healthy Hearts*, Pyramid House, 1969.

Warmbrand, Max, *Add Years to Your Heart*, Groton Press.

Clark, Michael, "Vitamin E – The Better Treatment for Angina", *Prevention*, December, 1972.

Alsleben, H. Rudolph and Shute, Wilfred E., *How to Survive the New Health Catastrophes*, Survival Publications, Inc., Anaheim, Ca. 1973.

ARTERIOSCLEROSIS

(Hardening of the Arteries)

DIETARY CONSIDERATIONS

The Airola Diet (see *Directions: 1*) with emphasis on raw foods. Several small meals, instead of a few large ones. Use plenty of raw seeds and nuts, also sprouted seeds. Cold-pressed vegetable oils, particularly safflower oil, flax seed oil and olive oil, should be used regularly. Make sure they are not rancid.

Avoid all hydrogenated fats and excess of saturated fats. Avoid meat, salt, and all refined and processed foods. Particularly avoid all white sugar and white flour and all products made with them. It has been clearly demonstrated that excessive consumption of white sugar and refined foods is one of the prime causes of hardening of the arteries and heart disease.

Avoid overeating and consequent obesity — a proven major cause of arteriosclerosis.

BIOLOGICAL TREATMENTS

1. Repeated short juice fasts (see *Directions: 3*), one week to ten days.
2. Plenty of outdoor exercise. Sedentary life is one of the major contributing causes of arteriosclerosis.
3. Eliminate all mental stresses and worries — also well-known contributing causes of arteriosclerosis.
4. Eliminate all environmental sources of metal poisoning, such as aluminum or copper cooking utensils, copper or lead plumbing, lead-glazed ceramics, contaminated water, etc. Toxic metals entering the body are known to be deposited on the walls of the aorta and the arteries.
5. Stop smoking. Smoking constricts the arteries and aggrevates the condition.

VITAMINS & SUPPLEMENTS (Daily)

C — in large doses up to 3,000 mg. Even more in severe cases.
Combined bioflavonoids (rutin, citrin, hesperidin) — 300-600 mg.
E — 600 to 1,200 IU.
Lecithin — 2 tbsp. of granules
Flax seed oil — 2 tsp.
B-complex, high potency, natural
Chromium (occurs in raw sugar, cane juice and in naturally hard water)
Niacin — 100-500 mg., preferably under doctor's supervision
B_6 — 50 mg.

Inositol — 500 mg.
Choline — 500 mg.
Brewer's yeast — 2-3 tbsp. a day
Magnesium — 400 mg.
Calcium — 500 mg.
Kelp — 1 tsp. granules or 5 tablets

JUICES

All available fresh, raw vegetable and fruit juices, in season. Grapefruit juice, pineapple juice, lemon juice, and green juice (see *Directions: 5*) are especially beneficial.

HERBS

Comfrey, garlic, cayenne, golden seal, mistletoe leaves, hawthorn berries, rose hips.

SPECIFICS

Vitamins C, E, B_6 lecithin niacin, chromium, magnesium, flax seed oil, garlic, systematic undereating, plenty of exercise.

REFERENTIAL READING

Ginter, E., *Science*, Vol. 179, February, 1973, pp. 702-709.
Schroeder, Henry A., *Journal of Chronic Diseases*, July, 1955.
Rodale, J. I. and Staff, *Encyclopedia of Common Diseases*, Rodale Books, Emmaus, Penna., 1970.
Airola, Paavo O., *Health Secrets from Europe*, Parker Publishing Co., West Nyack, N.Y., 1970. In paperback: Arco Publishing Co., N.Y., N.Y., 1971.
Alsleben, H. R., *Chelation Therapy*, 710 N. Euclid, Anaheim, California, 1972.
Alsleben, H. Rudolph and Shute, Wilfred E., *How to Survive the New Health Catastrophes*, Survival Publications, Inc. Anaheim, Ca. 1973.

NOTES:

1. Some biologically oriented doctors use chelation therapy in treatment of arteriosclerosis, with reported success.

2. Vitamin C helps in conversion of cholesterol into bile acids, as has been demonstrated in animal studies. This leads to the conclusion that vitamin C deficiency may cause elevated blood cholesterol and be involved in causation of arteriosclerosis.

DIETARY CONSIDERATIONS

A vegetarian diet with emphasis on *vegetables*, cooked and raw, particularly potatoes (raw and cooked) and all available greens. Alfalfa, fresh and tablets, is of specific benefit; also raw potato juice, freshly made. Eat alfalfa seed sprouts daily.

Most beneficial vegetables: alfalfa, wheat grass, watercress, potatoes, yams, celery, parsley, garlic, comfrey, endive.

Most beneficial fruits: bananas, sour cherries, pineapples, sour apples.

Avoid: meat, fish, fowl, cow's milk, cheese, bread (even whole grain), salt, sugar. Use honey for sweetener; kelp as a salt substitute. Raw goat's milk is excellent in fresh or soured form, up to a quart a day. I have known patients who cured themselves of arthritis by drinking one quart of goat's milk each day.

Yogurt, homemade cottage cheese and whole grain bread may be added to the diet when the patient is well on the way to recovery. Millet and rice are the best grains. Use sesame seeds, sunflower seeds and pumpkin seeds sparingly.

For complete details on the diet for arthritis, see my book, "There *IS* a Cure For Arthritis".

BIOLOGICAL TREATMENTS

1. All rheumatic diseases, including rheumatoid arthritis, are particularly responsive to vegetable juice therapy. Repeated juice fasts (see *Directions: 3*) of 4 to 6 weeks are recommended with about 2 months on the above diet between fasts. The alkaline action of raw juices and vegetable broth (see *Recipes*) dissolves the accumulation of deposits around the joints and in other tissues. Green juice (see *Directions: 5*) mixed with carrot, celery and red beet juice, and vegetable broth daily, are specifics for arthritis and other rheumatic diseases.

2. One of the most successful biological treatments for rheumatic and arthritic conditions is the *raw potato juice therapy*, used in folk medicine for centuries. The old way to make potato juice was as follows: take one medium size potato, wash it, cut it into thin slices (with the skin on) and place in a large glass. Fill glass with cold water and let it stand overnight. Drink the water in the morning on an empty stomach. Potato juice can also be made in an electric juicer. Make it fresh and drink diluted with water, 50-50, first thing in the morning.

3. It has been demonstrated that the administration of *bromelain* (pineapple enzyme), 6-8 tablets a day, helps reduce or eliminate swelling and inflamation in the soft tissues and the joints affected by rheumatoid arthritis.
4. Hot-and-cold showers, morning and evening (see *Directions: 7*).
5. Overheating baths (see *Directions: 7*), heat packs, mustard and castor oil packs regularly (see *Notes*).
6. Massage and individually adjusted exercises, regularly.
7. Acupuncture can be effective in relieving pain of arthritis.
   Note: For complete details on the biological treatment of arthritis, see my book, "There *IS* A Cure For Arthritis", available in book stores and health food stores, or from Health Plus Publishers, P.O. Box 22001, Phoenix, Arizona, 85028.

VITAMINS & SUPPLEMENTS (Daily)

C — 3,000 to 5,000 mg.
Bromelain — 6-8 tablets
Potassium — 500 mg.
Cod liver oil — 3 tsp.
Alfalfa tablets — up to 20 tablets, or 2 tsp. powder
Niacinamide — large doses up to 1,000 mg. (only under doctor's supervision)
Kelp — 5-10 tablets
Calcium-magnesium supplement — 500 mg. of each
B_6 — 50 to 100 mg.
Pantothenic acid — 100 mg.
B-complex with B_{12}, high potency, natural
Sprouts — alfalfa and mung bean
E — 600 to 1,000 IU
Brewer's yeast — 3 tbsp.
Sea water — 2-3 tbsp.

JUICES

Emphasis on raw vegetable juices: carrots, celery, red beets, parsley, alfalfa, raw potatoes. Citrus juices only sparingly. Sour cherry juice is specifically effective. Other fruit juices: fresh pineapple juice, black currant, sour apple juice. The enzyme in fresh pineapple juice, *bromelain*, reduces swelling and inflammation in rheumatoid arthritis, osteoarthritis and gout.

HERBS

Comfrey, alfalfa, parsley, poke berries, black cohosh, chaparral, buckthorn bark, sassafras, peppermint, slippery elm, ragwort, burdock root.

Vitamin C, bromelain, potassium, raw fresh cherries or cherry juice, (best cherries: sour, black, Royal Anne, Black Bing) raw pineapple, raw potatoes, alfalfa (plant and seeds), chaparral, mung bean and alfalfa sprouts, goat's milk.

REFERENTIAL READING

Airola, Paavo O., *There IS a Cure for Arthritis*, Parker Publishing Co., West Nyack, N.Y., 1968.

Airola, Paavo O., *How to Keep Slim, Healthy and Young with Juice Fasting*, Health Plus Publishers, P.O. Box 22001, Phoenix, Arizona., 85028, 1971.

Williams, Roger J., *Nutrition Against Disease*, Pitman Publishing Corp., N.Y., 1972.

Warmbrand, Max, *How Thousands of My Arthritis Patients Regained Their Health*, Arco Publishing Co., Inc., N.Y., N.Y.

Lancet, May 8, 1971.

Jennings, J., "A Pineapple Enzyme Reduces Inflamation", *Prevention*, February, 1972.

Wade, Carlson, *Helping Your Health With Enzymes*, Parker Publishing Col, N.Y. 1966.

Garten, M. O., *Health Secrets of A Naturopathic Doctor*, Parker Publishing Co., N.Y. 1967.

NOTES:

1.   If arthritis patient uses aspirin, cortisone, prednisone, or ACTH (the usual drugs prescribed by doctors for pain) he should take extra amounts of vitamin C (massive doses up to 5,000 mg. a day) because all the above-mentioned drugs significantly lower blood and tissue level of vitamin C, as shown in clinical studies.

2.   If arthritis patient has been taking cortisone or other corticosteroid drugs for a prolonged period (over a period of several years), such drugs cannot be withdrawn abruptly, but only gradually, and always under the supervision of a doctor. Such patients, even when they are put on a fast, should continue with medication, possibly on a reduced dosage.

3.   The following poultice for swollen joints has been used with good results: take 2 tbsp. mullein, 3 tbsp. granulated slippery elm bark, 1 tbsp. lobelia, 1 tsp. cayenne (red pepper powder). Mix ingredients in a bowl and add hot water to make a paste. Spread the paste on a cloth and cover the swollen joints with the poultice. Wrap the cloth with a plastic sheet and then with a dry towel. Leave for ½ to 1 hour, or less if burning sensation becomes unbearable.

4.   Castor oil packs are excellent for affected joints which are not in an inflamed condition (after the acute inflammation has subsided). The castor oil pack is made in the following manner: pour 3 to 4 tbsp. of castor oil in a pan and heat oil until it starts to simmer. Dip a flannel cloth into the oil until all the cloth is saturated. Place the cloth on the affected area and cover with a plastic sheet larger than the cloth, then cover with a thin towel and place an electric heating pad over it. Cover the whole pack

with a large towel or blanket. Keep on for ½-1 hour. Peanut oil can be used if castor oil is not available.

5. Mustard plasters on affected joints (not in an inflammatory condition) is an old time-proven remedy.

6. Excellent treatment for bursitis: peanut oil packs, as above, plus 2 tbsp. of peanut oil daily, internally. Diet: the same as above for arthritis.

7. There have been numerous reports by former arthritis patients who claim that they have cured their arthritis by drinking 2-3 tablespoons of sea water each day (or water from the Salt Lake).

8. It has been found in studies by Dr. Barton-Wright, et al., in England, that arthritis patients show always low blood levels of pantothenic acid. This could be due to dietary deficiencies, absorption difficulties or patient's inordinately high requirement of this vitamin. Clinical tests with intramuscular injections of pantothenic acid, in combination with sebacic acid and cysteine, were "remarkably successful." *(Prevention,* September, 1974)

ASTHMA

Extensive studies show that there are two basic causes of asthma: *one*, the typical allergic reaction to one or more allergens; *two*, psychic factors. Doctors agree that many young asthmatics (according to studies, about 25%) have in common a "deep-seated emotional insecurity and an intense need for parental love and protection". When emotional causes are suspected, these must be dealt with before biological and nutritional treatments can be effective.

DIETARY CONSIDERATIONS

There is a clear relationship between asthma and low blood sugar. Asthmatics have a consistently low blood sugar. (Note: diabetics, who have high blood sugar, hardly ever have asthma!) It is advisable, therefore, that asthma patients follow a special dietary program described in a section on *Hypoglycemia* (low blood sugar).

A vegetarian diet is best for asthma. Avoid all meat and fish. Avoid cow's milk. Goat's milk is well tolerated, mostly in soured form as yogurt or kefir. Lots of garlic, green vegetables and all available fruits; natural unfiltered honey; raw seeds and nuts; sprouted seeds and grains.

Diet should include manganese-rich foods, such as peas, beans, blueberries, nuts, buckwheat. Chronic manganese deficiency may be one of the contributing causes of asthma. Avoid sugar, ice-cream, and all refined and processed foods.

BIOLOGICAL TREATMENTS

1. Cleansing juice fast, one to two weeks, under doctor's supervision (see *Directions: 3*).
2. Alternating hot and cold showers each morning and evening (see *Directions: 7*).
3. Dry brush massage twice a day (see *Directions: 4*).
4. Chest pack according to Father Kneipp: wet pack over upper chest. (Place a wet towel over the chest and cover with a dry towel, then with a blanket. Leave on for ½ hour.
5. Plenty of exercise in fresh (non-smoggy) air. Deep breathing exercises several times a day.
6. Herbal vapor bath, for acute asthmatic attacks (see *Notes*).

VITAMINS & SUPPLEMENTS (Daily)

Manganese — 5 mg. taken twice a week for 10 weeks (Some biological doctors in Europe have treated asthma with manganese with excellent results)

E — 600 IU or more

C — 3,000 to 5,000 mg.

Pollen — 5 tablets or 2 tsp. crude pollen
A — up to 50,000 units
Bone meal — 2 to 3 grams
D — up to 10,000 units (after a few weeks, reduce to 2,000 units)
Garlic capsules — 3 with each meal
Alfalfa and comfrey tablets
Pantothenic acid — 100 mg.
B_6 — 50 mg. (B_6 is a natural antihistamine)
Kelp
Betaine hydrochloride — 1 tablet after each meal
Honey

JUICES

The best juices for asthma are: lime, comfrey, horseradish and garlic. Garlic and horseradish juices can be taken in small amounts mixed with the juices of carrots and red beets. Lime (or lemon) juice is best taken diluted with water first thing in the morning. Asthma patients should also take lime juice *plain*, 1 tsp. 2-3 times during the day, between meals.

HERBS

Comfrey (as tea, or comfrey leaves can be chewed fresh), mullein, sweet marjoram, lobelia, valerian root, ginseng, camomile, myrrh, coltsfoot, golden seal, hyssop, anise, wild plum.

SPECIFICS

Garlic, comfrey, manganese, vitamins C, B_6 and E, pollen, honey. Juice fast, vegetarian diet.

REFERENTIAL READING

Kamimura, Mitsuo, *Journal of Vitaminology*. 18, 1972, pp. 204-209.
Reich, Carl J., *Prevention* September, 1970.
Abrahamson, E. M., *Body, Mind, and Sugar*, Henry Holt and Co., N.Y., 1951.
Encyclopedia of Common Diseases, Rodale Books, Inc., Emmaus, Penna.
Nittler, Alan H., *A New Breed of Doctor*, Pyramid House, Publish., N.Y. 1972.
Kirschner, H. E., *Nature's Healing Grasses*, H. C. White Publications, Yuccaipa, Calif., 1960.
Warmbrand, Max., *The Encyclopedia of Natural Health*, Groton Press, Inc. 1962.
Brasher, G. W., "Infantile Asthma: Early Recognition and Management", *Texas Medicine*, Vol. 68, Nov., 1972.

NOTES:

1.   Although pollen is considered one of the commonest allergens of asthmatics, taken orally it has been shown to be an excellent remedy for asthma. Start with small doses and gradually increase to as much as possible, even several teaspoonfuls a day. Pollen is also available in tablet form.

2.   The Herbal Vapor Bath is taken as follows. Boil a quart of water in a pot. Put 1 ounce of each of the following herbs in the boiling water: ragwort, cudweed, wormwood. Bend over the pot, cover the head with a towel and inhale the steam for ½ hour, 2-3 times daily.

BALDNESS

The cause of so-called male pattern baldness, which is responsible for about 98% of all male baldness, is overproduction of male sex hormones. This results in the thickened galea (a sheet of tissue on the top of the scalp) and consequent constriction of blood capillaries in the scalp and impaired blood supply to hair roots. Programs outlined below are in regard to male pattern baldness, and hair loss caused by nutritional deficiencies only.

DIETARY CONSIDERATIONS

The Airola Diet (see *Directions: 1*) with an emphasis on raw vegetables, particularly silicon-rich plants such as alfalfa, comfrey, young horse tail plants, common nettle, onions and kelp. Whole grains, seeds and nuts, particularly oats (very rich in silicon), buckwheat, barley, sesame seeds, rye, millet, and rice. Goat's milk is preferable to cow's milk, mostly in soured form: yogurt, kefir, etc. Raw egg yolks, twice a week.

Diet should be adequate in high quality proteins, preferably of vegetable origin: sesame seeds, sunflower seeds, pumpkin seeds, buckwheat, almonds, and brewer's yeast and wheat germ (only if available fresh, not older than one week after it's made). It is erroneous to think that because hair is made of protein, those suffering from hair loss should eat *huge* amounts of protein. First, hair is not made of protein only, but of minerals as well, which are more important for hair health than proteins. Second, statistics show that Americans eat more protein than any other people in the world — and there is 50 times more baldness in the U.S. than in such countries with typically low-protein diets as China, Japan, Mexico, and India, to name a few.

Avoid salt, sugar, tobacco and alcohol — particularly salt and sugar. It has been demonstrated that overconsumption of salt and sugar are contributing causes of dandruff and hair loss.

BIOLOGICAL TREATMENTS

To increase circulation in the scalp and bring more blood to the hair roots, in addition to the nutritional program and special vitamins and supplements given below, the following measures have been found to be effective.

1. Headstands, two or three times a day (see illustrated instructions in my book, "Stop Hair Loss", available from health food stores, or from Health Plus Publishers, PO Box 22001, Phoenix, Ariz. 85028).

2. Regular use of a slant board, with head down, at least twice a day for 15 minutes.
3. Massage scalp with fingers or electric vibrator.
4. Avoid excessive shampooing.
5. Avoid prolonged mental work and mental stress, which constricts blood vessels in the scalp and impairs the circulation.

VITAMINS & SUPPLEMENTS (Daily)

Biotin — 25 mcg.
Inositol — 500-1,000 mg.
Niacin — 100-300 mg.
Choline — 500-1,000 mg.
Pantothenic acid — 50 mg.
B-complex, high potency, natural
Brewer's yeast — 3-5 tbsp.
Folic acid — 1 mg.
PABA — 50 mg.
B_6 — 50 mg.
E — up to 1,200 IU
C — 1,000 mg.
Bioflavonoids — 50-100 mg.
Lecithin — 2 tbsp.
Kelp — 1 tsp. of granules or 10 tablets
Silica — (from horse tail) 3 tablets
Cod liver oil — 2tsp.
Multi-mineral trace element supplement or 2 tbsp. pure sea water
Wheat germ (only if available fresh, less than one week after it is made)
Vegetable oils — 1-2 tbsp. Must be genuinely virgin, cold-pressed. Olive and sesame oils are best
Note: See *Directions: 2* regarding taking large doses of isolated B-vitamins for prolonged period of time

JUICES

Nettles, spinach, carrot, red beet, alfalfa. A little onion juice can be added to the vegetable juices.

HERBS

Horse tail (very young), nettles, alfalfa, parsley, kelp, birch leaves, fenugreek, onions, cayenne pepper. All the above can be used internally as tea or condiments. A strong tea of nettles, horsetail, camomile, rosemary, sage, burdock, Indian hemp and chaparral (singularly or in combination) can be used as hair rinses or conditioners. Nettles have been used for stimulating hair growth for centuries. Strong decoction of fresh or dry nettles is rubbed into the scalp once a day, after a preliminary wash with warm water (without soap).

SPECIFICS

Biotin, B$_6$, inositol, niacin, vitamin E, PABA, nettles, horsetail, brewer's yeast, silica. Headstand and scalp massage. Optimum diet with emphasis on silicon-rich foods.

REFERENTIAL READING

Airola, Paavo O., *Stop Hair Loss*, Health Plus Publishers, P.O. Box 22001, Phoenix, Ariz., 1965.

Airola, Paavo O., *Health Secrets From Europe*, Parker Publishing Co., West Nyack, N.Y., 1970. Paperback. Arco Pub. Co. N.Y., N.Y., 1971.

Yudkin, John, *Nature* (British Journal), Sept. 22, 1972.

Let's Live Magazine, Feb., 1971.

Davis, Adelle, *Let's Get Well*, Harcourt, Brace and World, Inc., 1965.

Lucas, Richard, *Nature's Medicines*, Parker Publishing Co., 1966.

Flesch, Peter, *Science News Letter*, Nov. 10, 1951.

Fox, DeWitt J., *Life and Health*, Vol. 86, No. 12.

NOTES:

The following "cures" for baldness and hair loss have been successfully used by some doctors and sufferers:

1. Mix 3 oz. of cayenne pepper (red pepper powder) with one fifth of Romanoff Vodka or pure alcohol. Leave for 2 weeks, agitating the bottle each day. Strain through several layers of fine cheesecloth. Rub a small amount into the scalp twice a day. KEEP AWAY FROM EYES!

2. Mix equal parts of castor oil and white iodine. Rub into the scalp and sit in the sun for 15 minutes. Treatment can be used once a day.

3. To restore natural color to gray hair, the following vitamins and supplements have been reported to be successful in some people: PABA, pantothenic acid, folic acid, brewer's yeast and blackstrap molasses. Also, a good multi-mineral and trace element formula or sea water (2 tbsp. a day).

BLADDER INFECTION

(Cystitis)

DIETARY CONSIDERATIONS

In chronic bladder infections, it is advisable to increase the acid content of the urine which helps to retard bacterial growth. It is important to keep a proper acid-base balance in the body, which must not become too alkaline. The patient should eat sparingly, with emphasis on whole grain products, cereals, and homemade cottage cheese, or other natural cheeses. For a week or two, a minimum of vegetables and fruits. When improvement is noticed, re-introduce vegetables and fruits to the diet. Take 2 tsp. of apple cider vinegar and 1 tsp. of natural honey in a glass of water with each meal. Also, cranberry juice daily (2 glasses) is very beneficial.

Watermelon seeds and pumpkin seeds are of specific benefit. Large doses of vitamins C and A are imperative.

Drink lots of liquids every day, especially medicinal herb teas (see *Herbs*).

BIOLOGICAL TREATMENTS

1. In acute condition, one week fast (see *Directions: 3*) on vegetable and fruit juices. Use juices and herbs suggested below. After the fast, follow the Airola Diet with emphasis on seeds, nuts, and grains. If condition persists, repeat juice fast after 2 weeks on suggested diet.
2. Hot sitz baths (see *Directions: 7*) 2 times a day in acute conditions.
3. If constipated, take daily enemas, using catnip tea in the enema. (Use 1 tbsp. of dried catnip to a quart of boiling water; cool down to body temperature before use.)

VITAMINS & SUPPLEMENTS (Daily)

C — in massive doses 5,000 to 10,000 mg. in acute cases. Reduce to 3,000 mg. when improvement is noticed

A — 25,000 to 50,000 units in acute condition. Reduce to 25,000 as maintenance dose

E — 600 IU

Betaine hydrochloride for older patients — 1 tablet after each meal with ½ glass water

Whey powder — 2 tsp. with each meal

Natural multi-vitamin-mineral formula

JUICES

Watermelon juice. Carrot, beet, cucumber, spinach or any other vegetable juice with small amounts of garlic or yellow onion juice added. Cranberry juice.

HERBS

Golden rod (Solidago), rose hips, burdock root, juniper berries (weak tea), shavegrass tea, parsley-mint, catnip, buchu leaves, clivers or stone root (for bladder stones), uva ursi.

SPECIFICS

Vitamin C and A, golden rod, whey, keeping pH of urine on acid side (with acid-forming foods, cranberry juice, apple cider vinegar, HCl) but only for the duration of the treatment.

REFERENTIAL READING

Walker, N. W., *Raw Vegetable Juices*, Norwalk Press, 1970.
Vogel, A., *The Nature Doctor*, Bioforce Verlag, Switzerland, 1960.
Rose, Mary Swartz, *Foundations of Nutrition*, Macmillan Co. 1944.
Schlegel, J. U., et al., *Journal of Urology*, 103, 155, 1970.
Evard, J. P., and Bollag, W., *Schweiz. Med. Wochenschr.*, Dec. 23, 1972, 102: 1880-82.

NOTES:

1. It has been clinically confirmed that cranberry juice increases the acidity of the urine, creating an unfavorable environment for pathogenic bacteria. Usual dosage: 2 or 3 glasses a day.

BURNS

The following biological treatments for thermal, X-ray, and sunburns have been found to be effective:

1. On fresh burns, immediately after the accident, squeeze a vitamin E capsule, or several capsules if the size requires, directly on the damaged area. Use as high potency E as available. If this treatment is given within a few seconds after the accident, it always prevents blistering, even in serious burns, and eliminates pain in a few minutes. On severe burns, repeat treatment every hour. Also take internally 600 IU vitamin E.

   If treatment is delayed and blisters are already formed, it will speed the healing considerably and prevent the development of scars.

2. One of the most effective treatments for burns on hands, feet or other limited area is to immerse burned part in iced or very cold water as soon after the accident as possible. Keep covered with water until the pain is gone. This treatment almost always prevents redness and blistering.

3. For protection against sunburns, PABA cream (available at health food stores) has been reported to be effective.

   For badly sunburned and inflamed skin, a *starch bath* (one pound cornstarch to a tubful of water) or a *vinegar bath* (two cups apple cider vinegar to a tubful of water) are useful and soothing. After bath, apply my *Formula F Plus* (see *Directions: 8*).

4. Vitamin C, taken orally and/or sprayed on the skin has been demonstrated in many major medical studies to be a most effective treatment for victims of severe burns.

5. Comfrey poultice from the fresh leaves or roots, applied over the infected sores of blisters, speeds the healing.

6. Liquid honey, used as an ointment, helps to heal burns.

7. For treatment of X-ray burns: apply fresh gel of Aloe Vera; repeat frequently. Promotes rapid healing without scars. Aloe Vera gel is extremely beneficial for all burns.

CANCER

Cancer is a disease of civilization. It is the end result of health-destroying living and eating habits, which result in a biochemical imbalance and physical and chemical irritation of the tissues. In addition to an abundance of carcinogens in today's food, water, air and environment, carcinogenic substances are also produced within the body as a result of deranged metabolism. Many biological and naturopathic doctors, both those who are active presently, as well as many great pioneers of the past, notably Drs. Bircher-Benner, Duncan Bulkley, A. Vogel, Max Gerson, Kristine Nolfi, Ragnar Berg, Are Waerland, Werner Zabel, J. H. Tilden, Alice Chase, to name a few, believed that faulty diet can be a basic cause of cancer. Based on their own extensive practice and by studying the eating habits of cancer-free natives and peoples around the world, their conclusions emphatically pointed to the fact that in addition to well-known environmental carcinogens, such as smoking, chemical poisons in foods and environment, etc., the cancer incidence is in direct proportion to the amount of animal proteins, particularly meat, in the diet. Racial groups and nations whose diet contains less meat, show less cancer incidence than groups consuming high-meat diets. Hospital records show that Seventh Day Adventists, Mormons and Navajo Indians, who eat little or no meat, suffer far less from cancer than the average meat-eating Americans. Recently, a link between excessive meat-eating and cancer has been explained by Dr. Willard J. Visek, research scientist at Cornell University. Dr. Visek says that the high-protein diet of Americans is linked to the high incidence of cancer in the U.S. The villain, according to Dr. Visek, is ammonia, the carcinogenic by-product of meat digestion.

Our actual daily protein requirement is only between 20 and 30 grams, as shown by numerous studies around the world. Protein eaten in excess of the actual need cannot be properly digested or utilized and acts in the body as a poison and carcinogen. In addition, overconsumption of protein taxes the pancreas and causes chronic deficiency of pancreatic enzymes, which are required for proper protein metabolism.

DIETARY CONSIDERATIONS

Therefore, the effective treatment for cancer must, in addition to any other internal or external specifics used (such as laetrile, tekarina, or hydrazine sulfate, for example), begin with total elimination of the basic causes of cancer — elimination of all environmental sources of carcinogens, such as smoking and carcinogenic chemicals in air, water and food. In addition, a complete change in diet is imperative. In the beginning, all animal proteins must be eliminated. As condition improves, some raw goat's milk, raw egg yokes and soured milk products, such as yogurt, kefir or acidophilous milk, made from goat's milk, may be added to the diet. The diet must be a 100% natural raw food diet, with emphasis on raw fruits and vegetables, particularly red beets, plus a minimum requirement of high quality proteins mostly from vegetable sources such as almonds, buckwheat, millet, sesame seeds, and sprouted seeds and grains. All foods must be natural, whole, unprocessed and *organically grown*, without man-made chemicals of any kind.

Pureed asparagus, four tablespoons a day, has been reported to be an effective addition to the anti-cancer diet.

Almonds, as a protein source, are particularly recommended. No proteins should be consumed before 11 a.m. Breakfast should consist of fresh fruits, fruit juices and herb teas. One pint of fresh or soured goat's milk can be used daily, plus 2 raw egg yokes *from fertile eggs* every second day. Lots of raw vegetable and fruit juices should be used daily. Green juices, made from alfalfa, comfrey, wheat grass, beet tops, etc., are excellent. (For a detailed description of the anti-cancer diet, see my book, "Cancer: Causes, Prevention and Treatment − The TOTAL Approach", available at health food stores or from the publisher: Health Plus Publishers, PO Box 22001, Phoenix, Arizona.)

Anti-cancer diet should contain a generous amount of foods rich in vitamins E and C and the trace mineral, selenium − all natural antioxidants, which can help prevent the chromosome damage caused by carcinogens that leads to cancer.

BIOLOGICAL TREATMENTS

1. If the patient is not too weak, a short 3-day cleansing fast on raw fruit and vegetable juices can be undertaken (see *Directions: 3*). To stimulate the liver and its detoxifying activity, red beet juice, or fermented beet juice, should be taken during fasting (½ glass three times a day) plus daily coffee enemas: one cup of strongly brewed coffee in 1 pint of water, used as a retention enema. Lactic acid fermented beet juice will markedly increase the oxygenation of the body cells.

    After a short fast, which can be repeated after 3 or 4 weeks, the Airola Diet of raw foods (see *Directions: 1*) should be maintained. Seed and grains are particularly useful, *especially in sprouted form.* As the patient improves, some cooked cereals, such as millet, whole rice, buckwheat, barley and oats can be included.

2. One of the most effective cancer treatments used in the famous Dr. Josef Issels' cancer clinic in Germany, as well as in many other biological clinics around the world, is *fever therapy* (see *Directions: 7*).

3. Plenty of rest, complete freedom from worries and mental stress, plenty of fresh, pure air day and night. If patient is strong, lots of exercise and walking; and generally health-strengthening mode of living.

4. In many countries of the world, but not in the United States, Laetrile (alias nitrilosides, amygdalin, or Vitamin B_{17}), a drug developed by Drs. Ernst Krebs Sr. and Jr., of the U.S., is used to treat cancer with reported success. Treatment is available in Mexico and many European countries.

5. Tekarina is another non-toxic injectable material, derived from seaweed, and developed by G. Lo Monaco, of Mexico, which, according to reports, has shown a remarkably high rate of success. Tekarina acts as a powerful detoxifier and, thus, is useful in biological treatment of many other ailments.

6. Many doctors and clinics which specialize in cancer use various vaccine-type drugs to stimulate the body's immunological response and increase its defensive and healing activity — thus helping the body to heal itself.

VITAMINS & SUPPLEMENTS (Daily)

Total vitamin and mineral supplementation is advised (see *Directions: 2*), but particularly the following anti-cancer vitamins:

C and A in Large doses:

C, up to 5,000 mg.

A, preventative dose 50,000 units

(If subjected to strong carcinogens — 100,000 units. In a short therapeutic program — up to 2 months — 250,000 units.)

B_3 — niacin or nicotinamide — 100 mg.

B-complex, high-potency, natural

E — up to 1,200 IU

Note: Vitamins E and B-complex are particularly important in cirrhosis of the liver.

Choline — 500 to 1,000 mg.

B_{15} — 100 mg. (50 mg. in morning; 50 mg. at bedtime)

Brewer's yeast — 3-4 tbsp.

Note: Recent studies, performed at Zurich University and in London Polytechnic, showed that brewer's or food yeast gives improved resistance against cancer development. Brewer's yeast is one of the best sources of selenium, an important anti-cancer mineral.

Multiple-enzyme digestive formula (including pancreatic enzymes, trypsin, chymotrypsin and pancreatin, plus betaine hydrochloric acid, ox bile, papain and pepsin.

Comprehensive mineral and trace element supplement, particularly rich in potassium.

JUICES

Red beet juice (from roots and tops), carrot, grape and generally all dark-colored juices, such as carrot, black cherries, black currants. Liver juice (liver extract "retine", as discovered by Dr. Szent-Gyorgyi – see *Referential Reading*).

Note: Fruit juices are best taken in the morning, and vegetable juices in the afternoon and evening.

HERBS

Chaparral tea, internally (particularly for skin cancer), eucalyptus oil (externally), milkweed plant (cancerillo), apricot pits, garlic, violet (viola odorata) in poultice form for skin cancer, also in form of tea. Red clover blossoms, as tea. Also, ginseng, golden seal, dandelion root and Irish sea moss.

SPECIFICS

Vitamins A and C, niacin, B-complex, almonds, apricot pits, chaparral, red beet juice, liver extract, brewer's yeast, raw foods, low animal protein diet, garlic.

Note: Cancer is a systemic disease and cannot be treated effectively with "Specifics". Only a *TOTAL* supportive and healing program, as outlined above, can be effective and help the body to heal itself. (See my book, "Cancer: Causes, Prevention and Treatment – The TOTAL Approach".)

REFERENTIAL READING

Airola, Paavo O., *Cancer: Causes, Prevention and Treatment – The TOTAL Approach*, Health Plus Publishers, PO Box 22001, Phoenix, Ariz., 1972.

Homburger, F. and Fishman, W. H., *The Physiopathology of Cancer*, Paul B. Haeber, New York, N.Y., 1953.

Bricklin, Mark, "Vitamin C, a Form of Cancer Insurance", *Prevention*, Oct. 1972.

Bush, Loraine, et al., *Biochemistry*, Feb. 1, 1972.

Williams, Roger, *Nutrition Against Disease*, Pitman Publishers Corp., N.Y. 1972.

Shamberger, Raymond J., report in the *Journal of The National Cancer Institute*, May, 1971.

Issels, Josef, "Nutritional Protection Against Cancer", *Tidskrift för Hälsa*, Nos. 2, 3, 4, 1972, Stockholm, Sweden.

Larson, Gena, "Is There An Anti-Cancer Food?", *Prevention*, April, 1972.

Oden, Max, *Vitalstoffe*, December, 1967.

Kelly, William Donald, *One Answer to Cancer*, The Kelly Research Foundation, Crepevine, Texas, 1969.

Prevention, April, 1972, "Vitamin A Fights Against Cancer".

Shamberger, Raymond J., et al., *Proceedings of the National Academy of Sciences*, May, 1973.

Krebs, Ernst T., Jr., "The Nitrilosides (Vitamin B_{17})" *Cancer News Journal*, Vol. 6, No. 1-4, Jan.-Apr., 1971.

"Liver May Hold the Secret of Cancer Prevention", Dr. Albert Szent-Gyorgyi's new discovery of anti-cancer substance extracted from the liver, "retine". *Prevention*, Nov., 1972, pp. 124-131.

March of Truth on Cancer, The Arlin J. Brown Information Center, PO Box 251, Fort Belvoir, Virginia.

Deråker, Ola, *Hälsa*, 7-8, 1972, Stockholm, Sweden.

Gerson, Max, "A Cancer Therapy – Fifty Case Histories", Dura Books, Inc., New York, N.Y.

Biochemical News, October, 1971.

NOTES:

1.   According to recent Swedish studies at Karolinska and Umeå Hospitals, vitamin C in large doses can be an effective prophylactic agent against cancer. It has been shown that abnormal metabolism of amino acid tryptophan, with consequent oxidation of its metabolites, can lead to the development of cancer in the bladder. Vitamin C, by preventing the oxidation process, can block cancer development. Swedish researchers suggest that vitamin C can be used as cancer preventative agent.

2.   Vitamins C and A in large doses are two natural substances used by the body to inhibit hyaluronidase, an enzyme found in cancerous tissues. Vitamin C effectively protects against carcinogenic effects of most poisons, including nitrates.

3.   According to several studies, vitamin A exerts an inhibiting effect on carcinogenesis. A recent study done by Dr. Raymond J. Shamberger, professor of the Department of Biochemistry, The Cleveland Clinic, Ohio, showed that vitamin A is one of the most important aids to the body's defensive system to fight and prevent cancer. When subjected to carcinogens, this vitamin has a remarkable ability to inhibit the induction and/or retard the growth of both malignant and non-malignant tumors.

4.   We strongly advise that when cancer is suspected, under no circumstances should "home remedies", nutritional or any other kind, be tried. Instead, a reliable doctor preferably a biologically oriented one, should be consulted immediately, and the patient should abide by the doctor's advice regarding most suitable therapies, including the therapies described in this book.

5.   Since it is not likely that the methods of treatment described in this section will be "in accord with the concensus of medical opinion", we are compelled to say that all information in this section is offered purely for educational and experimental purposes; as an objective scientific report, not as a recommendation or endorsement.

COLDS

(Acute or chronic infections: flu, grippe, tonsilitis, sinusitis, bronchial catarrh, chronic colds, virus-type infections)

DIETARY CONSIDERATIONS

In acute stage of disease, when fever is present in above-mentioned conditons, patient should abstain from all solid foods and only drink fresh fruit and vegetable juices, diluted with water, 50-50, plus herb teas from herbs recommended in this section. After fever subsides, a low calorie raw fruit and vegetable diet with plenty of raw juices and herb teas, sweetened with honey. Some raw seeds, nuts and sprouted seeds and grains. After the acute condition is over, the Airola Diet (see *Directions: 1*) with suggested supplements.

BIOLOGICAL TREATMENTS

1. In persistant chronic conditions, repeated short juice fasts (see *Directions: 3*), one week to 10 days.
2. Hot epsom salt baths, dry brush massage (see *Directions: 4*), plenty of rest, mild exercises and walking in *fresh* air.
3. Barefoot walking on sand, gravel and/or wet grass is strengthening in chronic conditions.
4. Once a week take sauna or Schlenz-bath, an over-heating bath (see *Directions: 7*).
5. In mouth and throat infections, keep clove of garlic or vitamin C tablet in the mouth.

VITAMINS & SUPPLEMENTS (Daily)

C — massive doses up to 5,000 mg. In acute condition, 1,000 mg. every second hour (vitamin C has an antibiotic action). In severe, acute conditions, 1,500 mg. ascorbic acid, intravenously, every second hour.

Bioflavonoids — rutin, hesperidin, citrin, — 200 to 600 mg.

Garlic — raw or garlic oil capsules. Garlic is a natural antibiotic.

A — 50,000 to 150,000 units (this dosage only for one month, reduced after that to 25,000 units a day).

Honey — natural, unheated, unfiltered, in herb teas.

Calcium lactate — 6 tablets

Pollen

Brewer's yeast

B_6 — 100 mg. (natural antihistamine)

B-complex — natural, high-potency

E — 600 IU

Zinc — 30 mg.

JUICES

Lemon, black currant, orange, pineapple, elderberries (particularly for bronchial catarrh), carrot, beet, tomato, green pepper, watercress, plus onion and garlic juice in small doses added to vegetable juices.

HERBS

Rose hips, golden seal, camomile, peppermint, lemon grass, slippery elm, ginger, chinchona bark, sage, desert tea (Ephedra Viridis).

SPECIFICS

Vitamins C, A, B_6, garlic, bioflavonoids, honey, rose hips, fresh juices. Optimum nutrition and repeated short juice fasts will increase body's resistance against colds.

REFERENTIAL READING

Pauling, Linus, *Vitamin C And The Common Cold*, W. H. Freeman & Co., San Francisco, 1970.

Klosa, J. *Report In German Medical Monthly*, March, 1950.

Andrewes, C., *The Common Cold*, W. W. Norton & Co., N.Y., 1965.

Airola, Paavo O., *How To Keep Slim, Healthy and Young With Juice Fasting*, Health Plus Publishers, P.O. Box 22001, Phoenix, Ariz., 1971.

Klenner, F. R., *The Key to Good Health: Vitamin C*, Graphic Aids Research Foundation, Chicago, Ill., 1969.

Alsaker, Rasmus, *Conquering Colds and Sinus Infections.*

NOTES:

1. *Garlic oil* combined with *onion juice*, diluted with water and drunk several times a day, has been found in several studies to be extremely effective to patients suffering from grippe, sore throat and rhinitis.

2. In so-called "intestinal flu", in addition to supplements mentioned above, *Betaine Hydrochloride* (2 tablets after each meal) helps in intestinal detoxification; also, pepsin is beneficial.

COLITIS

The underlying causes of colitis must be found before an effective corrective diet can be advised. Often, it is caused by an allergic sensitivity to certain foods — which must be eliminated from the diet (use Dr. Coca's pulse test to determine this — see *Referential Reading*). Often, it is poorly digested roughage, especially of cereals and carbohydrates, that cause bowel irritation. In such cases, the digestion should be improved, possibly with the help of digestive enzymes and small, frequent meals instead of a few large ones. Also, possible restriction of whole grains and whole grain products can be advisable, which, if not properly digested, cause fermentation in the bowels, with consequent gas and bowel irritation. Often, the intake of antibiotics may upset the bacterial flora in the intestines and interfere with proper digestion of food. In such case, plenty of yogurt, whey powder and acidophilus culture may be given to restore the proper bacterial balance in the intestines. Furthermore, mucous colitis is often of psychosomatic origin.

BIOLOGICAL TREATMENTS

1. In most cases of ulcerative as well as mucous colitis, one week juice fast is advisable (see *Directions: 3*). After the fast, a diet of *small, frequent meals* of raw and cooked organic foods should be given, with addition of generous amounts of yogurt, kefir, homemade cottage cheese and whey powder. *Sprouted* seeds and grains are usually well tolerated. Millet cereal is best. Bananas are very soothing and healing in ulcerative colitis. *All foods must be eaten slowly, chewed and salivated well.*
2. All refined carbohydrates should be avoided.
3. When there are *no* contraindications, such as open peptic or intestinal ulcers, 2 to 3 tablets of *Betaine Hydrochloride* should be given after each meal with a glass of water. Colitis is often caused by partially or incompletely digested animal proteins and carbohydrates in the colon and lower bowels.
4. In acute colitis caused by accumulation of gas, the following Kneipp wet pack is effective. Patient lays on his back with wet pack on his abdomen: first one wet towel, then slightly larger dry towel over it; finally, all wrapped with a thick flannel or a blanket.
5. Colonics once a week and daily enemas (with camomile tea) are advisable during treatment, but not longer than for one month.

VITAMINS & SUPPLEMENTS (Daily)

Comfrey-pepsin preparation
Betaine Hydrochloride tablets after each meal

Whey powder, 1 tbsp. with each meal, mixed with yogurt, kefir or
other soured milk

Vitamin K or vitamin K-rich foods (egg yolks, alfalfa tablets)

Calcium lactate — 3 tablets

B-complex, high potency, natural

Cod liver oil — 2 tsp.

Kelp

B_6 — 50 mg.

Cold-pressed vegetable oil, preferably olive oil — 2 tbsp. a day with
meals

JUICES

Papaya juice, raw cabbage juice. Avoid citrus juices.

HERBS

Peppermint, comfrey, cinnamon, camomile, caraway. In case of
chronic diarrhea, use dried blueberries, cinnamon and carob.

SPECIFICS

Whey powder, comfrey-pepsin, yogurt, papaya, millet cereal,
bananas, B-complex vitamins, small meals.

REFERENTIAL READING

Norman, N. Philip, *Ulcerative Colitis*, Lee foundation for Nutritional Research,
Milwaukee, Wisc.

Harrower, Henry R., *Practical Endocrinology*, Lee Foundation for Nutritional
Research, Milwaukee, Wisc.

Coca, Arthur F., *The Pulse Test*, Lyle Stuart, New York, N.Y.

Rodale & Staff, *Encyclopedia of Common Diseases*, Rodale Books, Inc., Emmaus,
Pa.

Sneddon, J. Russell, *The Natural Treatment of Liver Troubles and Associated
Ailments*, Health for All Publishing Co., London, 1966.

Lanyi, George, "Stomach Ache — What Can I Do", *Hälsa*, #7-8, 1972, Stockholm,
Sweden.

Hanson, Map, *Diet Management For Ulcerative Colitis*, Charles C. Thomas,
Springfield, Ill., 1972.

NOTES:

1.   Colitis-like symptoms may be caused by appendicitis. It is, therefore,
important that where there are doubts as to the origin of the symptoms
and pain, a physician is consulted without delay.

CONSTIPATION

Chronic constipation may result from a variety of physiological and psychological disturbances such as lack of sufficient exercise; hypothyroidism; dehydration (not enough water drinking); liver disfunction; specific food allergies (Dr. A. F. Coca); habitual neglect of the calls of nature; habitual use of laxatives; constant worries, nervousness or grief; over-refined foods; vitamin and mineral deficiencies, particularly of B, inositol and potassium; too much animal protein in the diet and resultant putrefaction in intestines, etc. These underlying causes must be eliminated before the condition can be corrected permanently, even with the biological means suggested in this section.

DIETARY CONSIDERATIONS

The Airola Diet (see *Directions: 1*) with emphasis on high residue vegetables and fruits, raw and cooked, plus whole grains, seeds and nuts. Sprouted seeds are of specific value.

The following foods should be used regularly: homemade sauerkraut (drink sauerkraut juice, too); sesame seeds (Tahini); soaked prunes and dried figs, taken morning and evening; yogurt, kefir or other soured milks; honey, natural, unfiltered; sprouted seeds such as alfalfa and mung beans; abundance of raw fruits, especially apples, and vegetables available in season. Take 2 tbsp. of cold-pressed vegetable oil (olive, sesame, safflower) each day. Morning and evening, drink 1 glass of Excelsior (see *Recipes*) made with vegetable broth plus flax seeds and wheat bran. Do not chew seeds, swallow them whole. Drink plenty of liquids: juices, herb teas, water, broths.

BIOLOGICAL TREATMENTS

1. In severe and persistant cases of constipation, 10-day juice fast is advisable (see *Directions: 3*). Begin fasting by taking 2 tbsp. of castor oil in a glass of orange juice. Take colonics twice a week during the fasting; take an enema every day. After the fast, follow vegetarian diet, as above.

2. Lack of sufficient exercise is one of the main causes of constipation. Exercise! Walk, swim, ride bicycle or horseback, dance, jog — anything! Plain walking, 2 or more hours a day, will remedy the problem in most cases. Do deep breathing exercises while walking.

3. Avoid all commercial laxatives. In emergency, use herbal laxatives sold in health food stores.

4. Avoid all refined and processed foods. Avoid salt, sugar and white flour in any form. Avoid coffee, tea and alcohol — all constipating beverages.

VITAMINS & SUPPLEMENTS (Daily)

Brewer's yeast — 3 to 4 tbsp. Take between meals with some sour fruit juice.

Whey powder — 2 tbsp.

Flax seed, wheat bran and/or rice bran, soaked in Excelsior (see *Recipes*)

Homemade sauerkraut

B-complex, natural, high potency

B_1 — 100 mg.

Choline — 500 mg.

Inositol — 500 mg.

A — 25,000 units

C — 1,000 mg.

Honey, natural, unprocessed

Yogurt or kefir, regularly

Vegetable oils, cold-pressed, 2 tbsp.

JUICES

Spinach, watercress, nettles, garlic and yellow onions (small amounts added to vegetable juices), black radish, dandelion, added to milder juices of carrots, cucumber, celery, cabbage, red beets and tomatoes. Fruit juices: apples, lemon. Sauerkraut juice is excellent if patient can tolerate it — some are bothered with gas. Use only homemade sauerkraut.

HERBS

Senna pod or senna leaf tea, alder buckthorn bark, dandelion, slippery elm bark, mandrake, licorice or licorice root tea, raspberry leaf, ginger, black root, mountain flax, psyllium seed, cascara sagrada (sacred bark).

SPECIFICS

Flax seed, psyllium seed, whey powder, brewer's yeast, B-complex vitamins, yogurt, soaked prunes and figs, licorice tea. High-residue diet. Plenty of exercise.

REFERENTIAL READING

Elwood, Catharyn, *Feel Like A Million*, Devin-Adair, New York, 1951.
Lee, Royal, "The Constipation Syndrome", *Applied Trophology*, Vol. 1, No. 6.
Rodale & Staff, *Encyclopedia of Healthful Living*, Rodale Books, Inc., Emmaus, Pa.
Airola, Paavo O., *How To Keep Slim, Healthy and Young With Juice Fasting*, Health Plus Publishers, PO Box 22001, Phoenix, Ariz.
Bogert, Jean, *Nutrition and Physical Fitness*, W. B. Saunders Co., 1971.
Nittler, Alan H., *A New Breed of Doctor*, Pyramid House, N.Y., 1972.

NOTES:

1. When enemas are used, add red raspberry leaf tea or wild cherry bark tea into enema water.

CRAMPS

(Muscle Spasms, Leg Cramps)

Muscle and leg cramps are usually due to dietary vitamin and mineral deficiencies, particularly of calcium, potassium, magnesium and vitamins D and B_6, or the body's inability to assimilate these nutrients from the diet. Symptoms of such cramps are usually aggravated at night and when inactive. The suggestions below are in regard to nutritional deficiency related cramps. For other causes and suggested treatments see *Notes* below.

DIETARY CONSIDERATIONS

The Airola Diet (see *Directions: 1*) with emphasis on calcium and magnesium-rich foods, such as leafy green vegetables, fruits, particularly apricots, and soured milk products (kefir, yogurt, clabbered milk). Avoid excess of citrus fruits and especially citrus juices. Avoid meat, liver and excess of grains, especially wheat (and wheat germ) which are all deficient in calcium. Millet is the best cereal; sesame seeds are excellent — use both in the daily diet. Almond and sesame seed milk (1 cup almonds, or sesame seeds, or one half cup of each, 4 cups water, 1 tbsp. honey, liquified in blender) is an excellent source of minerals and proteins.

BIOLOGICAL TREATMENTS

1. Massage, combined with heat pack, is the best treatment for acute spastic muscle cramps.

VITAMINS & SUPPLEMENTS (Daily)

Calcium lactate — 3 to 5 tablets
Magnesium (preferably magnesium chloride) — 2 tablets (800 mg.)
Vitamin D or fish liver oil
B_6 — up to 100 mg.
Pantothenic acid — 100 mg.
Vitamin E — 400 to 1,000 IU
Multi-mineral and trace element formula, or sea water — 2 tbsp.
Natural multi-vitamin formula

JUICES

Carrots, beet, cucumber, sweet fruit juices.

HERBS

Dandelion, alfalfa, belladonna, cayenne (for stomach cramps), blue cohosh, thyme.

SPECIFICS

Calcium-magnesium supplementation, cod liver oil, vitamins B_6, E, and D, sea water.

REFERENTIAL READING

Vogel, A., *The Nature Doctor*, Bioforce-Verlag, Switzerland, 1960.

Silver, Lewis J., *Doctor Silver's Extraordinary Remedies*, Prentice-Hall, Inc., 1964.

Ellis, John M., and Presley, James, *Vitamin B_6 : The Doctor's Report*, Harper and Row, N.Y., 1973.

Ayres, Samuel, and Mihan, Richard, *Journal of Applied Nutrition*, fall, 1973.

NOTES:

1. The above suggestions are in regard to cramps caused by metabolic insufficiency of calcium, magnesium, vitamins and trace elements, which is the most common cause of cramps and muscle spasms. There are several other causes, however. One is *the tissue oxygen debt*, or chronic oxygen deficiency in the tissues (symptoms aggravated at exertion). Vitamins C and E in large doses are helpful in such conditions.

    Muscle spasms in various organs (heart arteries, stomach, etc.) can be caused by mental stress, nervous irritability and other psychic factors. Organic minerals, particularly potassium, can be helpful in such cases, in addition to the other suggested programs. But the elimination of contributing psychic causes is imperative.

    Cramps associated with the menstrual cycle and menopause can be due to sex hormone influence on calcium metabolism, and due to endocrine insufficiency. Extra vitamin E, B_{12}, B_6, RNA (ribo-nucleic acid) and sarsaparilla and licorice (natural sources of sex hormones) can be helpful in such cases. Leg cramps during pregnancy are often relieved by giving vitamin B_6, in addition to calcium.

2. When leg cramps are associated with old age but *adequate* dietary calcium supply, the contributing underlying causes can be the lack of sufficient hydrochloric acid in the stomach, or lack of dietary magnesium or vitamin D, without which calcium cannot be properly utilized. In such case, the addition of magnesium, vitamin D and 2 tablets of betaine hydrochloride after each meal can be helpful.

3. In my experience, so-called "Fruitarians", who try to live on a fruit diet exclusively, often suffer from leg cramps and other symptoms of severe calcium deficiency (in addition to usual protein and fatty acid deficiencies). Not only are most fruits low in calcium, but they are even lower in magnesium, without which calcium cannot be utilized (seeds, nuts and beans are rich in magnesium). In addition, some fruits, especially those rich in citric acid, will rob the body of its own calcium storage, if eaten in excess. The best sources of calcium are most vegetables, cereals such as millet, oats, rice, sesame seeds, beans, and, of course, milk and homemade cottage cheese.

DENTAL CARIES

Dental caries, or tooth decay, is a "civilization disease", found only where refined, devitalized, processed and demineralized foods, grown on soils deficient in minerals, are eaten. To prevent dental caries, an early program, preferably during pregnancy, must be initiated. Expectant mother must see that her diet is adequate in vital nutrients, especially minerals, calcium, magnesium and phosphorus, and all the trace minerals. The baby must be breast-fed as long as possible, even over a year. After weaning, bone meal should be added to the child's food, first about ½ teaspoon, then at the age of 2, 1 tsp. a day (or 3-4 tablets). Child should drink milk, preferably goat's milk, at least until adolescence. Best form of milk is soured milk, such as yogurt, kefir or clabbered milk. All sweets and all refined foods, and anything made with white sugar and white flour, should be strictly avoided.

The Airola Diet (see *Directions: 1*) with suggested supplements will assure healthy teeth. Millet and sesame seeds are especially beneficial. Sesame seeds are extremely rich in calcium — twice as much calcium as phosphorus, this proportion being reversed in about all other cereals and seeds. Adults plagued with excessive caries should, in addition to bone meal and mineral supplements, take 1 tablet of hydrochloric acid after each meal which will help in mineral assimilation.

BIOLOGICAL TREATMENTS

1. Avoid all toothpastes and powders. Detergents in toothpastes are harmful to teeth and gums.
2. Brush teeth after each meal with plain, soft-bristled brush and water, possibly with fine salt powder. In the morning, also brush the top of the tongue, especially if it is coated. Massage gums with your fingers once a day.
3. Eat foods that require lots of chewing. Avoid soft, gooey foods.
4. To prevent and treat periodontal disease, sufficient dietary or supplementary calcium is a must. Calcium deficiency is a basic cause of periodontal disease.
5. An excellent treatment for gum problems, tenderness around teeth and periodontal disease is to rub the gums morning and evening with vitamin E, which can be squeezed from the capsules.

VITAMINS & SUPPLEMENTS (Daily)

Bone meal — 1 tsp. of powder, or 4-6 tablets (up to 1,500 mg.).
  Children, half dose
Magnesium — 500 mg.
A — 25,000 units

C — 1,000 mg.

F, unsaturated fatty acids — 3 capsules, or 1 tbsp. of vegetable oil

Comprehensive multi-mineral trace element formula — 3 tablets (or 2 tbsp. of sea water)

Betaine Hydrochloride — 1 tablet after each meal with ½ glass of water (only for adults over 40)

Regular use of soured milks, such as kefir, yogurt, acidolphilus milk or plain clabbered milk

Natural multi-vitamin formula

JUICES

All vegetable juices. Fruit juices only sparingly, and always diluted with water, 50-50; this especially applies to citrus juices.

SPECIFICS

Bone meal, sesame seeds, soured milks, vitamins A and C, mineral supplement with magnesium, Airola Diet.

REFERENTIAL READING

Miller, F. D., *Eating For Sound Teeth*, Lee Foundation For Nutritional Research, Milwaukee, Wisc.

Taub, Harald J., "Bone Meal For Sound Teeth", *Prevention*, Nov., 1972.

Rodale, J. I. & Staff, *Bone Meal For Good Teeth*, Rodale Books, Inc., Emmaus, Pa., 1972.

Lee, R., "The Systemic Causes of Dental Caries", reprint #30A, Lee Foundation of Nutritional Research, Milwaukee, Wisc.

Price, Weston A., *Nutrition and Physical Degeneration*, The Price-Pottenger Foundation, Inc., Monrovia, Calif.

Williams, R. J., *Nutrition Against Disease*, Pitman Publishing Co., New York, 1971.

Shaw, J. H., "Nutrition and Dental Caries", *SURVEY OF THE LITERATURE OF DENTAL CARIES*, National Academy of Sciences, National Research Council, Publ. #225, Washington, D.C.

DIABETES

Most biological doctors specializing in diabetes agree that diabetes is a "prosperity" disease, primarily caused by systematic overeating and resultant obesity. Four out of five diabetics were overweight before diabetes was diagnosed. Not only the overeating of sugar and refined carbohydrates, but also of protein and fats (which are transformed into sugar if eaten in excess), is harmful, and may lead to diabetes. Too much food taxes the pancreas and eventually paralyzes its normal activity. Diabetes is unknown in countries where people can't afford to overeat.

DIETARY CONSIDERATIONS

Consequently, the number one dietary consideration for diabetes must be a strict, *lacto-vegetarian, low calorie, alkaline diet* of high quality natural foods. Plenty of whole grains, especially buckwheat, and raw vegetables — especially Jerusalem artichokes and green beans — and fruits, especially grapefruits and bananas. Contrary to popular notion, fruits are beneficial in the diabetic's diet. Fresh fruits contain sugar, *fructose*, which does *not* need insulin for its metabolism, and is well tolerated by diabetics.

Natural carbohydrate foods are necessary in the diet of diabetics. The diabetic needs carbohydrates, but they must be *natural, unrefined, slow-digesting* carbohydrates, such as whole grains, especially buckwheat, millet and oats.

Emphasis should be on *raw* foods. About 80 percent of the diet should be raw. Raw foods stimulate the pancreas and increase insulin production. For protein, homemade cottage cheese and various forms of soured milks (yogurt, kefir, etc.) are best (see *Recipes*). Also, nuts and avocados.

Avoid overeating. Four to five small meals a day is better than a few large meals. Avoid all *refined* carbohydrates, such as sugar and white flour, and everything made with them. Avoid salt.

Diabetics have a tendency for overacidity because of slowed down protein and fat metabolism. Therefore, the diet should be *alkaline*, with emphasis on alkaline foods: vegetables, fruits and milk and milk products. Cucumbers, stringbeans, Jerusalem artichokes and garlic are especially beneficial. Garlic has been shown to be able to reduce blood sugar in diabetes.

BIOLOGICAL TREATMENTS

1. *Lots of exercise* is the most important single thing, aside from dietary restrictions, that a diabetic can do to help himself. Hard exercise in fresh air, such as sports, jogging, swimming, and hard physical labor will help to keep "the fire of the metabolic processes

burning fast". Heavy physical work and strenuous sports diminish the need for *insulin.*

2. Fasting is usually not advisable for diabetics. For obese diabetics, a short juice fast is possible, but only under a doctor's control.
3. Avoid all mental and nervous stresses and strains, which have a detrimental effect on the condition.
4. Avoid constipation (see section on *Constipation*).
5. Use dry brush massage twice a day (see *Directions: 4*). It will improve metabolism and circulation, so vital for diabetics.
6. Prevalence of diabetes is higher in soft water areas. Diabetics, and those who wish to prevent diabetes, should drink naturally hard, heavily mineralized water, which contains chromium and other trace elements. Clinical studies have demonstrated that an ample supply of trace minerals, particularly chromium and manganese, is important for effective glucose utilization. Chromium aids in metabolism of excess sugar. Two milligrams of supplementary chromium can be given for six months, preferably in combination with manganese and other trace elements.

VITAMINS & SUPPLEMENTS (Daily)

B-complex, natural, high potency. Must include min.25 mcg.B_{12}

Chromium supplement — 2 mg. for six months. If not available, brewer's yeast is a rich source

Manganese, or comprehensive trace element formula containing manganese

Brewer's yeast — 3 to 5 tbsp.

F, unsaturated fatty acids (extremely important) — 6 capsules or 2 tbsp. of cold-pressed vegetable oil

C — 1,000 to 3,000 mg.

E — 400 to 1,200 IU

A-D capsules

B_6 — 50 to 100 mg.

Niacin — up to 100 mg.

Lecithin — 2 tbsp.

Bone meal — 3 tablets

Potassium — 300 mg.

Kelp — 1 tsp. of granules or 3 tablets

Garlic capsules — 3 to 5

JUICES

Stringbean juice, parsley, Jerusalem artichoke, cucumber, celery, watercress, lettuce, sauerkraut juice. Juice of onions and garlic can be added to other vegetable juices. Best fruit juices: citrus. Cucumber contains a hormone needed by the cells of the pancreas in order to produce insulin. The natural hormones contained in onions and garlic are also beneficial in diabetes.

HERBS

Stringbeans, blueberry leaves, sinita (Sinita Organo), juniper berries (Juniperus Sabina Pinaceae), dandelion root, periwinkle, raspberry leaves, alfalfa, centaurea, comfrey root. Stringbean pod tea is excellent natural substitute for insulin and extremely beneficial in diabetes. The skins of the pods of green beans are very rich in silica and certain hormone substances which are closely related to insulin. One cup of stringbean skin tea is equal to at least one unit of insulin. The recommended dose: one cup of stringbean skin tea morning, noon and evening.

SPECIFICS

Stringbeans, cucumber, chromium, manganese, B-complex vitamins, brewer's yeast, vitamins C and E, garlic. Small meals, no refined or processed carbohydrate foods, and plenty of strenuous exercise or heavy physical work.

REFERENTIAL READING

Joslin, E. P., et al., *The Treatment of Diabetes Mellitus*, Lea & Febiger, 1952.
Diseases of Metabolism, edited by Garlield G. Duncan, M.D., W. B. Saunders Co.
Diabetes, Vol. 22, February, 1973.
Science Magazine, May 27, 1966.
Journal of Nutrition, 94, 89; 1968.
Shute, Wilfred E. *Vitamin E for Ailing and Healthy Hearts*, Pyramid House, 1969.
Alpert, Elmer. *New York State Journal of Medicine*, November 15, 1953.
Walczak, M., et al., *Journal of Applied Nutrition*, Spring 1972.
"New Concepts in Diabetic Dietetics," *Nutrition Today*, May-June, 1972.
Diabetes, Vol. 22, September, 1973.

NOTES:

1. One of the insidious side effects of diabetes is a threat of gangrene and possible amputation of the foot or lower leg. Dr. Wilfred E. Shute says that this can be successfully prevented, and the condition can even be corrected when the feet are already affected, with large doses of vitamin E, taken internally.

2. Blueberry leaf tea has been used for centuries in folk medicine for treatment of "sugar" diabetes. One cup of tea three times a day is the recommended dose.

3. Cactus pads ("de-spined" cactus leaves of Tuna and Nopal Cactus), are used by American desert Indians as a diabetes "cure." It has been reported that cactus pads contain a huge amount of natural, organic insulin. Cactus pads can be eaten raw or cooked. Mexicans eat these de-spined leaves, with chili sprinkled on them, as a part of their regular diet. Also, Sinita (Sinita Organo), cactus plant native to Sonora, Mexico, contains natural insulin and is used widely to treat diabetes.

4. To correct an advanced diabetes by biological, herbal and nutritional means may take a long time. Milder cases normally respond well in a shorter period of time. If patient is using insulin or other related drugs, they should not be withdrawn abruptly, but the drug dosage should be decreased gradually as the blood sugar values improve, and the reaction of insulin withdrawal should be closely supervised by a physician.

5. *Diabetic retinopathy*, diabetic vision problems and gradual deterioration of eyesight, is one of the most common complications of diabetes. Oral doses of thyroid hormone extract with large doses of B-complex vitamins, vitamin C and digestive enzymes have been used successfully to treat diabetic retinopathy (*Prevention*, May, 1973).

DIARRHEA

1. *Parasitic, bacterial diarrhea*

Parasitic diarrhea is caused by inflammation of the intestines and toxic effect of bacterial or mycotic action.

DIETARY CONSIDERATIONS

In acute condition, avoid all foods for three days, except cooked white rice with applesauce made from raw apples, and supplements suggested below. Use organic apples, if possible, and make fresh applesauce for each meal by mashing apples in the blender.

Drink 4 to 6 cups of herb tea each day, made from carob, dried blueberries, cinnamon or other herbs given below; but these three are the best.

After condition improves, meals can be enlarged gradually to contain cooked vegetables, millet, whole rice and soured milks, such as buttermilk, yogurt, etc. Add raw foods to the diet when condition is completely corrected.

Cultured milks, such as buttermilk, yogurt, kefir, etc., are very beneficial in diarrhea and dysentery, especially in infant diarrhea. Bananas are also an excellent food for infants suffering from diarrhea, as is ripe papaya fruit.

VITAMINS & SUPPLEMENTS (Daily)

Vitamin C — 100 mg. tablet every hour
Garlic — raw garlic clove chewed with or between meals
Pepsin tablets, or comfrey-pepsin tablets
Apple pectine or caoline-pectine preparation, like Kaopectate
Pulverized charcoal — 1 tsp. or 3 tablets every 2 hours

JUICES

No raw juices until acute condition is corrected. Then, papaya juice, lemon juice, fresh pineapple juice.

HERBS

Garlic, dried blueberries, cinnamon, amaranth, slippery elm bark, carob, comfrey, witch hazel, raspberry leaves, peppermint (the essence of peppermint is used, 15 drops in one cup of hot water, repeat every three hours).

SPECIFICS

Garlic, dried blueberries, cinnamon, pectine, rice-apple diet, peppermint essence, vitamin C, pulverized charcoal.

2. Metabolic Diarrhea

Metabolic diarrhea is due to digestive and assimilative disturbances, caused by a metabolic disorder, biochemical imbalance, weakened digestive organs, and nutritional deficiencies, often caused by prolonged deficiencies of B-complex vitamins, particularly of B_1.

DIETARY CONSIDERATIONS

The Airola Diet (see *Directions: 1*). Small frequent meals. Never overeat! Chew all foods extremely well. Do not drink liquids with meals — drink one hour before or two hours after the meal. Recommended cereals: brown rice, millet, oats and buckwheat.

BIOLOGICAL TREATMENTS
1. Initial juice fasting for one week, broken strictly according to instructions (see *Directions: 3*). Followed by the Airola Diet.
2. B-complex vitamins intravenously for two weeks, followed by high doses of natural B-complex orally.

VITAMINS & SUPPLEMENTS (Daily)

B-complex, natural, high potency

B_1 — 200 mg. for two weeks, then reduce to 50 mg.

B_3 — 300 mg. (100 mg. with each meal) for two weeks, then reduce to 100 mg.

B_6 — 50 mg.

Magnesium — 500 mg., preferably magnesium chloride

Pantothenic acid, 100 mg.

Potassium

Carob powder — 3 tsp. a day in hot water

Digestive enzyme formula, containing hydrochloric acid — 1 tablet with each meal

Vitamin C — 1,000 mg. to 3,000 mg.

Vitamin A — 25,000 units

JUICES

All available fresh vegetable and fruit juices.

HERBS

Carob, dried blueberry tea, ripe papaya fruit. Carob can be used as a chocolate-like beverage, sweetened with honey.

SPECIFICS

B-complex vitamins, B_1, carob, dried blueberries, small meals, Airola Diet.

REFERENTIAL READING

Wolfe, M. S., *The Journal of the American Medical Association*, Vol. 220, April 3, 1972, p. 275.

Hawkins, Harold F., DDS, *Applied Nutrition*, Lee Foundation for Nutritional Research, Milwaukee, Wisconsin.

La Rue, Antoine, *Canadian Medical Association Journal*, November 5, 1960.

International Medical Digest, 32:369, 1938.

Fries, J. H., *Journal of Pediatrics*, 37:367, 1950.

NOTES:

1. Diarrhea is often the result of antibiotic therapy. This is due to destruction of the friendly bacteria in intestines along with the pathogenic bacteria at which the antibiotic treatment was aimed. Yogurt, kefir or other cultured milks in daily diet is a good remedy in such cases.

2. Those who travel to Mexico and other countries where hygienic conditions and bacterial flora are different, often catch "turista," or bacterial dysentery. American travelers are often given by their doctors Entero-Vioform tablets which they take several times a day to prevent "turista." These tablets are now banned in several countries, notably in Japan and Sweden, after it has been found that they can cause severe nerve and eye damage. A much safer way to prevent "turista" when traveling in developing countries is to take two tablets of betaine hydrochloride after each meal. Hydrochloric acid kills bacteria in the stomach and prevents infection. Also, straight lemon or lime juice, taken on empty stomach, has an antiseptic sterilizing effect. Eating raw garlic daily is also an excellent preventative.

3. In some cases of non-bacterial chronic diarrhea, 3 tbsp. of raw, unprocessed wheat bran daily, taken in fruit juice, has been found to give a most instant relief.

4. For amoeba dysentery (chronic dysentery caused by amoeba parasite) the following herbs have been used successfully: golden seal, colchicum, peppermint and ginger. Also garlic and sulphur 6X (homeopathic preparation).

DIGESTIVE DISORDERS

(Indigestion, gas, flatulence, foul stool)

The main reasons for indigestion and gas are overeating, eating wrong food combinations, eating too fast, and neglecting proper mastication and salivation of food. In older persons, the most common cause of indigestion and flatulence is poorly digested and putrefying food (particularly proteins and carbohydrates) in the intestines due to deficiency of gastric digestive juices. Taking one or two tablets of hydrochloric acid and a few dolomite tablets with each meal usually remedies that.

DIETARY CONSIDERATIONS

In my research and clinical work I have made one discovery regarding digestive disorders which is as original as it is far reaching in its application. I have found that one of the prime reasons for this common disorder in the United States (one doctor told me that 90 percent of his patients complain of gas!) is the lopsided and totally unnatural American way of eating: a large vegetable salad in the beginning of each meal — *before* protein foods are eaten. Protein foods need lots of hydrochloric acid for proper digestion. If the stomach is first filled with predominantly carbohydrate foods, *which do not require hydrochloric acid for digestion*, and then the meal is finished with protein-rich food, *the protein will remain largely undigested* because there would be not enough hydrochloric acid in the stomach. Therefore, the large vegetable salad should be either eaten *with* protein food, or *after*, but *never before.* Try it and see what difference in your digestion it will make. In studying the eating habits of natives around the world I have found that if they eat protein at a meal, whether it is meat, fish, beans or cheese, they always eat *it first,* or *with* salads, but never *after.* The speculation that every meal should begin with raw foods because "you need enzymes of raw food to help digest other foods" is erroneous. There is absolutely no scientific evidence that enzymes in salad will help in digestion of proteins.

Of course, the ideal way of eating is to eat only *one* food at a meal, whether it is cereal, salad, fruit or protein meal. Such eating will help even further in eliminating gas and other digestive disorders.

Eating small meals, eating very slowly and chewing food extremely well are all very important rules. Never eat if not hungry. Never eat if emotionally upset. Do not mix too many different foods at the same meal. Never eat raw fruits and raw vegetables at the same meal — they require a different set of enzymes and will only "confuse" the digestive processes and cause indigestion. Avoid constipation (see section on *Constipation*).

Eat *yogurt* or other cultured milks with every meal, or at least some every day. Other *lactic acid foods*, such as sauerkraut, soured vegetables, sour bread, etc., will also help in digestion and can help prevent intestinal putrefaction (see *Recipes*).

For flatulence and gas, *garlic* is the supreme remedy. It neutralizes putrefactive toxins and kills undesirable bacteria, eliminating gas and helping digestion.

Pollen, in granular or tablet form, produces the same anti-putrefactive effect in the intestines and colon as lactic acid foods and garlic.

All refined carbohydrates such as sugar in every form and starchy refined cereal foods (white flour) should be strictly avoided.

BIOLOGICAL TREATMENTS

In persistent and chronic digestive problems, repeated short juice fasts (see *Directions: 3*) can help by giving the digestive organs time and opportunity to rest and regenerate.

VITAMINS & SUPPLEMENTS (Daily)

Hydrochloric acid, preferably Betaine HCl — 1 or 2 tablets after each meal with 1/2 glass of water. This is for older people or those who definitely show HCl deficiency

Comfrey-pepsin — 2 or 3 capsules

Plenty of lactic acid foods, such as soured milks, sauerkraut, lactic acid vegetables, etc.

Garlic, or garlic oil capsules

Multiple digestive enzymes, with bile, papain, pancreatin, and bromelain, with each meal

Magnesium, preferably in the form of dolomite or magnesium chloride

B-complex, natural, high potency

B_1 — 50 mg.

B_6 — 50 mg.

Niacin — 100 mg.

Vitamin F, essential fatty acids, from cold-pressed vegetable oils

JUICES

Raw, fresh juices of papaya, pineapple, lemon.

HERBS

Garlic, ginseng, slippery elm, peppermint, anise, dill, parsley, cayenne (red pepper), camomile, golden seal.

SPECIFICS

HCl, digestive enzymes, garlic, B-complex vitamins, dolomite, lactic acid foods, pollen. Eat *sparingly, slowly*, and *chew well.*

REFERENTIAL READING

Levitt, Michael D., "Intestinal Gas Production," *Journal of the American Dietetic Association*, June, 1972, Vol. 60, No. 6, p. 487.

McCarrison, Sir Robert, *Studies in Deficiency Diseases*

Warmbrand, Max, *The Encyclopedia of Natural Health*, Groton Press, New York, 1962.

Airola, Paavo O., *Are You Confused?*, Health Plus Publishers, P.O. Box 22001, Phoenix, Arizona, 1971.

Johnston, Edward A. *Vitamins and Their Relation to Deficiency Diseases of the Alimentary Tract*, Reprint from Lee Foundation for Nutritional Research, Milwaukee, Wisconsin.

Tebbel, John, *Your Body*, Harper and Brothers, New York.

Yudkin, J., et al., *The Proceedings of the Nutrition Society*, Vol. 31, May, 1972.

Nittler, Alan H., *A New Breed of Doctor*, Pyramid House, New York, 1972.

NOTES:

1. See *Directions: 1*, section 9.

2. Finely shredded raw apple mixed with raw honey and eaten slowly with raw goat's milk seem to be well digested even by those who are unable to digest any other kind of food.

DIVERTICULOSIS

According to the newest medical opinion, the prime cause of diverticulosis and diverticulitis is "low-residue diet" of western man. Disease is seldom encountered in the areas where people eat so-called "high-residue diet" of unrefined, whole, natural, bulky foods. Thus, diverticulosis is primarily a deficiency disease — the deficiency of high-residue foods.

DIETARY CONSIDERATIONS

Emphasis should be on high-residue foods, such as the Airola Diet (see *Directions: 1*) would supply: raw and cooked vegetables and raw fruits, seeds and nuts. Sprouted seeds are excellent (see *Recipes*). Sour rye bread and such cooked cereals as millet, brown rice, buckwheat and oats are beneficial (see *Recipes*).

Soured milks daily: yogurt, kefir, buttermilk or plain clabbered milk.

Potato-cereal with flax seed and bran is very beneficial (see *Recipes*) and should be eaten often.

Lactic acid foods, such as sauerkraut, sour bread, lactic acid juices, soured milks, are extremely beneficial (see *Recipes*).

Eat small, frequent meals. Avoid all refined and processed foods. Avoid all refined carbohydrates and animal foods, except soured milks.

Each morning, drink 1 glass of Excelsior (see *Recipes*). Also, several glasses of fresh juices and herb tea each day.

BIOLOGICAL TREATMENTS

1. If constipation or sluggish elimination accompany the condition, treat constipation as suggested in section on *Constipation*.
2. Maintenance of ideal body weight is important. Obese older persons have greater incidence of diverticulosis.

VITAMINS & SUPPLEMENTS (Daily)

Whey powder — 1 tbsp. with each meal
Garlic or garlic oil capsules
Folic acid — 1 mg.
Flax seed, whole, as in Excelsior (see *Recipes*)
Cold-pressed vegetable oils — 2 tbsp. (olive oil is best)
Natural multiple vitamin-mineral formula

JUICES

Carrot, beet, celery, green juices. Fermented lactic acid juices are especially beneficial (available at health stores). Best fruit juices: papaya, apple, pineapple, lemon.

HERBS

Flax seed, slippery elm, camomile, peppermint, aloe vera.

SPECIFICS

Whey powder, whole soaked flax seed, bran, garlic, high-residue foods. Soured milks.

REFERENTIAL READING

Painter, Neil S. and Burkitt, Denis P., Report in *British Medical Journal*, May 22, 1971 and June 29, 1971.

Berman, P. M. and Kirsner, J. B. *Geriatrics*, Vol. 27, April 1972, p. 117.

Prevention, March, 1967

Ellis, Harold, *Postgraduate Medicine*, Vol. 53, No. 6. May, 1973.

ECZEMA

*(Various forms of skin disorders and skin eruptions.
See special section on Psoriasis)*

DIETARY CONSIDERATIONS

The Airola Diet (see *Directions: 1*) from three basic food groups: seeds, nuts and grains; vegetables; and fruits, all 100 percent raw. Some seeds, grains and beans such as alfalfa seeds, wheat and mung and soy beans, can be sprouted. Complement this diet with cold-pressed vegetable oils (sesame seed oil or olive oil), honey and plenty of brewer's yeast.

No salt, coffee, chocolate or tea. No sugar in any form. No refined, processed or cooked foods. No meat, eggs, cow's milk or fish. Goat's milk is permitted, preferably in soured form (yogurt, kefir, etc.).

Raw potatoes have a specific beneficial effect.

BIOLOGICAL TREATMENTS

1. Juice fast, two to three weeks (see *Directions: 3*). After intermittent four weeks on raw food diet, juice fasting can be repeated if needed.
2. Avoid washing with soaps and shampoo. Bathe and wash affected parts often with plain water. After bath, rub the affected parts with a slice of cucumber. Acid-type soap, if available, can be used.
3. Use some of the following for external application:
   - Lanolin cream with vitamins A and E
   - Airola Formula F-Plus (see *Directions: 8*)
   - Aloe Vera, fresh jell or cream
   - Dust affected parts with whey powder each morning
4. If constipated, or suffering from sluggish elimination, follow anti-constipation program (see section on *Constipation* in this book). Chronic constipation is one of the main reasons for many skin disorders.
5. Emotional and nervous disorders — also common causes of skin disorders — must be corrected.

VITAMINS & SUPPLEMENTS (Daily)

C — up to 1,000 mg.

A — 50,000 to 75,000 units for 2 to 3 months; then, after a one month interval, continue with 25,000 units

B-complex, natural, high potency, with B_{12}

Cod liver oil — 1 to 2 tsp.

B_6 — 50 mg.

Biotin — 25 mcg.

PABA — 50 mg.

Inositol — 500 mg.

Calcium lactate — 4-6 tablets

Brewer's yeast — 2 to 3 tbsp.

Whey, 2-3 tbsp.

Lecithin — 2 to 3 tsp.

Kelp — 2 tsp. of granules or tablets

Cholorophyl tablets

Betaine Hydrochloride — 1 tablet after each meal

JUICES

Green vegetable juice, carrot, beet, celery, spinach, cucumber, black currants, red grapes.

HERBS

Comfrey, burdock, elecampane, juniper berry, Solidago (golden rod), wild pansies (Viola Tricolor), celandine, lavender, aloe vera, strawberry leaves, slippery elm bark, jimson weed.

SPECIFICS

Vitamins A, C and B-complex, brewer's yeast, carrots, green juices, kelp, raw potatoes, juice fasting.

REFERENTIAL READING

The Natural Way to Healthy Skin, Rodale Press, Emmaus, Pennsylvania.

Clark, Linda, *Secrets of Health & Beauty*, The Devin-Adair Co., N.Y., N.Y., 1969.

Rodale, J. I. & Staff. *The Encyclopedia for Healthful Living*, Rodale Press, Emmaus, Pennsylvania.

Clark, Michael, "A natural treatment for eczema", *Prevention*, October, 1973.

NOTES:

1. The most common causes of eczema and other skin diseases are found in faulty metabolism, constipation, poor elimination of toxic wastes and nutritional deficiencies. Juice fasting almost always results in marked improvement or complete remission of all symptoms. A certain worsening of the condition can be expected in some cases in the beginning or during the fast, due to the increased elimination of waste matter through the skin, but as fasting continues, the improvement will not fail to manifest itself.

2. French herbal healer, Maurice Mességué, developed a very successful natural treatment for eczema, which was used on thousands of patients with reported remarkable results — an estimated 98% rate of cure.

   Here is the Mességué treatment:

   Make an herbal extract in the following manner: boil a quart of water, using a glass or enameled pot, then let it cool until lukewarm. Drop in a handful of each of the following herbs: artichoke leaves, elecampane (flowers and leaves), celandine (leaves — fresh if possible), chicory (roots and tips), broom (flowers), lavender (flowers) and nettle (leaves — fresh if possible). Let the mixture soak for 4 to 5 hours. Strain and pour into a clean bottle for storage until use. Extract can be used for 8 days before a new one must be brewed.

The extract is then used for an 8-minute foot bath each morning before breakfast, and an 8-minute hand bath in the evening before dinner. The bath is made in the following manner: Boil 2 quarts of water and let stand for 5 minutes. Add 1/2 pint of plant extract to 2 quarts of boiled water. Take foot or hand bath as hot as you can tolerate. The bath preparation can be kept and warmed for the next bath, but without boiling or adding more water. (Maurice Mességué, "Of Men and Plant", Macmillan Company, 1973)

EDEMA

If edema is caused by heart failure, the patient should follow the dietary advice given in the section on *Heart Disease*. If edema is caused by kidney failure, which is another common cause, or by other causes, the following program is suggested.

DIETARY CONSIDERATIONS

Emphasis on raw vegetables and fruits, particularly cucumber, watermelon and pineapple, and all silicon-rich foods such as young green plants, alfalfa, common nettle, horsetail, garlic and onions, parsnips, asparagus, apples, strawberries, grapes, beets, coconuts.

Moderate amounts of raw nuts (almonds) and seeds (sesame seeds, sunflower seeds, flax seed, pumpkin seeds). Millet, rice and steel-cut oats are suitable cereals.

No animal proteins: no meat, eggs or fish. Small quantity of soured milks and homemade cottage cheese (see *Recipes*).

Salt intake should be reduced to minimum. Use only natural sea salt in small amounts.

BIOLOGICAL TREATMENTS

1. One or two-week juice fast (*Directions: 3*) using intermittently cucumber, pineapple and watermelon juice, six glasses total per day. Colonics once a week, enemas daily. Drink two glasses of kidney-bean pod tea each day. After the fast, a watermelon diet for an additional ten days. Eat nothing but ripe watermelon, as often as desired, but in small quantities each time. Continue with daily enema.

   After this, a lacto-vegetarian diet of raw and cooked vegetables, particularly green leafy vegetables, seeds, nuts and yogurt. Follow the diet suggestions given above.
2. Hot baths, preferably sauna, twice a week.
3. Lots of strenuous exercise, such as jogging, walking, playing tennis, etc., to induce perspiration.
4. Kidney bean pod treatment — see section on *Kidney Disease.*

VITAMINS & SUPPLEMENTS (Daily)

B_6 — 50 to 200 mg.
C — 2,000 to 5,000 mg.
Potassium (potassium gluconate)
Bromelain (pineapple enzyme) — 6 to 8 tablets
Silicon (natural diuretic), preferably in organic form of dried fresh plants, such as horsetail, or silica tablets, 2 to 3 tablets a day

JUICES

Cucumber, pineapple, watermelon, all green juices.

HERBS

Kidney bean pod tea (Phaseolus Vulgaris), lily-of-the-valley, juniper berry, garlic, jewel weed, parsley, horsetail.

SPECIFICS

Vitamins B_6 and C, kidney bean pod tea, horsetail, potassium, bromelain, cucumber, watermelon, garlic.

REFERENTIAL READING

Ellis, John M., *The Doctor Who Looked At Hands*, Vantage Press, N.Y., 1966.
Prevention, February, 1972.
Ellis, John M. and Presley, James, *Vitamin B_6: The Doctor's Report*, Harper and Row, New York, N.Y., 1973.

NOTES:

1. Edema associated with pregnancy is normally reduced by restricting salt intake and taking vitamin B_6, 50 to 150 mg. a day. Silica is also helpful — 2 to 3 tablets a day.
2. Edema associated with menstruation is helped by vitamin B_6, 50 to 100 mg. daily.

DIETARY CONSIDERATIONS

The Airola Diet (see *Directions: 1*) with all suggested supplements: vegetable oil, honey, brewer's yeast, kelp, lecithin and raw goat's milk, preferably in soured form; yogurt, kefir, acidophilus, etc. Emphasis on raw fruits and vegetables. Best vegetables are garlic and comfrey (both leaves and roots). Plenty of vegetable and fruit juices. Raw comfrey leaves should be chewed between meals. Also, 1 tsp. of fresh raw lemon (or lime) juice can be taken several times a day between or before meals.

BIOLOGICAL TREATMENTS

1. Short cleansing juice fast (see *Directions: 3*), one week to ten days. If patient is overweight, longer fast can be undertaken.
2. Lots of exercise and walking in fresh air. Walking up to 5-10 miles a day.
3. No smoking. If possible, move to a 100 percent smog-free environment.
4. Deep breathing exercises, several times a day, in fresh air.

VITAMINS & SUPPLEMENTS (Daily)

E — up to 1,600 IU

B_{15} — 100 to 150 mg. (50 mg. three times a day)

C — 3,000 to 5,000 mg.

A — 50,000 units. 100,000 units can be given for the period of 1 to 2 weeks.

Comfrey, fresh in salads, and dry (leaves and roots) in tea form

Brewer's yeast — 3 to 5 tbsp.

Lecithin — 1 tbsp.

Multi vitamin-mineral supplement, all natural

JUICES

Vegetable: green juice, carrot, parsnip, watercress, raw potato, with small amount of garlic juice added to vegetable juices.

Fruit: lemon, orange, black currants and rose hips.

HERBS

Comfrey, rose hips, licorice root, fennel seed, anise seed.

SPECIFICS

Vitamins E, B_{15} and C, comfrey, garlic, deep-breathing exercises in pure fresh air, lots of walking.

REFERENTIAL READING

Bass, Harry, *Journal of the American Medical Association*, December 23, 1969.
Menzel, D. B., et al. *Chemical and Engineering News*, June 29, 1970.
Clark, Michael, "Vitamin A (and E) Protect Against Emphysema," *Prevention*, May, 1973.

NOTES:

1.   An old emphysema "cure" from folk medicine with many favorable reports: 5 to 10 drops of anise seed oil on 1 tsp. of brown sugar taken 3 times daily before meals.

DIETARY CONSIDERATIONS

Three factors must be always considered in planning a diet for persons suffering from epilepsy:

1. elimination of all possible allergens, as allergic reaction to certain food substances or foods may be an underlying or triggering cause for epileptic seizures;

2. diet must be adequate in magnesium-rich foods, supplemented with magnesium supplements, as magnesium deficiency has been shown to be involved in epilepsy;

3. diet must be an anti-hypoglycemia diet, as, according to some researchers, low blood sugar, or hypoglycemia, is also involved in most cases of epilepsy. If hypoglycemia is present, follow the program suggested in section on *Hypoglycemia.*

Often, epileptics have deficient mineral assimilation, particularly of magnesium and calcium, especially if they are taken with meals. If magnesium deficiency is obvious, magnesium and calcium should be given on empty stomach, between meals, preferably with some sour fruit juice, apple cider vinegar and/or one tablet of betaine hydrochloride. For magnesium supplement, magnesium chloride, magnesium gluconate or magnesium oxide can be used.

It is important to eliminate completely all animal proteins, except milk, as they are not only lacking magnesium but will rob the body of its own magnesium storage as well as of vitamin B_6 reserves, both substances needed in large amounts by epileptics. Best food sources of magnesium are raw nuts, seeds, soybeans, cooked and green leafy vegetables, such as spinach, kale, chard, beettops etc. If vegetables are cooked, cooking water should be consumed.

The diet should be the Airola Diet (see *Directions: 1*) with as many raw foods as possible. Plenty of vegetable juices, particularly green juices (made from green leafy plants and vegetables). Sprouted seeds, such as alfalfa seeds and mung beans are recommended. Plenty of raw vegetables and fruits. At least 2 tbsp. of olive oil daily, preferably with food. A moderate amount of raw milk — preferably raw goat's milk — and milk products, including raw butter and unprocessed cheese, preferably homemade cottage cheese (see *Recipes*). Two or three raw egg yolks from fertile eggs can be taken each week.

Avoid all refined foods. No sugar or anything made with it. Use a little honey as sweetener.

Avoid overeating. Eat several small meals, instead of a few large ones.

Do not eat large meals before going to bed.

BIOLOGICAL TREATMENTS

1. Epileptics should strictly observe all the general rules of good health and build and maintain the highest level of general health possible.
2. Keep active mentally but avoid all severe mental or physical stresses. Avoid extreme excitations of all kinds, also situations where anger, fear or hate are provoked.
3. The Airola Diet and sufficient rest are especially required during periods of menstruation, pregnancy and menopause, as these seem to provoke seizures.
4. Plenty of fresh air is a must for epileptics. Do not live in a smoggy area. Sleep with windows open. If climate permits, live outdoors all of the time, day and night. A dry, warm climate is preferable for epileptics. Seizures seem to increase during cold winters and rain storms with high humidity.
5. As much as possible, physical activity in fresh air is advisable to oxygenate all the tissues, including the brain cells.
6. Plenty of rest and sound sleep are imperative, but do not go to bed immediately after a meal. One cup of herb tea (mistletoe, for example) sweetened with a little honey, is good.
7. Avoid constipation. If natural BM fails, take an enema before going to bed.
8. Epsom salts bath, twice a week, is beneficial.
9. Some practitioners have successfully used thyroid extract in the treatment of epilepsy, as epileptics tend to be low in thyroid.

VITAMINS & SUPPLEMENTS (Daily)

Magnesium — 500 mg. for children, 800 mg. for adults

E — start with 300 IU and gradually increase over period of several months to 1,600, even 2,000 IU

B_6 — 100 mg. Under doctor's supervision, up to 300 mg. daily

B_{15} — 100 mg., (50 mg. in the morning and 50 mg. before going to bed)

B-complex, natural, high potency, with 25 mcg. of B_{12}

Niacin — 50 mg.

Calcium — 1,000 mg.

A & D (10,000 A — 1,000 D) — 1 capsule

Folic acid — 0.5 mg.

Trace element formula with iron

C - 2,000 mg.

Betaine hydrochloride with other digestive enzymes (if not contraindicated) — 1 or 2 tablets after each meal with 1/2 glass of water

Yogurt or other soured milks

Zinc — 30 mg.

Whey powder — 2 tsp. with meals

Silica — 2-3 tablets

JUICES

Green vegetable juice, red beet, carrot, red grapes, figs.

HERBS

Mistletoe, hyssop, Irish moss, peruvian bark, black cohosh, horse nettle.

SPECIFICS

Magnesium supplement, vitamins E, B_6, B_{15}, elimination of allergens from diet and environment. Avoid emotional stresses.

REFERENTIAL READING

Abrahamson, E. M. and Pezet, A. W., *Body, Mind & Sugar*, Henry Holt and Company, N.Y.

Davidson, Hal M., article in *Quarterly Review of Allergy and Applied Immunology*, June, 1952.

Summary, June, 1961, published by Shute Foundation For Medical Research, London, Ontario, Canada.

Davis, Adelle, *Let's Eat Right to Keep Fit*, Harcourt, Brace Javanovich, Inc., N.Y., 1970.

Poole, M., "Research Offers New Hope For the Epileptic" (interview with Dr. S. T. Rich), *The Answer — Preventive Medicine*, Vol. 1, No. 3, 1972.

Vilter, Richard W., *Modern Nutrition in Health and Disease*, Wohl and Goodhart, ed., Lea & Febiger, 1964.

Keith, H. M., *Convulsive Disorders in Children with Reference to Treatment with Diet*, Little Brown & Co., Boston, 1963.

GALLBLADDER PROBLEMS

DIETARY CONSIDERATIONS

In acute state of gallbladder inflammation, *all eating should be avoided.* Patient should take nothing but water for two or three days, until acute condition is cleared. After this, patient should be put on juices for a few more days. Pear juice and beettop juice should be drunk intermittently.

The diet should be lacto-vegetarian, with emphasis on raw and cooked vegetables and vegetable juices. Moderate amount of fruits and seeds. Pears should be eaten generously, they have a specific healing effect on gallbladder. Include yogurt, homemade cottage cheese, two raw egg yolks twice a week, and 1 tbsp. of olive oil twice a day. Oil is necessary in the diet to stimulate the production of bile and the fat-digesting enzyme, lipase. High quality vegetable oil in the diet also prevents gallstone formation. Use butter in moderation. Avoid all meat and all animal fats, and all processed and denatured fats such as margarine and commerical oils.

Very important: do not overeat! Eat small meals. Remember: hospital records show that most gallbladder patients are overweight!

BIOLOGICAL TREATMENTS

1. In addition to total fasting in acute stages of disease, *cold milk compress* on higher abdomen, renewed every hour, was found to be of help. Dip flannel cloth in milk, place on abdomen, cover with piece of plastic, then cover with warm wool or wool blanket.

2. *For removal of gallstones*, the popular biological treatment is so-called *"oil cure."* Raw, natural, unrefined vegetable oils of olive, sunflower or walnut are used, olive oil being most common.

    Oil cure should be preceded by a two-day cleansing diet of vegetables and fruits (pears) plus soaked prunes, figs and psyllium seeds. Before beginning the cure, take a good enema to cleanse the bowels.

    Take 1/2 to 3/4 of a pint of oil at a time. After taking oil, lie down on your right side and remain in this position for two hours.

3. Another recommended oil treatment for gallbladder pain is as follows:

    First thing in the morning, on an empty stomach, take one ounce of vegetable oil, preferably olive oil, and follow immediately with four ounces of grapefruit juice. If grapefruit juice is not available, take lemon juice, or 1 tsp. apple cider vinegar in four ounces of water. Take this treatment each morning for several days, even weeks, if necessary.

4. Over 90 percent of human gallstones are composed chiefly of cholesterol. On the other hand, clinical studies show that the phospholipid concentration in the bile of patients with gallstones is significantly lower as compared with the patients with normal gallbladders. Giving gallstone patients two tbsp. of lecithin a day immediately results in increased phospholipid concentration in the bile. This will help to keep cholesterol dispersed and prevent the formation of gallstones.
5. Castor oil pack on the gallbladder area is helpful in acute inflammatory conditions (see section on *Arthritis*).
6. Retention coffee enema is effective in acute gallbladder colic: one cup of strong brewed (not instant or decaffeinated) coffee is added to one pint warm water. Retain as long as possible. Helps to relieve pain and relax the liver-gallbladder area.

VITAMINS & SUPPLEMENTS (Daily)

Lecithin – 2 tbsp. of granules, with meals (prevents formation of gallstones)

Choline – 500 mg. (essential for proper fat metabolism)

Inositol – 500 mg. (involved in cholesterol metabolism)

Biotin – 25 mcg.(involved in fat assimilation)

Beet leaf powder concentrate

B-complex, natural high potency, with B_{12}

B_6 – 50 mg.

Olive oil – 2 tbsp.

Comprehensive digestive enzyme formula with hydrochloric acid – 1 tablet after each meal

A – 10,000 to 25,000 units

C-complex (C with bioflavonoids) – 500 mg.

Brewer's yeast – 2 tbsp.

E – 600 IU

D – 5,000 units, once a week

JUICES

Pear juice, beettop juice, grapefruit, lemon, grape. Small amounts of dandelion and radish or black radish juice added to carrot or beettop juice. Pear and beettop juice are two specific juices that have a healing effect on gallbladder conditions, including the gallstones.

HERBS

Horsetail, dandelion, comfrey, fennel, parsley, white oak bark, peppermint oil (10 drops in a glass of hot water), dyer's root.

SPECIFICS

Pears, beettop juice or beet powder, olive oil, lecithin, B-complex vitamins, particularly choline, inositol and biotin. Eating small meals.

REFERENTIAL READING

Sturdevant, Richard A. L., *New England Journal of Medicine*, Vol. 288, No. 1, January 4, 1973.

McCormick, W. J., *Medical Record*, July, 1946.

Rodale, and Staff, *Encyclopedia of Common Diseases*, Rodale Book, Inc., Emmaus, Penna.

Donsbach, Kurt W. "How to Live with Your Gallbladder," *Let's Live*, December 1972.

Warmbrand, Max, *The Encyclopedia of Natural Health*, Groton Press, Inc., 1962.

Nittler, Alan H., *A New Breed of Doctor*, Pyramid House, N.Y., 1972.

Sneddon, J. Russell, *The Natural Treatment of Liver Troubles and Associated Ailments*, Health For All Publishing Co., London, 1960.

Vogel, A. *The Liver*, Bioforce-Verlag, Teufen, Switzerland, 1962.

GLAUCOMA

(Chronic glaucoma, or hypertension of the eye)

DIETARY CONSIDERATIONS

To date, it has not been shown that any particular diet is of specific value in prevention, treatment or control of glaucoma. It is generally believed that restoration of vision already lost due to nerve degeneration, caused by increased intraocular pressure, cannot occur. However, certain nutritional and other biological approaches have proven to be effective in controlling the condition and preserving the remaining sight.

Diet should be the Airola Diet (see *Directions: 1*) with emphasis on raw, *C-vitamin-rich foods*: fresh fruits and vegetables, in season.

Avoid such stimulants as coffee or tea. Caffein causes stimulation of the vasoconstrictors, elevating blood pressure and increasing blood flow to the eye.

Avoid excessive amount of fluid intake, whether it is juice, water or milk, *at any one time.* Drink small amounts several times with at least one hour intervals.

BIOLOGICAL TREATMENTS

1. Glaucoma is considered to be a "stress disease." Avoid emotional stresses and upheavals. Cultivate a tranquil, restful life style. Climate with great temperature changes (north) is detrimental. Southern temperate and more even climate is better tolerated.
2. Avoid prolonged eye stresses such as long movies, excessive TV watching, excessive reading, etc.
3. Avoid smoking. There is evidence indicating that smoking causes damage in glaucoma condition.
4. Avoid using sunglasses.
5. If using drugs for other conditions, always inform your doctor of your glaucoma condition; which will help him to avoid prescribing drugs which might adversely affect the glaucoma.

VITAMINS & SUPPLEMENTS (Daily)

C - 60 to 250 mg. per pound of body weight each day. That means, a 150 lb. person should receive about 7 grams of vitamin C, 3 to 5 times a day. It has been demonstrated in recent studies in Rome, Italy (and reported at the meeting of the Roman Ophthalmological Society) that the intraocular pressure in glaucomatous eyes can be dramatically reduced by the oral mega-doses of vitamin C.

Rutin — 150 mg. (50 mg. three times a day)

Vitamin A — 25,000 units

Choline — up to 2 grams

Comprehensive multi-vitamin-mineral formula

Pantothenic acid — up to 200 mg.

Lemon, grapefruit, orange, carrot, red beet and beettop juice.

Mega-doses of vitamin C, rutin, vitamin A, choline.

Cheraskin, E., and Ringsdorf, W. H. *New Hope for Incurable Diseases*, Exposition Press, 1971.
British Journal of Ophthalmology, Vol. 1, p. 42, 1958.
Health Bulletin, February 15, 1964.

NOTES:
1.   Due to the seriousness of the condition, glaucoma patients are advised not to experiment with self-treatments, but be under constant supervision of a sympathetic ophthalmologist, and abide by his advice as to the advisability of employing some of the suggestions listed above.

GOUT

DIETARY CONSIDERATIONS

The basic diet for gout is the same as for arthritis (see section on *Arthritis*) — a low-uric acid, low-purine diet. Foods high in potassium are protective against gout: potatoes, bananas, leafy green vegetables, beans, raw vegetable juices. Vegetable broth (see *Recipes*) is of exceptional value — take two glasses a day. Avoid all purine and uric acid producing foods: all meat, eggs, fish and milk. Glandular meats are especially bad. Raw goat's milk is beneficial, preferably in soured form. Avoid salt. Avoid wheat except in sprouted form. Peas should be avoided also.

Red sour cherries and strawberries are of specific value in gout, preferably eaten fresh, although canned or juiced are also beneficial. Make sure they are canned without sugar! Cherries have an exceptional ability to alkalize the system and neutralize uric acid. Take them in great amounts, especially in season, preferably on an empty stomach between meals. Sour cherries are best.

BIOLOGICAL TREATMENTS

Juice fast (see *Directions: 3*), one to two weeks. Sometimes, in cases of gout, a noticeable worsening of the condition may develop in the early stages of fasting when uric acid, dissolved by juices, is thrown into the blood stream for elimination. This usually clears up if fasting is continued. In severe cases it is advisable to have a series of short fasts, 3-4 days each, rather than one long fast.

VITAMINS & SUPPLEMENTS (Daily)

C — up to 5,000 mg.
E — 400 to 1,200 IU, depending on age and heart condition (higher dosage for older people)
B-complex, natural, high potency
Potassium — 2 tablets (use potassium bicarbonate)
Alfalfa tablets — 10 to 15 tablets
Natural multi-vitamin-mineral formula

JUICES

Red sour cherries, carrot, celery, parsley, alfalfa, raw potato juice, vegetable broth, green juice, fresh pineapple juice.

HERBS

Juniper berries, comfrey, alfalfa, sarsaparilla, birch leaves, ginger, parsley.

SPECIFICS

Animal-protein-free diet, red sour cherries or cherry juice, vitamin C, potassium-rich diet, juniper berries.

REFERENTIAL READING

Seegmiller, J. P., *Gout*, Grune and Stratton, 1967.

Airola, Paavo O., *There IS a Cure For Arthritis*, Parker Publishing Co., West Nyack, N.Y., 1968.

Williams, Roger J., *Nutrition Against Disease*, Pitman Publishing Co., New York

Warmbrand, Max, *New Hope For Arthritis Sufferers*, Groton Press, N.Y.

Blau, Ludwig W , *Texas Reports on Biology and Medicine*, Vol. 8, No. 3, Fall, 1950.

NOTES:

1.   A note of consolation to persons suffering with gout: it has been well established by many studies and clinical observations that a high blood level of uric acid is associated with a high level of intellectual attainment and such qualities as drive, leadership and high intelligence. (So, don't feel so bad! And, knowing this, perhaps you would rather live with painful toes than try to lower the uric acid level of your blood?!) However, it was *not* established whether the high blood level of uric acid contributes to the higher I.Q., or the intense intellectual activity leads to the elevation of blood uric acid.

HALITOSIS

If caused by tooth and gum conditions, tonsilitis, sinusitis, smoking or anemia, these conditions must be treated and eliminated before unpleasant breath will disappear. Most cases of bad breath, however, are caused by gastro-intestinal disorders, intestinal sluggishness and particularly by chronic constipation. The unpleasant odor is caused by an exceptionally large amount of waste matter expelled through the lungs. In such cases, the cause — internal sluggishness and constipation — must be corrected.

DIETARY CONSIDERATIONS

The Airola Diet (see *Directions: 1*) with emphasis on raw and cooked vegetables and fruits. Chew all food extremely well. Avoid constipating, refined carbohydrate foods, such as white sugar, white bread and baked goods. Even whole-grain bread should be eaten sparingly. Avoid meat and eggs. Faulty digestion of animal proteins (putrefaction of proteins due to overconsumption or deficiency of gastric enzymes and HCl) is a common cause of bad breath and unpleasant body odors.

Avoid overeating of any kind of foods.

Eat six to eight soaked prunes and/or a few dried (or soaked) figs with breakfast. Be sure to drink the water in which fruits were soaked.

Consume plenty of liquids — generous drinking of water (4-6 glasses a day) will often result in disappearance of bad breath.

BIOLOGICAL TREATMENTS

1. If constipated, follow anti-constipation program (see section on *Constipation*).
2. Get plenty of exercise! Lack of sufficient exercise is one of the main causes of constipation.
3. Take 1 tsp. of powdered charcoal in a glass of water first thing every morning.

VITAMINS & SUPPLEMENTS (Daily)

Alfalfa tablets, concentrated, defibred type — 6
Chlorophyl tablets — 3
Irish moss (Tillandsia) tablets — 1 or 2
Whey powder — 2 tbsp.
B_6 — 50 mg.
C — 1,000 mg. or more
Zinc — 30 - 60 mg.

Brewer's yeast — 2 to 5 tbsp. a day. Take brewer's yeast on an empty stomach mixed in with some sour fruit juice, water and apple cider vinegar or 1 tablet of hydrochloric acid

"Excelsior" — drink every morning (see *Recipes*)

Betaine hydrochloride — 1 tablet after each meal for people over 40

Multi-vitamin-mineral formula, natural

JUICES

Any available vegetable and fruit juices. Green juice is especially beneficial (see *Directions: 5*).

HERBS

Irish moss, alfalfa, peppermint, parsley, golden seal, rosemary.

SPECIFICS

Chlorophyl, Irish moss (Tillandsia), alfalfa, hydrochloric acid, vitamin C, plenty of liquids, anti-constipation diet.

REFERENTIAL READING

Young, R. A., "Bad Breath Doesn't Need Mouthwash," *Prevention*, January, 1969.

Airola, Paavo O., *Sex and Nutrition* (see Chapter 15 "If He Kissed You Once . . ."), Universal Publishing and Distributing Corp., New York, N.Y., 1970.

Waerland, Are, *Health is Your Birthright*, Humata Publishers, Bern, Switzerland.

HEART DISEASE

The basic causes of heart disease can be found in faulty eating and living habits and various mental and physical environmental stresses. The famous Framingham Heart Study of the National Heart and Lung Institutes, identified and qualified the following major risk factors in coronary heart disease:

    a. Elevated blood levels of cholesterol, triglycerides, and other fatty substances.

    b. Elevated blood pressure.

    c. Elevated blood uric acid levels (mainly caused by high protein diet).

    d. Certain metabolic disorders, notably diabetes.

    e. Obesity.

    f. Smoking.

    g. Lack of physical exercise.

Each, but especially a combination, of these risk factors can contribute to the development of heart disease. Most of them are of dietary origin. The successful treatment of heart disease is contingent on elimination of all the above risk factors — the underlying causes of the disease.

DIETARY CONSIDERATIONS

Lacto-vegetarian, low-sodium, low-calorie, low-animal-protein diet of high quality, natural organic foods with emphasis on whole grains, seeds and nuts, fresh fruits and vegetables with the addition of raw, unpasteurized milk and homemade cottage cheese (see *Recipes*).

Millet, buckwheat, sunflower seeds, sesame seeds, bananas, potatoes, okra, asparagus, apples, honey, brewer's yeast, flax seed oil, lecithin — these are specific nutritive factors beneficial in a heart condition. Buckwheat is rich in rutin which keeps arteries in good health. Potatoes and bananas are rich in potassium which is vital for healthy heart function. Okra, the slippery vegetable containing the viscous mucilage, is beneficial in atherosclerosis in that it helps to reduce blood vessel friction. It can be used in soups and stews, but also eaten raw or added to green juices (see *Recipes*). Apples contain pectin which is also of great benefit in atherosclerosis. Flax seed oil is rich in essential fatty acids, especially in *linolenic acid*, which is essential for a healthy heart. Lecithin can help to prevent fatty deposits in arteries that lead to heart attacks. Asparagus is beneficial for an enlarged heart.

No salt, no sugar, no alcohol, no coffee, no meat — all of these are definitely proven in reliable studies to be contributing causes to heart disease. Do not use any refined or processed foods. Avoid animal fats and processed fats, especially margarine and other hydrogenated fats. Small amounts of vegetable oils of highest quality, cold-pressed and unrefined, such as olive oil, flax seed oil, safflower oils, or sesame oil, are beneficial, even essential, *if supplemented with vitamin E.*

Do not overeat! Obesity is one of the main causes of heart disease. Statistics show that the obese have a 100 percent greater risk of developing heart disease or succumbing to a heart attack.

Do not drink *distilled water.* Avoid soft water. Naturally hard water contains minerals, especially chromium, which are vital for heart health. Naturally, your drinking water must be pure, uncontaminated, unchlorinated and non-flouridated natural spring or well water. Such drinking water is available now in most cities in bottled form.

Avoid all *refined carbohydrates*, such as white flour and white sugar and everything made with them. It has been conclusively demonstrated that excess sugar and refined foods in the diet is one of the main causes of arteriosclerosis and heart disease.

Do not drink *chlorinated water.* Chlorine destroys vitamin E in the body, which is absolutely essential for the health of the heart. *This is extremely important.*

BIOLOGICAL TREATMENTS

1. *Plenty of exercise*, both as preventative and therapeutic measures in heart disease, is imperative. Walking, jogging, jumping ropes, riding a horse or bicycle, swimming, etc. Not only would sufficient exercise in fresh air prevent most heart problems, but for those who survived a heart attack, exercise is singularly the most important measure to assure complete recovery and prolong life. There is a famous rehabilitation center for former heart attack victims in Yugoslavia where the only therapeutic program is gradually increased walks in hilly terrain. Patients, who could hardly walk 100 feet on arrival because of heart damage, walk and jog several miles in a few weeks, and leave the center able to continue with their normal work.

2. The second most important preventative and therapeutic factor in heart disease is *vitamin E*. Those who have a heart condition should take preventive doses, 600 up to 1,200 IU a day, and surviving heart attack patients should take 1,600 to 2,000 IU of vitamin E a day for the rest of their lives.

3. *Avoid smog.* Smoggy air definitely adversely affects a heart condition.

4. *Avoid emotional stresses and worries.* Severe emotional stress causes spasmatic constriction of arteries and may contribute to heart attack.

5. According to Dr. Royal Lee, the administration of *cytotrophic extract* of beef heart tissue is extremely effective in correction of heart abnormalities and in restoration of heart function after a heart attack.

6. *Do not smoke!* A recently completed ten-year study made in Stockholm, Sweden, shows that smoking is the surest way to become a heart attack candidate. Study shows that 82 percent of all men who died of a heart attack were smokers. The other important factors that contributed to heart attacks were: emotional stress, lack of regular exercise, alcohol and high cholesterol and lipid (fat) count in the blood.

7. If other measures fail, possibly periodic blood-letting can be considered, especially for those with high viscosity blood. Blood-letting is an ancient method, recently rediscovered by modern science (see *Notes*).

8. *Atherosclerosis*, with excessive cholesterol and lipids in the arteries, is one of the main causes of coronary heart disease. It has been clinically demonstrated that atherosclerosis may be caused largely by C-vitamin deficiency. Administration of large doses of vitamin C (1,000 to 3,000 mg.) daily resulted in drastic reduction of blood serum cholesterol. This has been clinically demonstrated by Dr. C. Spittle in England, Dr. Boris Sololoff in the United States, Dr. N. F. Zartsev in Russia, and Dr. Ginter of Czechoslovakia.

    Note: Administration of vitamin C to atherosclerotic patients may temporarily result in rise of serum cholesterol levels due to mobilization of the arterial cholesterol deposits. Although this is not serious and the continued treatment will eventually bring serum cholesterol level down, the phenomenon should be closely observed by a doctor, especially in coronary cases.

    There are eight other nutritional substances which play a vital role in maintaining proper levels of cholesterol and triglycerides in blood and arteries:

    a. *Vitamin F*, or unsaturated fatty acids. Sources are: crude, cold-pressed vegetable oils, raw seeds and nuts and grains. Also available in capsule form.

    b. *Lecithin*. Best food sources are unrefined, raw, crude vegetable oils, seeds, nuts and grains. Also available in granular, or liquid form, or in capsules.

    c. *Chromium*. The best natural food sources of chromium are: unsaturated cold-pressed oils, whole grains, organically grown fruits and vegetables, raw sugar and sugar cane, and brewer's yeast. Also in naturally hard drinking water.

d. *Niacin.* Normalizes blood clotting and markedly reduces cholesterol levels in arteries. Best food sources: brewer's yeast, whole grain products.

e. *Calcium.* Extra supplementary calcium reduces blood cholesterol. Best sources: milk, bone meal, sesame seeds, vegetables.

f. B_6 (pyrodoxine). It has been shown that prolonged deficiency of vitamin B_6 will lead to damage to arteries and consequent atherosclerotic development.

g. *Magnesium.* It has been shown that plentiful magnesium in the diet is imperative to health of the heart. Magnesium strengthens the heart muscle, and can prevent athero-sclerosis and heart attack.

h. *Zinc.* Recent research shows that low zinc values are associated with atherosclerosis (William Strain, et al.). Best food sources of zinc; seeds, nuts, grains, milk, eggs.

VITAMINS & SUPPLEMENTS (Daily)

E — up to 1,600 IU, depending on age and condition (in case of rheumatic heart disease not more than 175 IU). A doctor must determine the amount of vitamin E for each heart patient, especially in rheumatic heart damage, hypertension, cardiac decompensation or failure.

Magnesium — 500 mg. or more

Lecithin — 2 tbsp.

Calcium — 1,000 mg.

C — 1,000 to 3,000 mg.

Zinc — 30 mg., as zinc gluconate

Niacin — 100 mg.

B_6 — 100 mg.

Brewer's yeast — 3 tbsp.

Flax seed oil — 2 tsp.

Kelp — 1 tsp. of granules, or 3 tablets

Raw, unrefined honey

Wheat germ — only if available absolutely fresh, not older than one week after it is made

Natural multiple-vitamin-mineral formula

JUICES

Vegetables: carrot, beet, celery, asparagus, with small amount of garlic and onion juice added to vegetable juice.

Fruits: red grapes, black currants, rose hips, blueberries.

HERBS

Hawthorne berries, motherworth, horsetail, valerian root, black cohosh, mistletoe, melissa, rosemary. An excellent herb tea for heart diseases is made from the woody, interior walls of walnuts. Use the walls from 4 to 5 nuts for each cup. Soak them overnight, then boil them for 15 minutes the next morning. Take three cups a day. This tea alleviates the pressure and the pain in the chest. Tea can be sweetened with raw honey. Cinchona bark (the source of quinine and quinidine) is specific in the treatment of atrial fibrillation, a rhythm disorder of the heart.

SPECIFICS

Vitamins E, C, magnesium, lecithin, flax seed oil, okra, hawthorn berries. Low-protein, low-calorie, low-sodium diet. No smoking, no alcohol. Plenty of regular exercise.

REFERENTIAL READING

Shute, Wilfred E., *Vitamin E For Ailing and Healthy Hearts*, Pyramid House Publishers, New York, N.Y., 1969.

Sandler, Benjamin, *How to Prevent Heart Attacks*, published by Lee Foundation for Nutritional Research, Milwaukee, Wisconsin.

Marshal, Robert J. and Shepherd, John T., *Cardiac Function in Health and Disease*, W. B. Saunders Co., Philadelphia, 1968.

Alsleben, H. Rudolph and Shute, Wilfred E., *How To Survive the New Health Catastrophes*, Survival Publications, Inc. Anaheim, Ca., 1973.

Perry, H. M., "Minerals in Cardiovascular Disease", *Journal of American Diet. Association*, Vol. 62, June, 1973, p. 631.

Ginter, E., "Cholesterol: Vitamin C controls its transformation to bile acids." *Science*, Vol. 179, p. 702, February 2, 1973.

Bajusz, Eors, *Nutritional Aspects of Cardiovascular Disease*, J. B. Lippincott Co., 1965.

Bajusz, Eors, editor, *Electrolytes and Cardiovascular Disease*, Williams and Williams, 1966.

Yudkin, John, *Sweet and Dangerous*, Wyden, New York, 1972.

Spittle, C., Report on Atherosclerosis and Vitamin C, *The Lancet*, December 11, 1971.

Williams, Roger J., *Nutrition Against Disease*, Pitman, New York, 1971.

Witting, Lloyd A., *The American Journal of Clinical Nutrition*, March, 1972.

Medical Tribune, December 15, 1971.

"Atherosclerosis and Vitamin C Deficiency," *Prevention*, April, 1972.

Rodale & Staff, *Encyclopedia of Common Diseases*, Rodale Books, Emmaus, Pa.

Lee, R. S. and Wilson, D. E., "The Treatment of Hyperlipidemia," *New England Journal of Medicine*, 284:186-195, January, 1971.

Bailey, Herbert, *Vitamin E – Your Key to a Healthy Heart*, Arco Publishing Co., New York, N. Y., 1970.

Airola, Paavo O., "European System of Preventing Heart Attacks," in *Health Secrets From Europe*, Parker Publishing Co., West Nyack, N.Y., 1970. Paperback by ARCO Publishing Co., N.Y., 1972.

Browne, S. E., *British Medical Journal*, July 13, 1963.

Cheraskin E., et al., *Diet & Disease*, Rodale Press, 1968.

Warmbrand, Max, *Add Years to Your Heart*, Pyramid Books, N.Y., 1969.

Kochler, Milton, "Thick Blood Imperils the Heart," *Prevention*, September 1972.

Vroman, Leo, *Blood*, Doubleday, New York, 1971.

Selye, H. *The Chemical Prevention of Cardiac Necroses*, Ronald Press, 1958.

NOTES:

1.   It has been demonstrated in several American and Swedish studies that heart attack and stroke victims have often exceptionally high blood viscosity, or so-called thick blood, with larger than normal count of red blood corpuscles. Researchers concluded that a thousand-year old method, extensively used in folk medicine and by ancient doctors to prevent heart attacks – periodic blood-letting – was based on solid scientific grounds. Blood-letting "thins" the blood, lowers its viscosity, or hematocrit, and prevents the development of coronary thrombosis and blood clots. That women are not affected by strokes and heart attacks before the age of menopause to the same extent that men are, may depend on their usually much lower hemoglobin count. Needless to say, only qualified doctors should perform blood-letting, or decide on the advisability of such treatment in each individual case.

I dare to predict that this method of prevention of strokes and heart attacks may become widely used in the future medical practice – after it is given a little more scientific name, of course. By the way, periodic juice fasting also lowers blood viscosity and diminishes the risk of thrombosis and stroke.

2.   Since this book was published in 1974, more and more medical studies from around the world confirm that my dietary recommendations for the prevention of heart disease —low-animal-protein, low-fat diet of high-quality organic foods, with emphasis on whole grains, vegetables, and fruits — is the best nutritional protection against atherosclerosis, coronary heart disease, and heart attacks. Recent research at the University of California at Davis indicates that excessive free fats in the diet (free fats are any vegetable oils — even cold-pressed, butter, margarine, lard, fat cheeses, cream, bacon, and fatty meats) increase the likelihood of developing not only heart attacks, but also bowel cancer, breast cancer, and diabetes. Thus, a low-fat (any kind of fat) diet is a must for heart-disease and cancer prevention. Note that studies show that only so-called *free* fats are implicated; oil-rich whole, natural foods, such as nuts, and seeds, are not harmful at all.

3.   The currently-popular Pritikin Diet, which is very similar to the Airola Optimum Diet, and is based on the same low-protein, low-fat, low-calorie principle, has demonstrated its effectiveness to many who have adhered to it. It would be even more effective (especially in terms of recurrence on a long-term basis) if specific vitamins and supplements, as listed in this section, were incorporated into it. Although the Pritikin Diet can effect a rapid improvement in the condition of coronary heart disease, (mainly because, being extremely deficient in dietary fats, it causes the body to dissolve and metabolize arterial fat accumulations), it should be understood that it is a *strictly therapeutic diet*, which should not be adhered to for extensive periods of time. As soon as the condition for which the Pritikin Diet was used has been corrected, the individual should switch to the Optimum Diet, which is described in detail in this book. The Optimum Diet can assure that optimal health will be maintained and many future health problems prevented. The superiority of the Optimum Diet for the maintenance of the highest level of health, vitality, and prevention of disease, has been attested to by millions of people who adhere to it.

Notes #2 and 3 added July, 1980.

HEMORRHOIDS

DIETARY CONSIDERATIONS

Since chronic constipation is considered a major cause of hemorrhoids, the anti-constipation diet should be the first consideration (see section on *Constipation*).

Venous stasis, liver damage or sluggishness are other common causes. Pregnancy often aggravates hemorrhoids or causes them. A diet rich in fresh, raw fruits and vegetables and raw and sprouted seeds will improve circulation; an avoidance of animal proteins will help to correct venous stasis.

Foods rich in vitamin C, bioflavonoids and vitamin E are essential — fresh raw fruits and vegetables, especially cabbage, green peppers, citrus fruits, rose hips and black currants, and whole grains, seeds and nuts are such foods.

Plenty of liquids: water, herb teas, juices.

Avoid all refined foods and sugars.

BIOLOGICAL TREATMENTS

1. Achieving regular, frequent, soft and easy bowel movements is of essence. Proper diet (see above) and training can help to accomplish this.
2. Plenty of regular exercise, particularly *walking*, is imperative. Sedentary life, particularly lots of sitting, is one of the contributory causes.
3. Pollen suppositories, *Cernitory*, were shown to be effective in bringing relief even in advanced cases. *Cernitory* is available in Sweden and other European countries. According to a recent report, it is now imported into the United States.
4. Suppositories made from a peeled garlic bud or raw potato have been reported to bring relief.
5. Use my Formula F-Plus (see *Directions: 8*) for external application and lubrication.
6. Vitamin B_6, after each meal, has been shown in some studies to affect speedy recovery.
7. Sitz-bath daily (see *Directions: 7*).

VITAMINS & SUPPLEMENTS (Daily)

Bioflavonoid complex (citrin 100 mg., hesperidin 50 mg., rutin 50 mg.) 12-15 tablets

B_6 — 25 mg. after each meal

C — 1,000 to 2,000 mg.

Pollen or pollen extract

Collinsonia tablets, 3-6 tablets or more

B-complex, high potency, natural
Lecithin — 1 tbsp.
E — 600 IU
A — 25,000 units
K — especially in bleeding hemorrhoids

JUICES

Lemon, orange, grapefruit, papaya, pineapple.

HERBS

Collinsonia root (tea, tablets or capsules), witch hazel (to be rubbed externally), pollen, rose hips, yarrow, white oak bark.

SPECIFICS

Vitamins P (bioflavonoids) and B_6, pollen, collinsonia root. Cernitory (pollen suppository), raw garlic or raw potato suppository. Plenty of exercise, particularly walking.

REFERENTIAL READING

Nittler, Alan H., *A New Breed of Doctor*, Pyramid Publications, N.Y., 1972.
Rodale, & Staff, *Encyclopedia of Healthful Living*, Rodale Books, Inc., Emmaus, Pennsylvania.
Davis, Adelle, *Let's Get Well*, Harcourt, Brace and World, Inc. N.Y., 1965.
Airola, Paavo, *Health Secrets From Europe*, Parker Publishing Co., West Nyack, N.Y., 1970. Paperback by ARCO Publishing Co., 1972.

HIGH BLOOD PRESSURE

(Hypertension)

High blood pressure is *not a disease*, but a body's defensive and corrective measure, initiated to cope with pathological conditions in various functions of the body, such as general toxemia, impaired kidney function, glandular disturbances, defective calcium metabolism, degenerative changes in arteries (arteriosclerosis), overweight, emotionally caused disfunction in vaso-motor mechanism, etc. Thus, the objective of the biologically oriented doctor is not to lower the pressure with drugs or even with specific vitamins or foods, but to *eliminate the reasons for blood elevation*, i.e. to remove the causes of the condition. When these are removed, the blood pressure will go down to normal by itself. Nutritional or other programs suggested below are aimed at removing the causes of high blood pressure.

DIETARY CONSIDERATIONS

The Airola Diet (see *Directions: 1*) with emphasis on low sodium, high potassium foods: vegetables, fruits, seeds. Millet, buckwheat, oats and rice are best cereals. Raw goat's milk in small amounts.

Avoid all animal proteins (except goat's milk). Avoid coffee, alcohol, salt, and all strong spices, especially mustard, black and white pepper, ginger, nutmeg, etc. Such spices can be contributory causes of high blood pressure and heart disease.

Eat plenty of raw green leafy vegetables and raw fruits. Watermelons are beneficial. Garlic is specific for high blood pressure, eat a lot of it. Russian research showed that two foods are specific in reducing high blood pressure: garlic and buckwheat (rich in rutin).

Eat small meals — do not overeat. Remember, obesity is one of the main causes of high blood pressure.

BIOLOGICAL TREATMENTS

1. In my experience, *juice fasting* (see *Directions: 3*) is the most effective treatment for high blood pressure, bringing about in almost every case a sharp reduction in the systolic pressure in a short period of time. Vegetable and fruit juices and vegetable broth (see *Recipes*) will supply blood and tissues with the important mineral, potassium, which helps to eliminate accumulated sodium (salt) from the tissues. A juice fast also normalizes and corrects most other disturbances and malfunctions in the body which might be contributing causes to the elevated pressure.

   Recommended length of fast: 3 to 4 weeks, or several repeated one-week fasts if longer fast is inconvenient. The therapy can be repeated several times with an interval of 6 months between each long fast.

After the fast, a special diet, as outlined under *Dietary Considerations*, should be followed.

2. For those who for some reason cannot fast, a *watermelon diet* for a week (eat nothing but watermelon for one week) can be tried.

3. *Rice-fruit diet* is also shown to be effective: eat nothing but whole cooked rice and cooked and raw fruits for one or two weeks.

4. *Dry brush massage* morning and evening (*Directions: 4*). Lots of exercise, walking and deep-breathing exercises. Although strenuous exercises such as weight lifting or competitive sports are not advised, high blood pressure patients should exercise as much as possible, starting with mild exercises and walking, gradually increasing their length each day.

VITAMINS & SUPPLEMENTS (Daily)

Raw garlic, or garlic capsules -- several times a day
Rutin, or mixed bioflavonoids — 100 mg. to 300 mg.
C — 1,000 to 3,000 mg.
Choline (lecithin is a good source of choline)
Potassium — vegetable broth (see *Recipes*) is rich in potassium
Magnesium — 500 mg.
B-complex, natural, high potency
E — start with 100 IU and increase gradually to 400-600 IU. A doctor should observe the blood pressure closely as sometimes vitamin E tends to temporarily elevate blood pressure.
Natural multi-vitamin-mineral formula

JUICES

Vegetable juices: carrots, spinach, beet, comfrey, parsley, and small amounts of onion and garlic added to other juices.

Fruit juices: all citrus juices, black currants, grapes, cranberries.

HERBS

Hawthorn berries, mistletoe, valerian root, wild cherry bark.

SPECIFICS

Juice fast, raw garlic, vegetarian diet, systematic undereating, rutin, choline, potassium, magnesium, vitamin C.

REFERENTIAL READING

Sneddon, J. Russell, *Nature Cure for High Blood-Pressure*, Health For All Publishing Co., Croydon, Surrey, England, 1963.
Seelig, M., *American Journal of Clinical Nutrition*, June, 1964.
Airola, Paavo O. "How to Help Lower Your High Blood Pressure — Without Drugs," Chapter in my book, *Health Secrets From Europe*, Parker Publishing Co., West Nyack, N.Y., 1970.

Blair, Jackson, Report in *Medical Times*, November, 1966

Nolfi, Kristine, *My Experiences with Living Food.*

Allinson, Bertrand P., *Diet and High Blood Pressure*, Modern Publications, Reg:d, St. Catharines, Ontario, Canada.

Coca, Arthur F., *Medical Record*, December, 1950.

Seller, R. H. *Journal of American Medical Association*, February 22, 1965.

Rodale, J. I. & Staff, *Your Blood and Its Pressure*, Rodale Books, Emmaus, Pennsylvania.

NOTES:

1. High blood pressure can be of *emotional origin.* Several emotional stresses, worries, fears, pressures of competitive life, prolonged nervous tensions can raise blood pressure. These underlying causes of emotional origin must be removed before any nutritional or biological treatments can be successful.

2. *Low blood pressure* patients can also fast, but only under doctor's supervision. The best juices for low blood pressure are pineapple, celery, black radish, parsley, carrot, red beet, grapes and onion and garlic. The diet after the fast should be the Airola Diet (see *Directions: 1*), with emphasis on whole grain cereals, raw nuts and seeds, with milk and milk products, such as butter and cheese, preferably homemade cottage cheese (see *Recipes*). As supplements: B-complex, lots of brewer's yeast, B_1 (100 mg.) and vitamins E and K, in addition to general supplementation (see *Directions: 2*).

HYPOGLYCEMIA

(Low blood sugar)

DIETARY CONSIDERATIONS

The commonly recommended diet for hypoglycemia — high animal protein diet — is not advisable for this condition. Although it may help in controlling the condition, it is so harmful in many other aspects that using it would merely mean replacing one illness with a host of others. Continuous adherance to a high protein diet may lead to such serious conditions as kidney damage, heart disease, arthritis, cancer and even premature aging.

The best answer to effective control and remedy of hypoglycemia is the Airola Diet (see *Directions: 1*), or high *natural* carbohydrate-low animal protein diet based on three basic food groups: grains, seeds and nuts; vegetables; and fruits. This diet can be complemented with milk and milk products, brewer's yeast and vegetable oils.

Whole grains, seeds and nuts should form a base of this diet. Seeds and nuts should be consumed raw, mostly for breakfast, but also between meals as snacks. Grains should be cooked in the form of cereals. Cooked grains digest twice as slowly as raw grains — *this is important in hypoglycemia*. When you eat a good plateful of buckwheat, millet, wheat or oat cereal for breakfast or lunch, with a dash of butter or tablespoon of vegetable oil, and a glass of milk, such a meal will remain in your stomach for many hours — a half a day! — *slowly* releasing the nutrients and sugars into your bloodstream. The object of the diet we recommend here is to prevent blood sugar starvation by keeping a certain amount of usable sugars constantly going into the bloodstream. Animal proteins are digested relatively rapidly. Only the proteins needed by the body at the time of digestion are utilized as proteins — the rest are changed into sugar and burned as energy food, increasing blood sugar level. Cooked grains, on the other hand, digest very slowly and release sugars into the blood gradually during as much as 6-8 hours after the meal, keeping the blood sugar level normal and constant for a long period of time.

Hypoglycemics should eat 6 to 8 small meals a day, instead of only 2 or 3. In addition to regular breakfast, lunch and dinner, take snacks in between meals consisting of raw nuts, seeds such as sunflower or pumpkin seeds, or a glass of milk or yogurt, or a piece of fruit. Even any of the fresh sweet fruits can be eaten if you eat only *one*, and no more, at one time. Drinking fruit and vegetable juices between meals and one hour before meal is also advisable. Sweet fruit juice must be diluted with water, 50-50.

Natural unprocessed cheeses, especially homemade cottage cheese, (see *Recipes*) and soured milks, such as yogurt, kefir or plain clabbered milk, are excellent in anti-hypoglycemia diet.

Avoid completely: all refined and processed foods; white sugar, white flour and everything made with them; pastries, cookies, ice cream, etc. No coffee, alcohol, soft drinks or smoking. Natural honey is OK, in moderation.

Salt should be avoided too. Excessive salt consumption causes loss of blood potassium, which leads to a drop of blood sugar.

Here's a suggested diet, in a nutshell:

7 A.M. — Glass of fruit juice. Sweet juices must be diluted with water, 50-50.

8 A.M. — *Breakfast*: nuts, seeds, fruit, yogurt, cottage cheese
Or: cooked cereal with oil and raw milk.

10 A.M. — Snack: a few nuts, or glass of yogurt, or piece of fruit

12 Noon — Glass of fresh juice.

1 P.M. — *Lunch*: Cooked cereal: kruska, buckwheat, millet, etc. (see *Recipes*), with oil and milk, if not eaten for breakfast.
Or: fruit or vegetable salad with yogurt and 2 slices of whole grain bread with cheese and butter

3 P.M. — Glass of juice or kefir with 2 tbsp. of yeast.
Or: snack of nuts, fruit, halva (see *Recipes*), etc.

5 P.M. — Glass of fresh vegetable juice.

6 P.M. — *Dinner*: vegetable salad with cooked vegetable dish of: beans, tortillas, yams, green beans, baked potatoes, etc. Slice or two of whole grain bread. Cottage cheese, yogurt. Animal protein, if desired.

8 P.M. — Glass of milk or yogurt with 1 or 2 tbsp. of brewer's yeast.

VITAMINS & SUPPLEMENTS (Daily)

Persons with hypoglycemia should take the following supplements:

C — in large doses, 2,000 to 5,000 mg.

B-complex, natural, high potency

Pantothenic acid — 100 mg.

E — up to 1,600 IU

B_6 — 50 mg.

B_{12} — 25 to 50 mcg., even more under doctor's supervision

Magnesium chloride — 500 mg.

Potassium chloride — 200 mg.

Acidophilus yeast

Comprehensive, natural multi-vitamin-mineral formula

Brewer's yeast, 2 to 3 tbsp.

Concentrated sea water, for trace elements

Vitamins C and B increase tolerance to sugars and carbohydrates and help to normalize sugar metabolism. Pantothenic acid, B_6 and B-complex help to build up adrenals, which are often exhausted in persons with hypoglycemia. Vitamin E improves glycogen storage in the muscles and tissues. Potassium and sea water can help to normalize mineral balance and supply essential trace elements which are involved in sugar metabolism.

HERBS

Juniper (ceder) berries (Juniperus Sabina Pinaceae) have a nourishing regulating and stimulating effect on pancreas and are extremely useful in hypoglycemia and diabetes. Also: licorice root.

JUICES

Any fresh vegetable and fruit juices. Sweet juices should be diluted 50-50 with water, or drunk in small amounts only.

SPECIFICS

Vitamins C, E, and B-complex, Airola Diet, high in *natural* complex carbohydrates, such as whole grains, nuts, seeds and vegetables, and low in animal proteins. Frequent, small meals.

REFERENTIAL READING

Nittler, Alan H. "Hypoglycemia," *Let's Live*, April, 1972.
Nittler, Alan H. *A New Breed of Doctor*, Pyramid House, New York, 1972.
Roberts, Sam E. *Ear, Nose and Throat Disfunction Due to Deficiencies and Imbalances*, Charles C. Thomas, Publishers, Springville, Illinois.
Abrahamson, E. M., and Pezet, A. M. *Body, Mind and Sugar*, Henry Holt and Company, N.Y.
Martin, Clement G., *Low Blood Sugar and Your Health*, Arco Publishing Co., Inc., New York, N.Y.
Alsleben, H. Rudolph and Shute, Wilfred G., *How to Survive New Health Catastrophes*, Survival Publications, Inc., Anaheim, Ca. 1973.
Airola, Paavo, *Hypoglycemia: A Better Approach,* Health Plus Publishers, Phoenix, Az.

NOTES:

Dr. Alan H. Nittler, one of the leading experts on hypoglycemia, uses injections of complete adrenocortical extract (ACE), intramuscularly (in oil) or intravenously (aquaeous ACE), in addition to a nutritional program, which is a high natural carbohydrate diet, as suggested in this section.

The intravenous formula used by Dr. Nittler is as follows:

Aquaeous adrenocortical extract:	1,000 mcgm.
Vitamin B_{12} (cyanocobalamine):	1,000 mcgm.
Vitamin C (ascorbic acid):	250 mg.
Vitamin B_6 (pyridoxine):	100 mg.
Calcium glycerophosphate: (Calphosan®)	2 cc.
Dilute Hydrochloric acid 1:1,000	10 cc.

(From *The New Breed of Doctor* by Alan H. Nittler)

JAUNDICE

(Non-infectious kind. Discoloration of skin and eyes
the most prominent symptoms.)

DIETARY CONSIDERATIONS

In acute condition, no solid foods should be taken, instead the patient should be put on a one-week juice fast with special juices and medicinal herb teas. After fasting, the Airola Diet (see *Directions: 1*) with added raw *skim* milk and one cup of homemade skim milk cheese daily (see *Recipes*). Plenty of fresh vegetable and fruit juices. Add dandelion leaves, radishes (with leaves), endive, artichokes and watercress to the daily vegetable salad. Raw apples and pears are especially beneficial. Raw egg yolks, or whole eggs, can be taken twice a week.

Drink a glass of warm water with juice of 1/2 lemon each morning. Avoid all fats and fried foods.

BIOLOGICAL TREATMENTS

1. Juice fasting (see *Directions: 3*), one to two weeks. Use juices given below. Use retention coffee enema (see *Directions: 3*) every second day. Regular enemas on other days.
2. Warm packs or cabbage leaf compresses on the liver area (see *Directions: 6*).
3. Patient should have plenty of rest.
4. Barley water (1 cup of barley boiled in 6 pints of water and simmered for three hours) drunk several times during the day has been known to remedy jaundice.

VITAMINS & SUPPLEMENTS (Daily)

C — 1,000 mg. to 1,500 mg. every 3 hours in acute condition; given even during fasting. In chronic condition: 3,000 mg. to 5,000 mg. each day

E — 600 IU

B_6 — 50 mg.

Brewer's yeast — 3 to 5 tbsp.

Calcium-magnesium supplement

Natural multiple-mineral formula

JUICES

Lemon, grapes, pear. Small amounts of radish and dandelion juice added to carrot and beet juice.

HERBS

Irish moss (Tillandsia), dandelion, self-heal (Prunella Vulgaris) horsetail, birch leaves, rose hips, centaury, gentian, parsley, fennel, peach leaves, Dyer's root.

SPECIFICS

Juice fasting, vitamin C, Irish moss, dandelion, self-heal. Avoidance of fried and fatty foods. Plenty of rest.

REFERENTIAL READING

Warmbrand, Max, *Encyclopedia of Natural Health*, Groton Press, Inc., New York, 1962.

Davidson, C. S. "Dietary Treatment of Hepatic Diseases," *Journal of American Dietetic Association*, 62:515, 1973.

Vogel, A., *The Nature Doctor*, Bioforce-Verlag, Teufen, Switzerland, 1960.

Sneddon, J. Russell, *The Natural Treatment of Liver Troubles and Associated Ailments*, Health For All Publishing Company, London, 1960.

Vogel, A., *The Liver*, Bioforce-Verlag, Teufen, Switzerland, 1962.

NOTES:

1. Discoloration of the skin and eye whites may also occur as a result of excess of carotinoids in the diet, caused by such things as excessive drinking of carrot juice. This is completely harmless and disappears with dietary changes.

KIDNEY DISEASE

(Bright's Disease or Nephritis)

DIETARY CONSIDERATIONS

Low-protein vegetarian diet. Emphasis on raw and cooked vegetables and raw fruits. Avoid vegetables containing large quantities of oxalic acid, such as spinach and rhubarb. Chocolate and cocoa also contain oxalic acid and must not be used. Garlic, potatoes, asparagus, parsley, horse radish, watercress, cucumber and celery are excellent vegetables. Best fruits are papaya and bananas — both have healing effect on kidneys. Watermelon is excellent; it should be eaten by itself, not with any other food. A small amount of soured milks and homemade cottage cheese, preferably from raw goat's milk, can be included in the diet. Raw, unfiltered honey has medicinal value in treatment of kidney disorders. Brown rice is good.

Eat 5 or 6 small meals, in preference to a few large ones.

Eliminate all salt from the diet.

BIOLOGICAL TREATMENTS

1. In acute condition, *juice fast* (see *Directions: 3*), two to three weeks. Use mostly vegetable juices, such as cucumber, celery, watermelon, carrot. Add small amounts of horse radish, watercress, and garlic juice to other vegetable juices. Drink plenty of vegetable broth (see *Recipes*). Cranberry juice is excellent for kidney stones and bladder infections.

2. *Avoid smoking* — studies show that smoking impairs kidney function.

3. *Exercise!* Lack of exercise contributes to the development of kidney stones.

4. The following treatment for nephritis has been shown to be effective:

    One week of juice fasting, as above, followed by two weeks on *a diet of raw goat's milk*: consume nothing but 4 quarts of milk a day. Milk must be warmed up to body's temperature, and 1 tbsp. of crude blackstrap molasses added to each quart. During this treatment, take 1,000 IU of vitamin E and 75,000 units of vitamin A every day.

5. *Kidney bean pod treatment.* In European folk medicine, kidney bean pod (Phaseolus Vulgaris) treatment is considered most effective for all forms of kidney and bladder disorders, such as edema (due to kidney or heart condition), kidney inflammation, kidney and bladder stones, as well as in chronic gout and diabetes.

Kidney bean pod treatment is given as follows:

a. Follow the dietary suggestions given earlier.

b. Drink kidney bean pod decoction, 1 glass every 2 hours during the day. Decoction is made in the following manner. Use 2 oz. of *fresh* kidney bean pods (remove the seeds) for 4 quarts of water. Boil slowly (simmer) for 4 hours. Strain well through a fine cloth and let stand for 8 hours.

c. Decoction must be made *fresh* every day. If it is older than 24 hours it has lost its medicinal value.

d. Treatment length: 4 to 8 weeks.

6. *Corn silk tea* is another proven folk remedy. Drink a glass of corn silk tea several times a day. Treatment should continue for several months.

VITAMINS & SUPPLEMENTS (Daily)

A — 75,000 units (after 3 months, reduce to 10,000 units)

C — 1,000 to 3,000 mg. Deficiency of both vitamins A and C have been shown to contribute to the development of kidney stones.

E — up to 1,000 IU

Potassium chloride — 1 to 5 grams, for two weeks

Choline — 1,000 mg.

B_6 — 50 mg.

B_2 — 25 mg.

B-complex, natural, high potency

Lecithin — 1 tbsp.

Magnesium — calcium supplement

Honey

Kelp

JUICES

Watermelon, cucumber, celery. Small amounts of juice from horse radish, watercress and garlic added to carrot juice. Cranberry juice.

HERBS

Kidney bean pod tea, corn silk tea, birch leaves, Dyer's root (Rubia Tinctorum) shepherds-purse (diuretic), golden rod (solidago), dandelion (diuretic and kidney stimulator), uva ursi, kelp, spirea, juniper berry, catnip (for stones), parsley (diuretic and dissolves kidney stones), asparagus (diuretic), desert tea (Ephedra viridis), rose hip seeds.

SPECIFICS

Low-sodium, low-protein vegetarian diet, kidney bean pod tea, corn silk tea, vitamins A, C, B_6, choline, potassium, birch leaves, golden rod, watermelon, parsley, dandelion, Dyer's root, asparagus.

REFERENTIAL READING

Nittler, Alan H., *A New Breed of Doctor*, Pyramid House, N.Y., 1972.
Gershoff, S. N. et al., *American Journal of Clinical Nutrition*, May, 1967.
Warmbrand, Max, *Encyclopedia of Natural Health*, Groton Press, Inc., N.Y. 1962.
Garten, N. O., *The Health Secrets of a Naturopathic Doctor*, Parker Publishing Co., N.Y., 1967.
Scully, Virginia, *A Treasury of American Indian Herbs*, Crown, N.Y., 1970.
Dicker, S. E. et al., "Renal effects of protein-deficient vegetable diets", *Br. J. Exp. Pathology*, 27:158, 1946.
Laligh, J. J., "Protein overload nephropathy", *Arch. Pathol* 89:548, 1970.
Moise, T. S. and Smith, A. H., "Effects of high protein diet on kidneys", *Arch. Pathol.* 4:530, 1927.
Dougherty, J. C., "Influence of high-protein diets on renal function", *Journal of American Dietetic Association*, 63:392, October, 1973.

NOTES:

1. *For kidney stones*: in addition to above, 500 mg. magnesium oxide. *For severe nephritis*: massive doses of vitamin C, up to 5,000 mg., plus 500 mg. bioflavonoid complex, in addition to above.

2. Harvard University studies showed that supplementary B_6 and magnesium can help to prevent kidney stone formation.

3. Herbal remedy, which is claimed to be able to dissolve kidney stones, is called Dyer's root, also known as madder or as Rubia Tinctorum. (Dr. A. Vogel.)

4. Cranberry juice is an old folk remedy — also used by some doctors and clinics today — for kidney stones and pyelonephritis. Cranberries contain quinic and benzoic acids, as well as bacteriostatic substances that pass unchanged through the kidneys and urinary tract. Cranberry juice raises the acidity of the urine, creating an unfavorable environment for pathogenic bacteria.

LEG ULCERS

(Varicose and Diabetic Ulcers)

DIETARY CONSIDERATIONS

After an initial cleansing juice fast, a *raw food diet*, with emphasis on vegetables and fruits, with a few almonds, sesame seeds and sunflower seeds. Lots of raw vegetable and fruit juices, especially green juices. Fresh comfrey and alfalfa are excellent healers. Garlic and onions should be included generously in the diet.

BIOLOGICAL TREATMENTS

1. Two-week cleansing juice fast (see *Directions: 3*). Use juices given below. Green juice, made largely from comfrey, is especially healing.
2. For dressing: Formula F-Plus (see *Directions: 8*), used intermittently with a dressing of pure d-alpha tocopherol (vitamin E), squeezed from capsules directly on the ulcers several times a day. Vitamin E speeds healing and prevents scarring.
3. A poultice of macerated comfrey leaves and/or roots, speeds healing processes. Comfrey contains allantoin, the healing component that has the ability to remove the necrotic tissue, clean the area and induce the growth of healthy new tissue by stimulating leukocytic activity and promoting granulation and the formation of epithelian cells.
4. The following herbs, in the form of decoction or tea, can be used for washing, topical application or dressing: strong comfrey tea, chaparral tea (could also be taken internally), golden seal and myrrh tea (1 tsp. golden seal, 1/2 tsp. myrrh), or plain myrrh decoction.
5. A dressing of crushed yellow onions is also extremely effective in killing pathogenic bacteria and speeding the healing.

VITAMINS & SUPPLEMENTS (Daily)

E-complex — up to 1,600 IU
C — up to 3,000 mg.
A — 100,000 units for 3 months, then reduce to a maintenance dosage of 25,000 units
B-complex, natural, high potency
Zinc — up to 60 mg.
Bone meal or other mineral supplement
Multi-vitamin-mineral formula

JUICES

Green juice with plenty of comfrey leaves (see *Directions: 5*). Juice of onions and garlic added to carrot and green juice. Fruit juices: apple, pineapple and citrus juices.

HERBS

Comfrey (for tea, juice, poultice or dressing), chaparral (for tea, poultice and dressing), myrrh (externally), golden seal (internally and externally as dressing).

SPECIFICS

Vitamins E, C and A, comfrey, juice fast, raw vegetarian diet.

REFERENTIAL READING

Kirschner, H. E., *Nature's Healing Grasses*, H. C. White Publications, Yucaipa, Calif., 1960.

Vogel, Alfred, *The Nature Doctor*, Bioforce Verlag, Teufen (AR) Switzerland, 1960.

Jennings, Joan, "Comfrey – The Gourmet's Medicine," *Prevention*, April, 1972.

Bourne, G. H., "The Effect of Vitamin C on the Healing of Wounds," *Proceedings of the Nutrition Society*, 4, 204, 1946.

LIVER TROUBLE

(Congestion, Fatty Degeneration, Sluggishness, Enlargement)

DIETARY CONSIDERATIONS

After an initial liver cleansing program (see below), the Airola Diet (see *Directions: 1*) of raw, organically grown foods. Adequate high quality protein is essential in liver diseases. The best complete proteins for liver patients are obtained from brewer's yeast (also rich in B-vitamins, which are vital for liver health), raw goat's milk, homemade raw cottage cheese (see *Recipes*), sprouted seeds and grains, and raw nuts, especially almonds. Sesame seed butter (Tahini) is especially beneficial in liver disorders because of its unusually high content of methionine, unsaturated oils, calcium and high quality proteins.

Do not overeat — eat small frequent meals.

Exclude all fats and oils for several weeks.

Exclude all processed, canned and refined foods. Avoid all chemical additives in foods and poisons in air, water and environment. Environmental poisons damage liver. Avoid synthetic vitamins — they also are harmful and prolonged ingestion may damage liver. Avoid drugs.

No salt, no strong spices (like mustard, black and white pepper), no sugar in any form, no alcohol — all these can damage liver. Alcohol robs liver of B-vitamins. Use honey as sweetener.

Red beets, red beet juice or beet powder are especially beneficial in liver disorders. Also endive, artichoke, cucumber, garlic and lemon.

BIOLOGICAL TREATMENTS

1. Juice fast (see *Directions: 3*), 7 to 10 days, with emphasis on beet juice.
2. For congested, "clogged" and "toxic" liver, a special liver detoxifying juice fast for 3 days, as follows:

    Mix fresh juice of 10 lemons in two quarts of water, sweeten with natural honey. Drink one glass every two hours. Also, twice daily drink a green vegetable juice mixed with about 50 percent red beet juice.

    After the juice fast, two weeks of the Airola Diet as above. Repeat the fast if necessary.
3. Another widely used liver cleansing method is as follows:

    On two evenings, take one cup made of equal parts of fresh lemon juice and olive oil (2 oz. of each). On third evening take a double dose (4 oz. of each). On the following morning, take an enema. Follow it with a second enema to which 1 cup freshly brewed coffee has been added. This coffee enema should be retained for as long as possible — up to 20 minutes. Repeat coffee enema in the evening.

This method effectively cleanses out both liver and gall bladder. Especially recommended in cases of gallstones.

4. Many biologically-oriented doctors recommend using animal liver, liver tablets or liver extract in the treatment of liver disorders. This treatment was beneficial a few decades back when healthy animal livers were obtainable. In view of the fact that presently available animal livers are all loaded with poisons (liver is the detoxifying organ which filters and stores poisons), we cannot recommend such treatment, unless totally poison-free liver can be obtained. Some manufacturers sell dessicated reindeer liver tablets from Alaskan deer, which are supposed to be relatively free from poisons. A specially low-heat processed dessicated liver from Argentine animals may be OK.

VITAMINS & SUPPLEMENTS (Daily)
Brewer's yeast — 3 to 5 tbsp.
B-complex, natural, high potency
C — large doses up to 3,000 mg.
Choline — up to 10 grams a day for two weeks
B_6 — 50 mg.
B_{12} — 50 mcg.
E — up to 600 IU
A — 25,000 units
Lecithin — 2 tbsp.
Niacin — 100 mg.

JUICES
Red beet juice made from tops and roots, lemon juice, papaya juice (specific for enlarged liver), grape juice; radish, black radish and dandelion juice added in small amounts to beet juice.

HERBS
Dandelion, horsetail, bolbo leaves, birch leaves, St. John's Wort, wahoo, lobelia, barberry, balmony, parsley, sarsaparilla, liverworth leaves, centaury, golden rod.

SPECIFICS
Red beet juice, juice fasting, vitamins B-complex and C, choline, brewer's yeast, lemon juice, dandelion, artichokes. Airola Diet with adequate amount of high quality proteins, preferably from homemade raw skim milk cheese, kvark (see *Recipes*), and sesame seed butter.

REFERENTIAL READING

Davidson, C. S., "Dietary Treatment of Hepatic Diseases," *Journal of American Dietetic Association*, 62:515, 1973.

Willis, G. C., *Canadian Medical Association Journal*, June 15, 1957.

Sneddon, J. Russell, *The Natural Treatment of Liver Troubles and Associated Ailments*, Health For All Publishing Co., London, 1960.

Warmbrand, Max, *Encyclopedia of Natural Health*, Groton Press, New York.

Airola, Paavo O., *How to Keep Slim, Healthy and Young with Juice Fasting*, Health Plus Publishers, Box 22001, Phoenix, Arizona, 1971.

Vogel, A. *The Liver*, Bioforce-Verlag, Switzerland, 1962.

Bircher, Ruth, *Eating Your Way to Health*, Faber and Faber, London, 1961.

Fredericks, Carlton, *Prevention*, April 1973.

NOTES:

1.   The liver is involved in almost all conditions of ill health. Therefore, liver cleansing programs can be of benefit in the treatment of virtually every chronic condition. When there is serious liver damage, it takes a long time to recuperate. Patient should not expect momentary results and should have the patience to remain on the special diet and other programs for a long time, often as much as 3 months to a year.

MALE IMPOTENCE

Impotence is becoming "epidemic" in the United States, even among young men. Although most psychiatrists try to explain the "impotence boom" by psychological causes, inhibitions, fears of failure, feelings of inadequacy aggravated by increased demands of the liberated women, etc. — all valid factors, indeed! — it is becoming more and more evident that the causes of impotence are more dietary than psychic. Fears of failure become psychological and deep-seated only after the occurrence of several initial failures caused usually by physical inadequacy.

Programs outlined below are aimed at correcting dietary and physiological causes of impotence.

DIETARY CONSIDERATIONS

Special high virility diet as described in my books *Rejuvenation Secrets From Around the World — That "Work"* and *Sex and Nutrition* (see *Referential Reading*). Emphasis on whole, raw seeds and nuts, especially sesame seeds, pumpkin seeds, sunflower seeds, almonds and peanuts. Buckwheat, millet and oats are excellent cereals. Plenty of raw milk, fresh and in sour form, plus homemade cottage cheese (see *Recipes*). Also, regular, unprocessed cheese and butter are beneficial. Twice a week, fertile eggs which can be eaten raw. Halva is a special virility food from the Orient (see *Recipes*). Two tablespoons of cold-pressed vegetable oils each day: olive oil, soy oil, sunflower oil, sesame seed oil. Abundance of sprouted seeds and grains, such as mungbeans, soybeans, wheat and alfalfa seeds. Avocado is an excellent virility food.

Brewer's yeast, kelp, lecithin and other supplements listed below.

Zinc-rich foods are vital for virility. Many studies indicate that a deficiency of *zinc* in diet is associated not only with diminished potency, but also with dwindling fertility and with prostate disorders. Zinc is lacking in processed foods. The best dietary sources of zinc are whole, unrefined grains and seeds, brewer's yeast, oysters, eggs and onions. Sunflower and pumpkin seeds are excellent sources.

Most meat and poultry today contain the growth hormone, dietylstilbestrol, which is definitely destroying virility in men.

The following "Pep-up Cocktail" is recommended in my book *Sex and Nutrition*:

Pep-up Cocktail
(makes two glasses)

1 1/2 glasses whole, raw, unpasteurized milk
2 tbsp. non-instant skim milk powder

2 egg yolks, raw (also whole eggs can be used)

1 tbsp. wheat germ oil — only if available fresh, non-rancid

Otherwise use cold-pressed sesame seed oil or olive oil

2 tbsp. wheat germ — if available fresh,
   not more than one week old

1 tbsp. sesame seeds

2 tbsp. pumpkin seeds

2 tsp. lecithin granules

1 tbsp. natural, raw honey

1 tbsp. crushed ice

Grind sesame seeds and pumpkin seeds in seed grinder first. Then blend all ingredients in the blender. Eat slowly with a spoon, or sip with a straw.

This is a perfect lunch for a busy, tired husband. A perfect revitalizing drink for tired wife, too.

BIOLOGICAL TREATMENTS

1. Avoid smoking and alcohol — both are detrimental to virility. Good wine in small amounts has a relaxing effect, but any alcohol in large doses has a detrimental effect on sexual performance.
2. Avoid all refined, denatured and devitalized foods.
3. Avoid smog — lead in smog kills virility.
4. Cold local bath on genitals (Sitz-bath) once a day is stimulating (see *Directions: 7*). Rub genitals warm after each bath. Swimming in cold ocean water is also effective.
5. In Europe, KH-3 (Gerovital) is popular and widely acclaimed as general and sexual rejuvenator. Presently, it is not available in the U.S., but is sold in Mexico and in most European countries.

VITAMINS & SUPPLEMENTS (Daily)

E — up to 1,600 IU

Wheat germ oil — 2 tbsp. a day (only if available fresh, non-rancid, otherwise use sesame seed oil or olive oil)

Wheat germ — one half cup (only if available fresh, not more than one week old)

PABA (Para-amino-benzoic acid) — 100 mg.

Folic acid — 1.0 mg.

Lecithin — 3 tbsp.

Kelp — 2 tsp. of granules or 10 tablets

C — up to 3,000 mg.

Fish liver oil, plain, unfortified, 3 tsp.

Brewer's yeast — 2 tbsp.

B-complex, high potency, natural

Zinc supplement — up to 30 mg.

Multi-vitamin-mineral formula, all natural

JUICES

Any available fresh fruit and vegetable juices.

HERBS

Ginseng, damiana, Gotu-Kola, sarsaparilla, golden seal.

SPECIFICS

Vitamins E, PABA, folic acid, lecithin, zinc-rich foods, sesame seeds, Airola Diet, ginseng, damiana, high quality vegetable oils, fertile eggs, raw milk.

REFERENTIAL READING

Airola, Paavo O., *Sex and Nutrition*, Award paperback, Universal Publishing and Distributing Co., New York, 1970.

Airola, Paavo O., *Rejuvenation Secrets From Around the World — That "Work,"* Health Plus Publishers, P.O. Box 22001, Phoenix, Arizona, 1973.

Shute, Evan *Urological and Cutaneous Reveiw*, Vol. 48.

The Complete Book on Minerals for Health, Rodale Books, Inc. Emmaus, Pennsylvania, 1972.

Kinderlehrer, Jane, "Impotence, More Dietary than Psychic," *Prevention*, January, 1973.

Walton, Alan Hull, *Food For Love*, Paperback Library, Inc., New York, 1963.

MENOPAUSAL SYMPTOMS

Hot flashes, disturbances in calcium metabolism, insomnia, diminished interest in sex, irritability and mental instability are typical symptoms of hormone starvation due to menopause. Although menopause cannot be avoided, it can be postponed for as long as 10-20 years with proper nutritional program, special supplements and the right mental attitude.

DIETARY CONSIDERATIONS

The Airola Diet and all the general supplements (see *Directions: 1*). Emphasis on vitamin E-rich raw and sprouted seeds and nuts, unpasteurized high quality milk and homemade cottage cheese (see *Recipes*), abundance of raw, organically grown fruits and vegetables.

Total elimination of all processed, refined and denatured foods, such as white sugar and white flour, and everything made with them.

Brewer's yeast, lecithin, cold-pressed vegetable oils and kelp are essential supplements. Plenty of raw juices every day.

BIOLOGICAL TREATMENTS

1. Plenty of outdoor exercise, such as walking, jogging, swimming, riding horse or bicycle, sports, etc., is imperative to postpone menopause.
2. Avoid mental and emotional stresses and worries – do not even *worry* about *getting* old, just *do* something to postpone aging!
3. Get sufficient sleep and relaxation. Develop a habit of having a siesta each afternoon.
4. Follow all general rules of maintaining a high level of health. The healthier you are, the less menopausal symptoms you'll experience.
5. Take special supplements such as vitamins E, C, B_6 PABA and pantothenic acid, which have a specific property of stimulating the body's own production of estrogen or enhancing the effect of existing estrogen.

VITAMINS & SUPPLEMENTS (Daily)

E – up to 1,200 IU (stimulates production of estrogen)
B_6 – up to 100 mg.
Brewer's yeast – 3 to 4 tbsp.
A – 50,000 units
B_1 – 50 mg.
Calcium lactate – 3 tablets
PABA – up to 100 mg. (natural substitute for estrogen)
B-complex, natural, high potency
Pantothenic acid – up to 100 mg. (can help delay menopause)

Bonemeal — 3 tablets
Kelp — 3 tablets or 1 tsp. of granules
Betaine Hydrochloride — 1 tablet after each meal
Whey powder — 2 tsp.
C — up to 3,000 mg.
Cod liver oil — 2 tsp. or 4 capsules
Cold-pressed vegetable oils, such as sesame or olive oil

JUICES

Freshly made juices of fruits and vegetables, in season.

HERBS

Honduras sarsaparilla, licorice (Aletris Farinosa), unicorn roots (Helonias Dioica), elder. All these herbs contain the natural female sex hormone, *estrogen*, which to some degree can help compensate for diminished hormone supply due to menopause.

SPECIFICS

Vitamins E, C, A, B, and B_6, brewer's yeast, PABA, pantothenic acid, mineral supplement, licorice, unicorn roots, elder.

REFERENTIAL READING

Airola, Paavo O., *Sex and Nutrition*, (see page 39), Award paperback, Universal Publishing Co., N.Y., 1970.
Raffy, A., Report to International Congress on Vitamin E, Venice, 1955 (see Rodale, *Encyclopedia of Healthful Living*).
Fredericks, Carlton, "Hotline to Health," *Prevention*, August, 1973.
Ellis, Jonn M. and Presley, James, *Vitamin B_6 : The Doctor's Report*, Harper and Row, New York, 1973.

NOTES:

1.   Lately, it has become popular to take estrogen (female sex hormone) to prevent or postpone menopausal symptoms. Although hormone therapy is apparently quite successful and will, in many cases, help the patient to feel and act younger, the majority of biological doctors do not recommend it, mainly because of its possible carcinogenic effect. If, however, estrogen therapy *is* undertaken, it should never be administered at the same time as vitamin E therapy, which is recommended in this section — ingestion of estrogen and vitamin E should be separated by several hours. Also, generous amounts of vitamins B_6, C, PABA, folic acid, pantothenic acid and B_{12} will render estrogenic hormones more effective.

MENSTRUAL DISORDERS

Many hormonal and metabolic changes occur before and during menstrual periods, which can cause such unpleasant symptoms as depression, tension, cramps, fainting spells, melancholia, tenderness of breasts, water retention, tachycardia, backache, etc. Although these symptoms are common, they are not normal. Healthy women, living close to nature and eating good diets of natural foods (such as women in Hunza, China, Russia, and Central American Indians) do not suffer from the monthly ordeal that women in Western countries do. Most menstrual symptoms are caused by nutritional deficiencies which lead to deficiency and/or improper metabolism of female sex hormones which abound during menstrual period. Vitamins E and B_6 are particularly involved, as well as minerals calcium and iodine.

DIETARY CONSIDERATIONS

Diet should contain an adequate, but not excessive, amount of high quality proteins, preferably from raw, unpasteurized milk and sour milks, such as yogurt, kefir, clabbered milk, etc., plus one cup of kvark, homemade cottage cheese (see *Recipes*), daily.

Whole grains, nuts and seeds, especially in sprouted form, should form the basis of the diet. Almonds, buckwheat, millet, oats, sesame seeds, sunflower seeds – these will supply not only high quality proteins, but also essential minerals and vitamins, particularly the all-important vitamins E and B-complex.

Brewer's yeast (or food yeast), cold-pressed vegetable oils, kelp, rose hips, lecithin and vitamins E and B_6 are important supplements.

Iron-rich foods should be emphasized: blackstrap molasses, apricots, milk, eggs, whole grains and nuts. Plenty of raw vegetables and fruits, particularly grapes and red beets. Vitamin C helps to absorb iron from food sources. Eat frequent small meals, instead of few large ones, to prevent low blood sugar, which is common during menstruation (see section on *Hypoglycemia*).

BIOLOGICAL TREATMENTS

1. Absolutely no smoking – smoking aggravates menstrual disorders.
2. Take daily hot Sitz bath (see *Directions: 7*) with camomile or juniper needles added to the water.

VITAMINS & SUPPLEMENTS (Daily)

B-complex, natural, high potency

B_{12} – up to 50 mcg. Under doctor's supervision, up to 200 mcg. a day

Brewer's yeast – 2-3 tbsp.

Calcium lactate or bonemeal — 6 tablets (excellent for menstrual cramps)

B_6 — 50 to 100 mg.

C — up to 1,000 mg. (helps to absorb iron)

E — up to 600 IU (helps to restore menstrual regularity)

Kelp — 3 tablets or 1 tsp. of granules

F, essential fatty acids — 3 capsules

Natural multi-vitamin-mineral formula

JUICES

Green juice (see *Directions: 5*), red beet juice, dark fruit juices such as grape juice, prune juice, cherry juice, black currant juice.

HERBS

Ladies mantle and amaranth (in excessive menstruation), life root (in suppressed menstruation), black cohosh (in obstructed menstruation), blue cohosh and yarrow (in mentrual difficulties), motherwort (promotes menstrual flow). Garlic also encourages the menstrual flow. Wormwood and pennyroyal (in painful menstruation), desert tea (Ephedra Viridis), for delayed or difficult menstruation.

SPECIFICS

The Airola Diet, adequate in high quality milk and vegetable proteins and iron-rich foods. Vitamins B-complex, C, B_6, B_{12} and E, brewer's yeast, calcium supplement. Herbs as above.

REFERENTIAL READING

Ellis, John M., and Presley, James, *Vitamin B_6: The Doctor's Report*, Harper and Row, New York, 1973.

Fredericks, Carlton, *Eating Right For You*, Grosset and Dunlap, 1972.

Garten, M. O., *The Health Secrets of a Naturopathic Doctor*, Parker Publications Co., New York, 1967.

Davis, Adelle, *Let's Get Well*, A Signet Paperback, New American Library, New York, 1973.

NOTES:

1. Premenstrual edema, swellings and soreness are often relieved by administration of vitamin B_6, 50 to 150 mg. a day, especially during 10 days preceding menstruation.

2. Vitamin B_{12} is helpful in restoring normal menstrual cycle. 25 to 100 mcg. daily is usually recommended.

3. Irregular and/or profuse menstruation can be caused by thyroid deficiency. Kelp is of specific importance in such condition.

MIGRAINE HEADACHE

DIETARY CONSIDERATIONS

The Airola Diet (see *Directions: 1*) with emphasis on alkaline raw foods, fruits and vegetables and sprouted seeds.

Avoid salt and acid-producing foods such as meat and too much cereal and bread, even whole grain cereals.

Eat small frequent meals. Avoid overeating. (See diet for *Hypoglycemia.*)

BIOLOGICAL TREATMENTS

1. Plenty of rest during the night and possibly a nap every afternoon. Sleep with windows open.
2. Plenty of exercise and walking in fresh air. Deep-breathing exercises are of special importance.
3. If constipated, follow anti-constipation program (see section on *Constipation*).

VITAMINS & SUPPLEMENTS (Daily)

Niacin — 300 mg., 100 mg. 3 times a day. In acute condition, 200 mg. three times a day. A doctor must determine the proper dosage.

Rutin — 200 mg.

B_{15} — 100 mg.

E — up to 1,200 IU

B-complex, natural, high potency, with B_{12}

B_6 — 50 mg.

Pantothenic acid — 100 mg.

Calcium supplement

C — up to 1,000 mg.

Brewer's yeast — 2 tbsp.

Multi-vitamin-mineral formula

JUICES

Fresh fruit juices in season.

HERBS

Rosemary, peppermint, blue violet.

SPECIFICS

Niacin (for acute condition), Airola Diet, rutin, B_{15}, B-complex, calcium.

REFERENTIAL READING

Dalessio, D. J., "Dietary Migraine," *American Family Physician*, Vol. 6, December 1972, p. 60.

Vogel, A., *Nature Doctor*, Bioforce Verlag, Teufen, Switzerland, 1962.

MULTIPLE SCLEROSIS

DIETARY CONSIDERATIONS

Only organically grown, poison-free, whole, unprocessed raw foods: raw fruits and mainly root vegetables, raw milk (preferably goat's milk), raw fertile eggs, raw seeds and nuts, raw rolled oats (freshly made and not steamed).

Raw, unpasteurized homemade cottage cheese (see *Recipes*) and homemade soured milk.

Raw, unsalted, fresh butter (must be from "organic" sources).

Crude cereal germ oils (such as wheat germ oil) — unprocessed, cold-pressed, non-rancid — as sources of arachidonic acid, an unsaturated fatty acid, which is of specific value in treatment of MS.

Raw sprouted seeds and grains, particularly sprouted wheat and rye (see *Recipes*), several times a day.

Daily use of fermented lactic-acid foods, such as sauerkraut, sour pickles and lactic acid vegetables, all homemade (see *Recipes*). Health food stores carry some lactic acid foods and juices, imported from Europe, which are of special value for MS patients.

Raw unfiltered honey is the only sweetener allowed.

No coffee, tea, chocolate, salt, spices (mustard, pepper and vinegar), sugar or any refined, processed, canned or frozen foods. Especially avoid all refined carbohydrates.

All fruits and berries are beneficial. Best vegetables for MS are: carrots, cabbage, radishes, kohlrabi, cucumbers, red beets and tomatoes.

Liquid whey (the liquid portion of soured or curdled milk) contains orotic acid (vitamin B_{13}) which has been shown to be of special value in treatment of multiple sclerosis. When raw cottage cheese is made at home, liquid whey should not be thrown away but used for drinks.

BIOLOGICAL TREATMENTS

1. Short juice fast (see *Directions: 3*), 4 to 5 days. After the fast, a strict raw lacto-vegetarian diet of raw fruits and vegetables, milk, seeds, sprouts and lactic acid foods, as suggested above.

2. Extensive physiotherapeutic and hydrotherapeutic programs: massage, exercises, swimming, cold showers morning and evening, hot baths, hot mineral baths, if possible (see *Directions: 7* for therapeutic baths).

3. Vitamin supplementation is vital in treatment of MS. Dr. Frederick Klenner, Riedsville, N.C., uses large doses of B_1, B_3 and B_6 with reported success. Vitamin F (essential fatty acids) and vitamin E are also specific.

VITAMINS & SUPPLEMENTS (Daily)

E — up to 1,800 IU

F, essential fatty acids — 6 capsules

B-complex, natural, high potency, with B_{12}

B_1 — 100 mg.

B_6 — 100 mg.

B_3 — 100 mg.

B_2 — 100 mg.

B_{12} — 100 mcg.

Inositol — 500 mg.

C — up to 1,000 mg.

Lecithin — 3 tbsp. of granules

Pantothenic acid — 100 mg.

Raw saturated and unsaturated fatty acids for carbon[20] fat (from crude, cold-pressed oils, also from fresh, non-rancid wheat germ oil)

Brewer's yeast — 2 to 3 tbsp.

Magnesium supplement

Bone meal — 3 tablets

Liquid whey from soured milk

Natural multi-vitamin-mineral formula

JUICES

Any available raw vegetable and fruit juices from organically grown fruits and vegetables.

HERBS

Evening Primrose, sarsaprilla

SPECIFICS

Raw, organically grown foods, sprouted wheat, lecithin, vitamins B_1, B_3, B_6, F and E, fermented lactic acid foods, fresh unsalted farm butter.

REFERENTIAL READING

Airola, Paavo O., "Good News For Victims of Multiple Sclerosis," Chapter 12 in the book *Health Secrets From Europe*, Parker Publishing Co., West Nyack, New York. Paperback published by Arco Publishing Co., Inc., New York, N.Y., 1970.

Evers, Joseph, *Directions for Treatment of Multiple Sclerosis*, Karl F. Haug, Ulm/Donau, West Germany.

Waerland, Ebba, *Waerland Therapies*, Ny Nord Förlag, Stockholm, Sweden, 1955.

Clark, Michael, "Saved From MS by Organic Food," *Prevention*, November, 1972, pp. 92-98.

Alsleben, H. Rudolph and Shute, Wilfred E., *How to Survive the New Health Catastrophes*, Survival Publications, Inc. Anaheim, Ca. 1973.

(Nerve irritation and pain)

Neuritis can be caused by a variety of nutritional deficiencies and metabolic disturbances, such as faulty calcium metabolism, deficiencies of several B-vitamins (B_{12}, B_6, B_1, pantothenic acid, B_2), general toxemia, chronic acidosis, faulty phospholipid metabolism, etc. The best treatment for neuritis is to make sure that the patient gets optimum nutrition (well assimilated) with all the general vitamins and other supplements, but particularly the specific supplements which are listed below.

DIETARY CONSIDERATIONS

The Airola Optimum Diet (see *Directions: 1*) with emphasis on whole grains, particularly wheat, buckwheat and brown rice, raw seeds and nuts, especially almonds. Raw fruits and vegetables. Sprouted seeds, artichokes, raw milk, especially in soured form, and 1 cup of homemade cottage cheese (see *Recipes*) a day.

BIOLOGICAL TREATMENTS

1. Dry brush massage (see *Directions: 4*) and intermittent hot and cold showers (see *Directions: 7*), daily.
2. Daily walks and exercises, if patient is able to.
3. Constipation, or any other disorder, if present, must be corrected.

VITAMINS & SUPPLEMENTS (Daily)

B-compex, natural, high potency, large doses
Vitamins, B_1, B_2, B_3, B_6, B_{12} and pantothenic acid should be all represented in high potencies in this formula, or they could be taken separately
Brewer's yeast — 3 to 5 tbsp.
Magnesium chloride — 400 mg.
Calcium lactate — 6 tablets
Silica — 3 tablets
Multi-vitamin-mineral formula, all natural

JUICES

Carrot, beet, citrus fruit, apple, pineapple.

SPECIFICS

B-complex vitamins in large doses. Brewer's yeast, or other food yeast. Optimum Diet. Calcium, magnesium, silica.

REFERENTIAL READING

Bicknell, F., and Prescott, F., *The Vitamins in Medicine*, Lee Foundation for Nutritional Research, Milwaukee, Wis., 1953.
Davis, Adelle, *Let's Get Well*, New American Library, Inc., N.Y., 1972.
Stone, S., *Disorders of Nervous System*, 11, 131, 1950.
Ropert, R., *Nutritional Abstracts Review*, 29, 273, 1959.

OBESITY

(Chronic overweight)

All experts agree that, with the rare exceptions of thyroid insufficiency and defective metabolism, the number one cause of obesity is overeating. But what causes overeating?

The basic cause of overeating (and consequent obesity) is a disordered appestat mechanism which controls the appetite. Nutritional deficiencies caused by denatured foods disrupt the work of the appestat. Plenty of physical activity and/or exercise is required to keep the appestat working well. Also, appestat function can be disrupted by negative emotions, such as anxiety, fear, hostility, insecurity, etc. Thus, obese persons should make every effort to avoid such feelings and foster a positive outlook on life.

DIETARY CONSIDERATIONS

Low calorie Airola Diet of nutritious foods (see *Directions: 1*) with emphasis on 5 or 6 small meals, instead of two big meals a day. Plenty of raw fruits, vegetables and fresh juices.

Avoid all sugar and white flour, and everything made with them. Avoid salt, coffee, tea, alcohol. Avoid all refined and denatured foods.

Take 2 tsp. of apple cider vinegar in glass of water with every meal.

Low protein diet (35 grams a day) has been found to lead to safe weight reduction without the health damaging side-effects of a high protein diet.

BIOLOGICAL TREATMENTS

1. Repeated short juice fasts, one week to 10 days (see *Directions: 3*). Long juice fast, up to 40 days, or more, can also be undertaken, but only under expert supervision. For all details on fasting see my book *How to Keep Slim, Healthy and Young with Juice Fasting* (see *Referential Reading*).
2. Lots of physical work or exercise, especially walking, jogging, swimming, sports like tennis, etc. Strenuous exercise and/or physical activity are imperative for effective weight control.
3. Dry brush massage, twice a day (see *Directions: 4*) and intermittent hot-and-cold shower every morning (see *Directions: 7*).

VITAMINS & SUPPLEMENTS (Daily)

Multi-vitamin-mineral formula, all natural
Kelp — 5 to 10 tablets, or 2 tsp. of granules
B_6 — up to 100 mg.
Brewer's yeast — 2 to 3 tbsp.
B-complex, with B_6 and B_{12}, high potency

Inositol — 500 mg.

C — up to 1,000 mg.

E — up to 600 IU

Calcium-magnesium supplement (about 500 mg. of each)

Lecithin — 2 tsp.

Cold-pressed vegetable oil (olive, sesame, safflower) — 1 tsp. with each meal (3 times a day)

JUICES

Fruit: lemon, grapefruit, orange, cherry, pineapple, papaya.

Vegetable: cabbage, celery, green juice (see *Directions: 5*).

HERBS

Kelp, chaparral, chickweed, Irish moss, sassafras.

SPECIFICS

Low-calorie optimum diet of high quality natural, whole, unprocessed foods. Several small meals in preference of a few large ones. Periodic juice fasting. Plenty of physical work and/or exercise. B-complex, brewer's yeast, kelp, cold-pressed vegetable oil.

REFERENTIAL READING

Lincoln, J. E., "Calorie Intake, Obesity and Physical Activity," *The American Journal of Clinical Nutrition*, Vol. 25, March 1972, p. 390.

Yudkin, J., "The Practical Treatment of Obesity," *Proceedings of Royal Society of Medicine*, 58:200, 1965.

Airola, Paavo O., *How To Keep Slim, Healthy and Young with Juice Fasting*, Health Plus Publishers, Box 22001, Phoenix, Arizona, 1971.

Alsleben, H. Rudolph and Shute, Wilfred E., *How To Survive the New Health Catastrophes*, Survival Publications, Inc. Anaheim, Ca. 1973.

Williams, Roger, *Nutrition Against Disease*, Pitman Publishing Corp., New York, 1971.

Dole, V. P., *American Journal of Clinical Nutrition*, 5:591, 1957.

The American Journal of Clinical Nutrition, November, 1962.

Schachter, S. "Obesity and Eating," *Science*, 161:751, 1968.

Postgraduate Medicine, May, 1972 (special issue on Obesity).

NOTES:

1. Persons with a tendency for overweight should take all their vitamins and food supplements *after meals*, to minimize the appetite-stimulating effect of some vitamins, notably vitamins from a B-complex.

2. Most so-called reducing diets are harmful, and although some may help to take pounds off, they do so at the cost of damaged health. High protein diet and low or no carbohydrate diets are especially harmful. Severe restriction of carbohydrates with no restriction of fats and proteins may take weight off effectively, but can have the disastrous effect of causing irreparable damage to brain, nerve system and heart. A high-protein diet, always popular with reducers, will admittedly help to reduce, but always with severe health damage as the result.

Overindulgence in proteins is one of the prime causes of such dreaded diseases as arthritis, osteoporosis, heart disease and cancer.

3. Those who have "tried everything" and cannot reduce, should check the condition of their liver. Liver damage is common among overweight persons and can be a major cause of obesity. A damaged liver is unable to synthesize an adequate amount of energy-producing enzymes. Such a person should restore the health of his liver (see section on *Liver*) before reducing by a proper diet can be made possible.

4. Since the appestat workings can be disrupted by negative emotions, hostility, insecurity, hate, fear, etc., the reducing program which does not take into consideration *mental discipline* and the correction of mental attitudes is doomed to fail.

5. Because each obese person has different underlying causes for the condition — emotional, glandular, metabolic, nutritional or psychosomatic — and because obesity is often associated with many other specific conditions of ill health, we advise that each person who wishes to go on a reducing program should do so in collaboration with his own doctor, preferably a nutritionally-educated doctor, who knows a little more about health, obesity and nutrition than just an orthodox line on a "high protein diet."

OSTEOPOROSIS

Abnormal porosity of bones in older people is usually caused by nutritional deficiencies (vitamin and mineral deficient diet), the body's inability to properly absorb and utilize nutrients, overconsumption of meat, post-menopausal hormonal imbalances and diminished physical activity with age. Separately or combined, the above-mentioned causes can lead to development of osteoporosis. Prolonged cortisone treatment, by blocking the bone-building activity and decreasing the intestinal absorption of calcium, also may cause osteoporosis.

DIETARY CONSIDERATIONS

The Airola Diet (see *Directions: 1*) with emphasis on mineral-rich foods, such as whole grains, seeds, nuts, cooked and raw vegetables and fruits, raw milk and milk products, such as homemade cottage cheese (see *Recipes*). Foods rich in minerals, especially calcium, magnesium, potassium and silicon, such as green vegetables, cabbage, carrots, fruits and berries of all kinds — strawberries, raspberries, blueberries, etc., — should be eaten often. Sesame seeds and sunflower seeds are excellent foods.

Also an abundance of lactic acid foods, such as sauerkraut, lactic acid vegetables, sour bread and soured milk products (see *Recipes*). Oats, barley, buckwheat, millet and rice are the best grains.

The Airola Diet should be supplemented with a good all-inclusive mineral and trace mineral supplement and *Betaine Hydrochloride* tablets with each meal to assure proper assimilation.

Avoid large meals and overeating. Eat slowly and chew food extremely well. Avoid white sugar and white flour products. Avoid processed, refined and denatured foods. Avoid meat, especially beef which contains 25 times as much phosphorus as calcium; a high meat diet will invariably lead to calcium and magnesium deficiencies.

BIOLOGICAL TREATMENTS

1. Diminished physical activity and loss of muscle strength are contributing factors in senile osteoporosis. Plenty of regular physical activity and/or sufficient regular exercise is necessary, both for prevention and treatment of osteoporosis.

VITAMINS & SUPPLEMENTS (Daily)

Horsetail (a rich source of silicon) — extract or tea
   Available now in capsule form or as silica tablets
Bone meal — 3 tablets
Calcium-magnesium supplement — 500 mg. of eaeh
Magnesium chloride — 400 mg.
D — up to 5,000 units. Or cod liver oil — natural, unfortified, 3 tsp.
C — up to 1,000 mg.

Potassium iodine

Sea water — 2 tbsp.

Betaine Hydrochloride — 1 or 2 tablets after each meal with 1/2 glass water

Multi-mineral and trace element supplement, possibly in form of sea water

E - 600 IU

Alfalfa tablets

Apple cider vinegar with meals — 1 tsp. in glass of water with 1 tsp. honey

Multi-vitamin supplement, all natural

JUICES

Raw vegetable juices: green juice with turnip tops, alfalfa and comfrey, red beet, carrot, celery. Fruit juices: pineapple, lemon, papaya.

HERBS

Horsetail, nettles, comfrey, parsley, alfalfa.

SPECIFICS

Bone meal, silica, avoidance of high-phosphorus foods (beef, liver), magnesium, vitamins D, C, E, HCl.

REFERENTIAL READING

Selye, Hans, *Calciphylasis*, University of Chicago Press, Chicago, Ill., 1962.

Hegsted, D. M., *Modern Nutrition in Health and Disease*, Wohl and Goodhart, ed., 1955.

Nature, Vol. 241, Jan. 3, 1973, pp. 59-60.

Nordin, B. E. C., *Medical Press*, February 10, 1960.

Kervran, Louis C., *Biological Transmutations*, Swan House Publishing Co., Binghampton, N.Y., 1972.

Cecil-Loeb Textbook of Medicine, W. B. Saunders, 1971.

Hahn, Theodore, *Jewish Hospital of St. Louis, Newsletter*, February, 1974.

NOTES:

1. According to Dr. L. C. Kervran, the exponent of the biological transmutation concept, administration of calcium-rich foods or calcium supplements is *not* advisable in osteoporosis, calcium deficiency or decalcification for any reason. He advises the use of *silica, magnesium* and *potassium*, as a much more effective way of improving mineral metabolism and getting calcium into bones and other tissues. By the process of "biological transmutation," silica is changed into easy-assimilable calcium in the body. He particularly recommends using extract or tea, made of young plants of horsetail, as the best source of silica.

2. Drinking distilled water for prolonged periods often leads to the development of osteoporosis, because distilled water not only lacks the much needed minerals, but also leaches the minerals out of the body. Those who insist on drinking distilled water should fortify it with sea water to restore the lost minerals.

PARKINSON'S DISEASE

DIETARY CONSIDERATIONS

One hundred percent raw food diet of organically grown foods. Emphasis on raw seeds, nuts and grains, plenty of sprouts, raw milk, preferably goat's milk, and raw fruits and vegetables. Green, leafy vegetables and yellow turnips (rutabaga) are especially beneficial. Sesame seeds and sesame seed butter are excellent. Once or twice a week, take 1/2 tsp. of pure gelatin — use with foods or mix with citrus or tomato juice.

In general, a low-protein diet of raw, organically grown foods is best for patients with Parkinson's Disease.

BIOLOGICAL TREATMENTS

1. Short, repeated cleansing juice fasts, 6 to 10 days each (see *Directions: 3*).

VITAMINS & SUPPLEMENTS (Daily)

B_6 — 200 mg. Up to 2,000 mg. can be used under doctor's supervision. Some doctors have used successfully injections of B_6 together with magnesium

B_2 — up to 100 mg. (improves circulation)

B-complex, with high content of niacin — natural, high potency

Glutamic acid — up to 8 tablets

Magnesium — 500 mg.

Calcium lactate — 3 tablets

Brewer's yeast — 3-4 tbsp.

E — 600 IU

C — up to 1,000 mg.

Pure sea water — 1 to 2 tbsp.

Lecithin — 2 tbsp. granules

(Nerve cytotrophin is used by some doctors with reported good results)

JUICES

Any raw vegetable and fruit juices, in season.

HERBS

Ginseng, damiana, cayenne.

SPECIFICS

B-complex, B_6, glutamic acid, magnesium, sea water, Optimum Diet of raw organically grown foods, with plenty of sprouts and raw goat's milk.

REFERENTIAL READING

Gillespie, N. G., et al., *Journal of American Dietetic Association*, 62:525, 1973.
Nittler, A. *The New Breed of Doctor*, Pyramid Publishing Co., 1973.
Lancet, May, 1971.
Journal of American Medical Association, June, 1971.
Cotzias, G. C. et al., *Ann. Rev. Med.*, 22:305, 1971.

NOTES:

1.	In early stages of the disease, good results can be obtained with nutritional and biological therapies. In chronic, advanced cases, especially if the origin of the disease is emotional, or if the nerve tissue is destroyed, a notable improvement is difficult to obtain. However, good optimal nutrition and other measures suggested above will at least prevent the condition from getting worse — which can be considered an achievement in such a condition as Parkinsonism.

2.	Some biologically-oriented practitioners use "Nerve Cytotrophin" in Parkinson's Disease with reported good results.

3.	Treatment with L-dopa (levodopa, an amino acid, precursor of dopamine) has been shown to be effective in many studies and clinical use. L-dopa treatment must be accompanied with a low-protein diet (0.5 gm. protein per kilogram body weight per day). A high-protein intake interferes with the beneficial action of L-dopa (J. Am. Dietetic Assoc. 82:520, 1973).

PROSTATE PROBLEMS

(Chronic Prostatitis)

DIETARY CONSIDERATIONS

The Airola Diet (see *Directions: 1*) with emphasis on raw seeds and nuts, especially pumpkin and squash seeds, sunflower seeds, almonds and sesame seeds. All of these foods are rich in high quality proteins, unsaturated fatty acids, and *zinc* — food elements that are essential for the health of the prostate.

Plenty of raw vegetables and fruits, plus fresh juices.

Use cold-pressed vegetable oils, such as sunflower oil, sesame seed oil or olive oil for fatty acids, lecithin, brewer's yeast, and vitamin E — all important factors for prostate health.

Avoid coffee, alcohol, and all strong spices — all considered to be contributing causes of prostatitis predisposition.

Deficiencies of zinc and vitamin F (essential fatty acids) have been shown to be contributing causes of prostate disorders. Inclusion of these nutrients in the diet has brought great improvements in prostate condition.

BIOLOGICAL TREATMENTS

1. Avoid sexual excitation without a natural conclusion in the form of ejaculation, or orgasm. Such practices as advanced petting and withdrawal, without orgasm, leads to a prolonged engorgement and suppressed or incomplete ejaculation, which may lead to functional and even structural damage.

2. Avoid deliberate prolongation of the sexual act, during which the approaching ejaculation is suppressed.

3. Avoid undue abstinence from sexual gratification. Develop "sexual regularity" and do not deviate from the established rhythm, if possible.

4. See that your general health status is high. Optimum health is imperative for healthy sex organs and glands.

5. Exercise! Walking is the best possible form of exercise for keeping the prostate gland in good shape. One or two hours a day is not too much.

6. Another effective exercise (prostate massage) is done as follows: Lie flat on back, pull knees up as far as possible, then press the soles of both feet together. Holding soles pressed together, lower the legs as far as possible with a forceful movement. Repeat as many times as possible.

7. In acute conditions, hot sitz baths daily, with camomile tea added to the water (see *Directions: 7*).

VITAMINS & SUPPLEMENTS (Daily)

Pollen, or pollen extract — 6 tablets or 2 tsp. of crude pollen

F, essential fatty acids — 6 capsules

E — 600 IU or more

Chlorophyll perls (sex hormone precursor)

Zinc supplement, organic, 30 mg.

Lecithin — 1 or 2 tbsp.

C — 1,000 mg. In acute condition, up to 5,000 mg.

B_6 — 50 mg.

Fish liver oil, natural, unfortified — 2 tsp.

Multi-mineral-vitamin supplement, natural

Kelp — 2 tsp. of granules or 6 tablets

Brewer's yeast — 2 tbsp. (good source of organic zinc)

JUICES

Any raw vegetable and fruit juices, in season.

HERBS

Juniper berry, ginseng, damiana, kelp, echinacea (for enlargement and weakness), ergot (claviceps purpurea), birch leaf.

SPECIFICS

Pollen, zinc, pumpkin seeds, vitamins E and F, regularity in sexual habits, lots of walking and other exercises.

REFERENTIAL READING

Airola, Paavo O., *Sex and Nutrition*, see Chapter 13, "Can Prostate Problems be Prevented by Nutritional Means?", Award paperback, Available from Health Plus Publishers, P.O. Box 22001, Phoenix, Arizona, 1970.

Taub, J. Harald, "Pollen and Your Prostate," *Prevention*, February, 1972.

Hart and Cooper, *Vitamin F in the Treatment of Prostate Hypertrophy*, Report #1, Lee Foundation for Nutritional Research, Milwaukee, Wis.

Voisin, Andre, *Soil, Grass and Cancer*, Philosophical Press, Phila.

Nittler, Alan H., *A New Breed of Doctor*, Pyramid House, N.Y., 1972.

Willy, A., et al., *The Illustrated Encyclopedia of Sex*, Cadillac Publishing Co., Inc., N.Y.

Kenyon, Herbert R. *The Prostate Gland*, Random House, N.Y.,

Tobe, John H., *Your Prostate*, The Provoker Press, St. Catharines, Ontario, Canada, 1950.

Rodale, J. I., *Prostate*, Rodale Books, Inc., Emmaus, Pennsylvania.

DIETARY CONSIDERATIONS

The Airola Diet, with emphasis on raw seeds and nuts, especially sesame seeds, flaxseeds, pumpkin seeds, and sunflower seeds. Plenty of raw vegetables and fruits, organically grown, in season.

Cold-pressed vegetable oils, such as sesame oil and flaxseed oil, 2 tbsp. a day. Vegetable oils must be virgin, genuinely cold-pressed by hydraulic press, unrefined and unheated.

Avoidance of all animal fats (saturated fats) — pork, milk, butter, eggs. No refined or processed foods. No foods containing hydrogenated fats or white sugar.

Avoidance of citrus fruits, especially citrus juices. Cranberry or apple juice are permitted.

When the improvement is obvious, goat's milk, yogurt and homemade cottage cheese (kvark) may be added to the diet.

BIOLOGICAL TREATMENTS

1. Since psoriasis is a metabolic disease, a cleansing juice fast, 2 to 3 weeks, is always advisable in the beginning of treatment. Fast can be repeated after 4 weeks on diet.
2. Avoid too frequent bathing. Do not use soap.
3. Mineral baths are extremely beneficial, especially hot mineral baths; also, regular sea water baths.
4. Sea water can be applied externally over affected parts with a cotton ball once a day.
5. Frequent exposure of affected parts to the sun, particularly in a combination with ocean swimming is extremely beneficial and often results in a striking improvement.
6. For external application: Formula F-Plus (see *Directions: 8*).
7. Plenty of regular exercise in fresh air, especially exposing the affected parts. Deep-breathing exercises.
8. If regular bathing in ocean is not possible, take a homemade salt water bath once a week (see *Directions: 7*). Or take an acid bath once a week. Add one-half cup of apple cider vinegar to your bath water. This helps to restore acidity to the skin, which is imperative for restoration of health.

VITAMINS & SUPPLEMENTS (Daily)

E — up to 1,600 IU

A — up to 100,000 units for one month, then reduce to 25,000 daily for 3 months; and repeat

Lecithin — 4 tbsp. of granules, after 2 months reduce to 2 tbsp.

Calcium-magnesium supplement — 500 mg. of each

F (essential fatty acids) in capsule form or in form of flaxseed, sesame seed, or soy oil — 2 tbsp. a day

B-complex, natural, high potency, with B_{12}, B_6 and folic acid

Brewer's yeast — 2-3 tbsp.

Kelp — 5 tablets or 1 to 2 tsp. of granules

C with bioflavonoids, up to 3,000 mg.

Whey powder

Sea water, 2-3 tbsp. a day, for trace minerals

JUICES

Carrots, beets, cucumber, grapes, black currants. Avoid citrus juices.

HERBS

Sarsaparilla, burdock, elm bark, saffron, chaparral, dandelion, sassafras, mullein.

SPECIFICS

Lecithin, vitamins E, A, B-complex, sesame seeds, sesame oil. Frequent exposure to sun and mineral or sea water. Specific herb teas.

REFERENTIAL READING

Klein, Jill, "A Diet for Psoriasis," *Prevention*, January 1973.

Hoffman, R., et al., *New England Journal of Medicine*, 236:933, 1947.

Vogel, A., *The Nature Doctor*, Bioforce-Verlag, Teufen, Switzerland, 1960.

REJUVENATIVE TREATMENT

*(For prevention and treatment of premature aging
and sexual senility)*

DIETARY CONSIDERATIONS

The Airola Diet (see *Directions: 1*) with generous use of special rejuvenative foods, which have been empirically and scientifically shown to be factors in prevention of mental, physical and sexual senility and in prolongation of youthful vitality and appearance. Some of the foods or food substances specifically noted for such properties are: rose hips; whey; soured milks, such as yogurt, kefir or clabber milk, particularly made from goat's milk; kvark; buckwheat; millet; garlic; lecithin; vitamins E, A, C· and rutin; lactic acid foods, such as homemade sauerkraut, lactic acid vegetables, soured milks and sour bread; honey, pollen; halva (made from sesame seeds and honey); cayenne pepper; ginseng; sarsaparilla; kelp; cold-pressed vegetable oils and brewer's yeast.

For complete details on nutritional approach to rejuvenation, see my book, *Worldwide Secrets for Staying Young.*

BIOLOGICAL TREATMENTS

1. Physical activity in fresh air and/or sufficient exercise is imperative for preservation of youth and prevention of aging processes.
2. Systematic *undereating* is one of the prime secrets of long life in youthful vitality. *Keep slim* — extra weight rapidly ages you — mentally, physically and sexually.
3. Avoid: smoking, coffee, tea, salt, and all processed, canned refined and denatured foods, especially white sugar and white flour, and everything made with them.
4. Think young! Be active! Keep up with a regular sex life! Sexual inactivity causes atrophy of the sex glands. And you are only as young as your endocrine and sex glands!
5. Periodic juice fasting (see *Directions: 3*) can help you to stay younger longer.
6. Gerovital, or KH-3, developed by a Rumanian, Dr. Ana Aslan, is used extensively in Europe as a rejuvenative and revitalizing drug. It is a procaine-based formula fortified with B-complex vitamins. Not presently available in the U.S.

VITAMINS & SUPPLEMENTS (Daily)

Brewer's yeast — up to 5 tbsp.

E, d-alpha tocopherol — up to 1,200 IU. Twice as much if mixed tocopherols are used

A, natural, from fish liver oils — up to 100,000 units (see *Directions: 2* on taking high doses of vitamins)

Rutin — up to 200 mg.

C - up to 3,000 mg.

B-complex, natural, high potency

RNA, ribo-nucleic acid — 30 to 300 mg. in tablets; or obtain by using plenty of brewer's yeast

B_6 — up to 100 mg.

Lecithin — 2 tbsp.

Kelp — 5 tablets, or 2 tsp. of granules

Garlic, or garlic oil capsules

Whey powder or tablets

Natural multi-vitamin-mineral formula

Multi-enzyme digestive formula for older people

All the above vitamins and supplements have been shown by numerous clinical and other studies to be potent rejuvenative factors, which can prolong life and extend youthful vitality into old age. Two other supplements, which I deliberately left off the list, because of virtual impossibility to obtain them fresh, are *wheat germ* and *wheat germ oil.* They can be marvelous rejuvenative foods, *if they are absolutely fresh and non-rancid.*

JUICES

Fresh pineapple, papaya, lemon, lime, apricot and other fresh vegetable and fruit juices, in season.

HERBS

Ginseng, Hydrocotyle Asiatica (minor), damiana (for males), licorice (for females), sarsaparilla, Gotu-Kola (Hydrocotyle Asiatica, major), falce unicorn, elder, garlic.

SPECIFICS

Brewer's yeast, vitamins E, A, C and B-complex, RNA, ginseng and other rejuvenative herbs, garlic, rutin, Airola Diet of special rejuvenative foods (see *Dietary Considerations*).

REFERENTIAL READING

McCay, C. M., "Diet and Aging," *Vitamins and Hormones*, 7:147, 1949.

Sokoloff, B., et al., "Aging, Atherosclerosis and Ascorbic Acid Metabolism," *Journal of the American Geriatric Society*, 14, 1239, 1966.

Airola, Paavo O., *Rejuvenation Secrets From Around the World — That "Work,"* Health Plus Publishers, P.O. Box 22001, Phoenix, Arizona, 1974.

Airola, Paavo O., *How to Keep Slim, Healthy and Young with Juice Fasting*, Health Plus Publishers, P.O. Box 22001, Phoenix, Arizona, 1971.

Airola, Paavo O., *Sex and Nutrition*, Award paperback, Universal Publishing & Distributing Co., N.Y., 1970.

Clark, Linda, *Stay Young Longer*, Pyramid Books, N.Y., 1968.

Frank, Benjamin, *Nucleic Acid Therapy in Aging and Degenerative Diseases*, Psychological Library, 1969.
Tappel, A. L., *Geriatrics*, October 1968, p. 97.
Lucas, Richard, *Nature's Medicines*, Parker Publishing Co., West Nyack, N.Y., 1968.
Trimmer, Eric J., *Rejuvenation*, Award Books, N.Y., 1970.
Newman, Barkeley, *Must We Grow Old?*, G. B. Putnam's Sons, 1959.
Verzar, F. "Aging of Collagen," *Scientific American*, 208:110, 1963.
Searcy, R., *Diagnostic Biochemistry*, McGraw-Hill, 1969.
Wade, Carlson, *The Rejuvenation Vitamin*, Award Books, N.Y., 1970.

NOTES:

1.   The single most potent rejuvenative food is brewer's yeast. With its rich source of rejuvenative nucleic acids (15% of its weight!), and all the anti-aging B-vitamins, including B_6, organic zinc — plus 40% of highest quality proteins! — brewer's yeast consumed regularly can help to keep you young, prevent degenerative diseases and halt aging processes.

2.   Vitamin E — by preventing oxidation processes in the body, increasing cell oxygenation, keeping endocrine glands, including sex glands, in excellent working condition and in aiding in sex hormone production — is a powerful rejuvenator.

3.   Regular use of licorice, falce unicorn, elder, and vitamin E can help to postpone female menopause by supplying natural hormone substances and/or helping the body in hormone production.

4.   Vitamin B_6 decreases in our system with age, increasing the body's susceptibility to infections and illnesses of advanced age. Therefore, the dietary supplementation of B_6 is imperative for prevention of premature aging. Brewer's yeast is the best source of vitamin B_6.

SCHIZOPHRENIA

DIETARY CONSIDERATIONS

Hypoglycemia is almost always involved in schizophrenia, possibly being one of its contributing causes, together with many dietary deficiencies and biochemical imbalances. The ultimate cause of schizophrenia is chronic undersupply of oxygen to the brain. Therefore, it is extremely important that the blood sugar level is kept constant at all times and not allowed to drop too low. Frequent small meals of high quality natural foods, with emphasis on slow-to-digest whole grain products, such as buckwheat, millet, oats, brown rice, barley, etc., plus an abundance of whole raw and sprouted seeds and nuts. Almonds, peanuts, sesame seeds, sunflower seeds and pumpkin seeds are especially beneficial. (See anti-hypoglycemia diet in section on *Hypoglycemia*.)

An adequate amount of high quality protein is necessary, but complete proteins of vegetable origin are preferable to animal proteins. Soybeans, almonds, peanuts, buckwheat, sesame seeds, sunflower seeds and all sprouted seeds, plus all vegetables and brewer's yeast supply easily digested proteins of highest biological value. These foods are also rich in E and B vitamins, zinc, and other trace minerals needed by schizophrenia patients.

According to Dr. Carl Pfeiffer, of the New Jersey Neuropsychiatric Institute in Princeton, schizophrenia is primarily a biochemical disorder in the brain, caused mainly by mineral and trace element imbalance. He names particularly the *deficiency of zinc* combined with an *excess of copper*. His studies showed that 80 percent of the patients suffering from schizophrenia were found to have a deficiency of zinc and an excess of copper and iron in their body tissues. He suggested dietary supplementation of zinc and manganese, which apparently helps to displace copper in the body and eliminates the deficiency of zinc. According to Dr. Pfeiffer, 95 percent of the schizophrenic patients showed marked improvement after the trace element therapy.

Avoid all refined and devitalized foods. Total ban on sugar, white flour, and all foods and drinks that contain them. No animal proteins — they rob the body of much needed niacin, B_6 and magnesium.

BIOLOGICAL TREATMENTS

1. By far, the best biological treatment for schizophrenia is juice fasting (see *Directions: 3*). Repeated short juice fasts, or one long fast (4 to 6 weeks) usually normalize all body functions, eliminate biochemical disorder and imbalances and restore the patient to excellent health. Several of my patients have had excellent results with such treatment. Needless to say, fasting for schizophrenia, in each case,

should be undertaken only on advice of an expert practitioner and done under constant supervision, preferably in a fasting clinic. Note that the blood sugar level, which is so important for patients with schizophrenia, *remains normal during the fast*, if the fast is administered correctly. The cleansing and normalizing effect of fasting on all body functions is responsible for its healing effect. Fasting patients should take juices and broths every 2 hours. After the fast, patients should be put on the Airola Diet with vitamin supplementation as suggested in this section.

2. Schizophrenia has been successfully treated by Drs. A. Hoffer, H. Osmond, et al., with massive doses of niacin in the form of niacinamide; 1,000 mg. to 3,000 mg. of niacinamide are given with each meal; often as much as 25,000-30,000 mg. per day! This should be accompanied by an equal amount of vitamin C, high potency B-complex vitamins, especially pantothenic acid, and 3 to 5 tbsp. of brewer's yeast. After recovery, a large maintenance dose of niacin must continue indefinitely to keep the disease under control.

The schizophrenic apparently lacks the enzyme NAD (Nicotinamide Adenide Dinucleotide) which is needed for proper metabolism of adrenalin. Deficiency of NAD causes a build-up of certain metabolic toxins which react chemically on nerves and brain. Niacin neutralizes the toxins and helps the body to produce its own NAD.

Although *niacinamide* appears not to be toxic even in extremely high doses (Dr. Hoffer, the discoverer of niacin treatment for schizophrenia, gave doses as high as 24,000 mg. daily for a short period of time), massive doses of *niacin* should not be given for prolonged periods of time — not longer than for one to three months. In a few cases, massive doses, given for more than a year, caused stomach ulcers, jaundice, liver damage and sexual impotency, possibly by creating an imbalance in the other B-complex vitamins. The amount of niacin needed by different individuals varies widely. Persons with schizophrenia show an unusual need for this vitamin, and seem to tolerate niacinamide well, even in massive doses, for as long as 10 to 15 years. In spite of this, taking into consideration the widely individualized requirements, any person who wishes to try mega-vitamin therapy should have his dosage prescribed for him by an expert practitioner. Only the niacinamide form of niacin should be used, although a small amount of plain niacin or nicotinic acid may be added to the massive dose of niacinamide.

VITAMINS & SUPPLEMENTS (Daily)

Niacin or niacinamide — see Biological Treatments. Maintenance or preventive dose: 100 to 300 mg. daily

Zinc and manganese supplement, possibly in combination with other trace elements

B-complex, natural, high potency, with B_{12}

C — massive doses to equal niacinamide dosage

B_1 — 100 to 300 mg.

Brewer's yeast — 3 to 5 tbsp.

Inositol — 500 mg.

B_6 — 100 to 300 mg.

E — up to 1,000 IU

B_{15} — 100 mg.

Lithium carbonate, therapeutic doses. Available on prescription only.

Multi-vitamin-mineral formula, natural

JUICES

All fruit and vegetable juices, in season. Overly sweet juices should be diluted with water, 50-50.

SPECIFICS

Niacin, niacinamide, vitamins C, B-complex, B_1, B_6, B_{15}, zinc, manganese, brewer's yeast. Frequent small meals. Airola Diet of optimal nutrition.

REFERENTIAL READING

Hoffer, A., and Osmond H., *How To Live with Schizophrenia*, University Books, New Hyde Park, New York, 1966.

Hoffer, A., *Niacin Therapy in Psychiatry*, Charles C. Thomas, Springville, Ill., 1962.

Clark, Linda, "How To Avoid Contamination by Toxic Metals," *Let's Live*, November 1972, p. 72.

Orthomolecular Psychiatry: Treatment of Schizophrenia, edited by David Hawkins and Linus Pauling, Freeman and Co., 1972.

Watson, G., and Currier, W. D., *Journal of Psychology*, 49, 1960.

Cott, Allan, *Schizophrenia*, 3:2, 1971.

Kubala, A. L., et al., "Nutritional Factors in Psychological Test Behavior, *Journal of Genetic Psychology*, 96, 343, 1960.

Plante, Elizabeth A., "A Bio-Chemical Approach to Mental Disease, *The Answer: Preventive Medicine*, Vol. 1 No. 6, 1972.

NOTES:

Further comments regarding the toxicity of niacinamide and niacin mentioned on the previous page:

According to Doctors Harvey Ross ("Orthomolecular Psychiatry") and Carl Pfeiffer ("Mental and Elemental Nutrients"), niacinamide can be toxic in large doses and should only rarely be administered in doses over 3 grams per day, as it can cause liver damage and possibly other side effects. Niacin, on the other hand, seems seldom to be contraindicated, except for those with stomach ulcers.

Note added July, 1980.

I am including smoking in this section of ailments because so many people have asked me if there is anything that can be done to help an addicted smoker to lose his taste for cigarettes.

In my experience, there is a 100 percent effective way of breaking the habit of smoking, drinking alcohol or coffee, or using addictive drugs. *This method is:* JUICE FASTING (see *Directions: 3*).

Tobacco-, alcohol-, coffee- or drug-addict's "craving" is brought about by a certain physiological body dependence on the poison which develops during prolonged use. The addict's blood poison level must remain high at all times. As it drops down, he feels "desire" to light another cigarette, or drink another cup of coffee, to bring the toxic level up again.

The only way this physiological dependence can be broken is by *cleansing* the body completely of all the accumulated poisons, be it nicotine, caffeine, alcohol or heroin. During the juice fasting, all the toxins will be effectively excreted, all the tissues cleansed and freed from the poison, the blood will be completely purified — *and all the "craving" will be gone!*

I have had numerous patients who have successfully broken the habit of smoking or drinking with juice fasting. Normally, after two to three weeks of juice fasting, all the *physiological* desires have disappeared, which means that the body has been cleansed from all the poisons, and the patient is free from his addiction. A certain amount of *psychological* desire, a habit to hold something between your fingers, will linger for a few months, but will gradually also disappear.

Naturally, after the fasting a 100 percent health-building diet of natural foods — the Airola Diet (see *Directions: 1*) of optimal nutrition through unrefined, whole, poison-free foods — must be maintained.

NOTES:

1.   Women who smoke, age *twice* as fast as their non-smoking female friends — especially by external signs of aging, such as wrinkles, and dull, lifeless, gray, deteriorating complexion. I can spot any woman, who has smoked for more than five years, just by looking at her complexion — provided it is not hidden by a thick layer of make-up. Smoking is not only about the most unfeminine thing a woman can do, but it also causes what most women dread most — premature aging . . . not to mention cancer! Juice fasting is a simple and effective solution.

STOMACH ULCERS

(Gastric or duodenal)

Both gastric and duodenal ulcers can be caused by, in addition to the usual nutritional or metabolic causes, severe nervous and mental stress. Therefore, before the nutritional or biological treatment can be successful, the psychological causes must be solved or removed. Persons with a predisposition for peptic ulcers should avoid all situations resulting in mental stress and prolonged nervous strain or irritability. Complete rest and relaxation from all pressing problems and worries is imperative.

DIETARY CONSIDERATIONS

Anything that can irritate the mucous membranes of the stomach and duodenum must be eliminated from the diet. Meals must be small and frequent, possibly six to eight times a day. Food must be chewed extremely well, 40 times each mouthful — fletcherised! It is important that all food is well salivated. If the patient cannot chew well, food should be liquified or pureed in a blender, then chewed as if it were whole.

In an acute case of active ulcers, whole grains, nuts and whole-grain breads and cereals should be avoided in the beginning of the treatment. Well cooked millet cereal, with milk, is the best, and can be given even in the beginning of the treatment in small amounts. Also cooked white rice, with milk, is well tolerated. Almond milk made from blanched almonds in a blender, is very beneficial, as it binds the excess of acid in the stomach and supplies high quality proteins. Also regular milk, warmed-up to body temperature, is well tolerated, particularly raw goat's milk. Raw goat's milk actually helps to heal stomach ulcers. Soured milks, such as yogurt, kefir or clabbered milk, can be included. Brewer's yeast, mixed with soured milk, can be taken on an empty stomach between meals.

Raw fruits and vegetables should be avoided for a few weeks, as many of these are especially irritating. Potatoes, squashes, yams, avocados, and raw bananas are, however, well tolerated.

All sour fruits should be avoided, especially citrus fruits. Sweet fruits can be eaten in moderation.

All fried foods must be eliminated. It has been shown that heated vegetable oils can be a contributing factor in development of ulcers.

The following must be strictly avoided: tobacco, alcohol, coffee, tea, chocolate, salt, and all strong spices such as white and black pepper, mustard, vinegar, chili, etc. All these are known to cause an increase in the flow of digestive juices which irritate the stomach lining. Also white sugar and soft drinks should be avoided.

Avoid food and drink that is either too hot or too cold — all drinks and foods should be consumed preferably at room or body temperature.

BIOLOGICAL TREATMENTS

1. The most effective biological treatments for peptic ulcers are as follows:

   FOR DUODENAL ULCERS

   Raw, freshly made cabbage juice, 1/2 glass several times during the day. If the patient has difficulty taking cabbage juice straight — it has a rather pungent taste — it can be mixed 50-50 with carrot and/or celery juice.

   Raw potato juice is also excellent for duodenal ulcers.

   FOR STOMACH ULCERS

   Raw, freshly made potato juice, possibly with a small addition of cabbage juice, 1/2 glass several times a day on empty stomach.

   Note: Both cabbage and potato juice *must be freshly made* on your own juicer and drunk *immediately after it is made.* I mean, *right there and then*! Even after one minute of waiting, the medicinal value disappears. Both juices contain medicinal, healing factors (vitamin U in cabbage juice) which are lost in storage because of rapid oxidation.

2. Strong tea, made from dried comfrey roots and leaves, taken several times a day on an empty stomach (at body temperature, of course), is also a very effective treatment for peptic and duodenal ulcers.

3. When desperate, one may just drink copious amounts of water to ease ulcer pain.

VITAMINS & SUPPLEMENTS (Daily)

E — 600 to 1,200 IU

Brewer's yeast, 2-3 tbsp. a day, mixed with soured milk, taken on an empty stomach between meals

A — 25,000 to 50,000 units

B-complex, *natural*, including B_{12}. Make sure the product contains *only* B-vitamins from natural sources — no synthetics

Chlorophyll tablets — 3

Halibut liver oil — 2-3 tsp.

When the patient is on the way to recovery, a maintenance dose of all other vitamins can be added to the diet (see *Directions: 2*)

JUICES

Raw cabbage juice (vitamin U) for duodenal ulcers.

Raw potato juice for gastric (stomach) ulcers.

HERBS

Comfrey root, cinita organo (Mexican plant), slippery elm, licorice, violet, golden seal, cloves, camomile, flaxseed, chaparral, canagra (Kanagra). Tea must not be drunk hot, but at body temperature.

SPECIFICS

Raw cabbage and potato juice; vitamins E and A, comfrey tea; goat's milk; brewer's yeast; frequent small meals; complete relaxation and avoidance of all mental stress and worries; strict avoidance of tobacco, alcohol, coffee, tea, salt and all strong spices.

REFERENTIAL READING

Kangas, Jon A., et al., *The American Journal of Clinical Nutrition*, Sept., 1972.
California Medicine, January 1956.
Cheney, Garnett, *Journal of the American Dietetic Association*, Sept., 1950.
Lanyi, George, "Stomach ache – What Can I Do," *Hälsa*, No. 7-8, 1972, Stockholm (Swedish)
Rodale, J. I., *The Encyclopedia for Healthful Living*, Rodale Books, Inc., Emmaus, Penn.
Clark, Mikael, "Vitamins A and E Protect Against Ulcers," *Prevention*, April, 1973.
Sapp, O. L., "Treatment of Duodenal Ulcer," *American Family Physician*, Vol. 7, February, 1973.
Domz, C. A., *Life and Health*, Vol. 86, No. 3.

NOTES:

1.   To determine if ulcers are gastric or duodenal, x-rays are usually used. If you wish to avoid x-rays, the following symptomatic signs can be of help: gastric ulcers cause pain *after* the meal, while duodenal ulcers cause pain *before or between* meals (so-called "hunger pain").

2.   Note that complete fasting, even juice fasting, is *not advised* for stomach ulcers. It is best to combine raw cabbage and raw potato juice therapies with restricted diet as suggested above.

3.   Low blood sugar (hypoglycemia) is often connected with peptic ulcers. Studies show that 75 percent of patients with peptic ulcers also have hypoglycemia. Follow the anti-hypoglycemia diet (see section on *Hypoglycemia*) if this is one of the contributing causes.

4.   Several studies show that vitamins E and A, especially taken together, have not only a protective effect against development of ulcers caused by stress, but also a curative effect on existing ulcers.

THROMBOPHLEBITIS

DIETARY CONSIDERATIONS

Strict natural raw food diet, with emphasis on sprouted seeds and grains, such as sprouted wheat, alfalfa seeds and soy or mung beans, raw fruits and vegetables and fresh juices. Especially beneficial foods are: pineapple, citrus fruits, papaya, alfalfa, comfrey and sesame seeds.

BIOLOGICAL TREATMENTS

1. Avoid prolonged inactivity. Beginning slowly, develop a regular program of outdoor activity, particularly walking, gradually increasing the length each day.
2. Hot-and-cold shower morning and evening (see *Directions: 7*).
3. Dry brush massage, 15 minutes morning and evening (see *Directions: 4*).

VITAMINS & SUPPLEMENTS (Daily)

E — 600 to 800 IU, even more, up to 1,600 IU, if necessary
Bromelain (pineapple enzyme) — 6 to 8 tablets
Rutin — 100 to 200 mg.
C — large doses up to 5,000 mg.
B-complex, natural, high potency
Pantothenic acid — 100 mg.
Natural multi-vitamin-mineral supplement

JUICES

Pineapple juice, lemon juice, green juice (see *Directions: 5*).

HERBS

White oak bark, lobelia, marigold.

SPECIFICS

Vitamins E and C, bromelain, rutin, raw food diet.

REFERENTIAL READING

Cirelli, M. G., *Clinical Medicine*, June, 1967.
Prevention, February, 1972. See "Pineapple Enzyme Reduces Inflamation."
Shute, W. E. and E. V., *Your Health and Vitamin E.*
Sneddon, J. Russell, *The Natural Treatment of Liver Troubles and Associated Ailments*, Health For All Publishing Co., London, 1960.

NOTES:

1. Thrombophlebitis can be associated with serious consequences if blood clots (emboli) form in the vein, break off and are carried to the heart or lungs. Therefore, we discourage all self-treatment of thrombophlebitis, nutritional or otherwise, and advise patients suffering from the condition to remain under their doctor's supervision and follow his advice in regard to most suitable treatment in their case, including the nutritional approach.

VARICOSE VEINS

DIETARY CONSIDERATIONS

The Airola Diet (see *Directions: 1*) with emphasis on whole grains, seeds, nuts, vegetables and fruits, 75 to 80 percent raw. Especially beneficial grains: wheat, buckwheat, millet. Take all general supplements recommended in *Directions: 2*.

Avoid constipation, which is often a contributing cause to varicose veins (see anti-constipation diet in section on *Constipation*).

BIOLOGICAL TREATMENTS

1. Daily exercises on a slant board, with head down. Also, headstand, twice a day, if possible.
2. Foot of bed should be elevated slightly — 3 to 4 inches (one brick on flat side).
3. In severe cases, wearing elastic stockings occasionally to force blood into deeper veins can be advisable.
4. Sitting in chairs is considered to be one of the main causes of varicose veins, according to studies made at the Auckland Medical School. Therefore, avoid sitting as much as possible. Walking and riding bicycle are good exercises. Swimming is extremely beneficial.

VITAMINS & SUPPLEMENTS (Daily)

Rutin and/or mixed bioflavonoids — 300 mg. to 500 mgs.
C — up to 3,000 mg.
E — 600 to 1,200 IU
B-complex, high potency, natural
Calcium lactate — 1,000 mg.
Brewer's yeast — 2 to 3 tbsp.
Kelp — 1 tsp. of granules or 5 tablets
Natural multi-vitamin-mineral formula
Lecithin — 2 tsp.

JUICES

Pineapple, rose hips, black currants, grapes, citrus juices, carrot, comfrey, spinach and small amounts of garlic and onion juice added to vegetable juices.

HERBS

White oak bark, marigold, witch hazel, yarrow, mistletoe.

SPECIFICS

Vitamins E and C, rutin, pineapple juice, buckwheat.

REFERENTIAL READING

Shute, Wilfred, *Vitamin E for Ailing and Healthy Hearts*, Pyramid House, 1969.
Davis, Adelle, *Let's Get Well*, Harcourt Brace Javanovich, Inc., N.Y., 1968.

NOTES:

The following biological methods have been reported to be effective in removing warts:

1. *Vitamin E.* Squeeze the contents of one 100 IU capsule of vitamin E on non-medicated band-aid and place over the wart. Repeat continuously for 2 to 3 weeks.

2. *Castor oil.* Apply generously over wart every night and morning for several months.

3. *Vitamin A and E, internally.* Take 100,000 units of A, and 600 IU of E, for one month.

4. *Vitamin G-complex* (Dr. Royal Lee's formula) — 6 tablets a day.

5. *Celandine.* The juice is squeezed out of fresh plant and applied to warts or corns.

6. *Figs.* Milky juice of fresh, barely ripe figs, applied directly on warts several times a day for a couple of weeks.

7. *Papaya.* The juice of *green* papaya applied to the warts several times a day.

8. *Potato.* Cut raw potato and rub it on. Repeat several times a day for a couple of weeks.

9. *Asparagus.* Eat 4 tbsp. of asparagus pureé twice a day. Canned puree or home-made pureé of cooked asparagus in blender (use both asparagus and the liquid).

Note: It is my opinion, based on a life-time of experience, that *the patient's faith* in the treatment, whether it is one of the above-mentioned, or any of the hundreds of other popular wart remedies, plays a most important role in achieving results. This is, of course, true in regard to any disease or treatment, but seems to be more so in regard to warts.

WORMS

(Intestinal worms, pinworms, tapeworms)

The following harmless biological treatments, both ancient and modern, have been reported to be effective in removing intestinal worms:

1. *GARLIC* — Garlic has been used for this purpose since in early history by Chinese, Greeks, Romans, Hindus, Babylonians, as well as by many modern biological practitioners. Both fresh garlic and garlic oil (now available in capsule form) are effective. For those who do not like the taste of garlic and refuse to eat it (children especially), an ancient method of garlic medication may be the answer: place a couple of cloves of fresh garlic in each shoe — yes, *shoe*! As child walks, garlic is crushed and the worm-killing garlic oil is absorbed by the skin and carried by the blood into intestines. Garlic possesses a powerful penetrative force. Within 10 minutes of its being rubbed on unbroken skin it can be detected in the breath.

2. *PAPAYA SEEDS* — Fresh papaya seeds, about 1 tbsp., should be chewed and swallowed on empty stomach. They can be mixed with honey to improve the taste. Repeat several times. Also dried papaya seeds can be used. Crush them well and swallow with a little water.

3. *ALMOND BRAN AND FIG JUICE* — This is Dr. Royal Lee's formula in tablet form, available through health food stores. Dosage: 4 to 6 tablets. Children, 1/2 dose.

4. *SODIUM CHLORIDE* — Sodium chloride, or common salt, is a time-proven remedy for pinworms. Children, who develop worms, are often deficient in salt. Heavily salted diet for a week or two has been known to effectively remove pinworms.

5. *CHAPARRAL TEA OR TABLETS* — Taken on empty stomach, 3 times a day.

6. *ARECA NUT (BETELNUT)* — This herb has been used by prominent herbalists for tapeworm. Dose: 2 to 4 drachms. Also, MALE FERN is used for the expulsion of tapeworm.

7. *PINKROOT, WORMSEED AND WORMWOOD* — These herbs are commonly used for expelling all types of intestinal worms.

8. *PUMPKIN SEEDS* — This completely harmless and beneficial food has been used in folk medicine for expelling worms.

9. *MALE FERN (Aspidium)* — This herb is used for the expulsion of worms, especially tapeworms. One tsp. of fern roots is steeped in 1 cup of boiling water for half an hour. Cool it and drink 1 or 2 cupfuls a day, a good mouthful at a time.

IN A NUTSHELL

Here are a few of the herbal, nutritional and other biological treatments for conditions not covered *in preceding sections on common diseases. Please understand that these are just a few specifics — in a nutshell format — not comprehensive or complete treatments in any sense. In alphabetical order:*

ANXIETY, tension: Bone meal, 5 to 10 tablets a day, with 2 capsules of fish liver oil (for vitamin D); B-complex vitamins; brewer's yeast.

ATHLETE'S FOOT: Mutton tallow. To make tallow, take mutton fat (preferably from lamb kidney — ask your butcher) and cook it over a slow fire. Strain and store in clean jar. Wash feet and apply at night. Change socks every day. Dust feet with garlic powder.

BACK PAIN: Vitamins E and C, calcium, magnesium, manganese.

BED SORES: Topically: Vitamin E. Orally: E, A, C, zinc. Also: honey topically.

BEDWETTING: Cinnamon bark tea. Chewing cinnamon bark is even better.

BEE STING: Antidote for: Acid-forming minerals such as calcium chloride, hydrochloric acid, ammonium chloride.

BOILS: Tea of sarsaparilla, red clover, nettle; carrot and beet juice.

BRONCHITIS: Tea of chickweed, slippery elm, mullein. Breathe the steam from hot catnip tea.

BUERGER'S DISEASE: Vitamin E, large doses up to 2,400 IU; lecithin; vitamin C.

BURNING FEET: Vitamin B_6.

BURNING MOUTH: B-complex, B_{12}, niacin, folic acid.

BURSITIS: Peanut oil, internally, 1 tbsp. a day; alkaline diet. Chloride-rich foods: kelp, watercress, avocado, endive, tomatoes, celery, oats, etc.

CANKER SORES (Fever blisters): Yogurt or Lactobacillus Acidolphilus culture, in tablet form or liquid. Lots of vitamin C. Burdock root tea. Avoid sweets and citrus fruits.

CATARACTS: Vitamin B_2. Chaparral tea taken internally. A drop of liquid honey in corner of eye at night.

COLD EXTREMETIES (cold feet and hands): Niacin, RNA (ribo-nucleic acid), B_2.

CONGESTION, bruises: Witch hazel decoction, rubbed externally.

CRACKED LIPS: Vitamin B_2, brewer's yeast.

CUSHING'S DISEASE: Potassium in large doses.

CYSTITIS: Corn silk tea, steamed egg plant, apple cider vinegar.

DANDRUFF: Nettle and chaparral tea, internally and externally. Rinse with vinegar added to the water. Castor oil, topically. Elimination of all sugar from the diet. B-complex vitamins.

DIZZINESS (Vertigo, Meniere's Disease): Niacin; B_1, B_2, B_6, pantothenic acid. Vitamin C. Catnip tea.

DRY SKIN: Almond oil; sesame oil; Formula F-Plus (see *Directions: 8*).

EAR ACHE: A few drops of warm castor oil in ear; plug with cotton.

EYES: To strengthen eyes, especially in weakness resulting from diabetes: chaparral tea, internally; vitamin A.

FEVER: Vitamin C. Chinchona bark tea. Lemon or grapefruit juice.

GAS: Garlic, papaya juice, hydrochloric acid with meals. Herbs: calamus (Sweet Flag), peppermint, slippery elm bark.

GOUT: Cherries — raw, juiced or frozen. Purine-free (low animal protein, low grain) diet.

GRAY HAIR: To restore natural color: PABA, pantothenic acid, folic acid, brewer's yeast, blackstrap molasses. Also, multiple mineral and trace element formula, or seawater (2 to 3 tbsp. a day).

HAYFEVER: Pollen (granules or tablets), pollen-rich (unprocessed, raw) honey. Herbs: black cohosh, jimson weed.

HORNET STINGS: 1. Honey; dab raw, untreated honey several times on the sting areas. Relieves pain and prevents or minimizes swelling. 2. A third of a teaspoon of unseasoned meat tenderizer in a teaspoon of water. Apply to insect stings (hornets, bees, mosquito, etc.). It will relieve pain and may minimize the allergic reaction.

HYPERKINETIC CHILDREN: Large doses of minerals: calcium, magnesium and potassium; balanced high potency B-complex formula: 30 mg. of B_1, B_2, B_6, 100 mg. niacin, PABA and pantothenic acid, 500 mg. inositol and choline, plus B_{12} and folic acid. Avoid all foods with artificial flavorings and colorings.

IMPETIGO: Garlic oil, squeezed from capsules, on irritated area.

INFECTIONS (colds, flu, etc.): Vitamins C, A, B_6 (B_6 acts as natural antihistamine).

INSOMNIA: Magnesium chloride, calcium, B_6, pantothenic acid, B_{15}. Before going to bed, one cup of chaparral, licorice root, peppermint, valerian, lady's-slipper or hops tea. Hops tea and licorice root tea are especially effective.

ITCHY SKIN: Add vinegar to bathing water. Take 2 tbsp. of vegetable oil daily. Herbs: yarrow, marjoram, violet. Dry brush massage (see *Directions: 4*).

LEG CRAMPS (at night): Magnesium, calcium lactate, B_6, silica. B_6 is also good for tingling and numbness in fingers and toes.

LENTIGOS (liver spots, brown skin marks): Dandelion root tea, avoid excessive exposure to sun.

LUPUS ERYTHEMATOSUS: Externally: PABA cream. Internally: carrot juice, vitamin A, manganese supplement. Avoid sunbathing.

LUPUS VULGARIS: Vitamin D_2 (isoniazid), vitamin C.

MOSQUITO BITES: 1. *To prevent:* Eat lots of raw garlic; avoid all sugar and white flour in any form; supplement diet with vitamin B-complex and/or brewer's yeast. 2. *To relieve itching of mosquito bites:* (a) Rub with raw garlic or fresh lime (or lemon) juice. Repeat as often as possible. (b) Rub with damp salt. (c) Rub with vitamin C tablet or powder.

MOTION SICKNESS: Large doses of brewer's yeast plus B-complex vitamins several weeks prior to exposure.

MUSCLE SPASMS: Calcium lactate, honey, magnesium chloride, silica, chaparral tablets or tea.

MUSCLE STIFFNESS (after unaccustomed exercise or heavy work): For prevention and treatment: massive doses of vitamin C.

MUSCULAR WEAKNESS: Vitamin B_6, potassium (best sources: bananas, potatoes, beans, raisins, green leafy vegetables, vegetable juices).

MYASTHENIA GRAVIS: Arachidonic acid (present in cereal grain oils), liquid lecithin, calcium, vitamin D, choline, manganese.

MYOPIA (nearsightedness): Vitamin D (large doses) plus calcium.

NAILS (brittle, thin, peeling fingernails): Brewer's yeast, bone meal, gelatin, silica, horsetail tea or extract, hydrochloric acid. White spots on finger and toe nails: zinc supplement.

NATURAL CONTRACEPTIVE: Stoneseed, infusion made of the plant's roots, drunk as tea (used by Nevada Indian tribes).
    WARNING: In giving this information, the author and publisher do not prescribe or recommend, and assume no responsibility. Information is given strictly for educational and research purposes.

NEURALGIA: B-complex, B_{12}, B_6, pantothenic acid, lecithin, calcium, sesame seeds, yeast.

NEURASTHENIA: Niacin, B-complex.

NUMBNESS ("going to sleep" peripheral nerves in toes, fingers or other parts of the body): Vitamin B_6.

OSTEOMALACIA: Vitamin D (up to 50,000 units a week for short periods), plenty of sunshine, HCl for older patients.

PARALYSIS (due to nerve interference, strokes, brain misfunction, etc.): B_6, up to 2,000 mg., injected or orally, under doctor's supervision only.

PELLAGRA: Niacin in large doses, B-complex.

THE PILL (to counteract carcinogenic effect of estrogen): Iodine (kelp). B-complex vitamins. Vitamin C. To counteract pill-induced pyridoxine deficiency and resultant depression: B_6 supplement. To counteract deficiencies caused by birth control pills: B-complex vitamins, specifically B_{12} and folic acid.

POISON IVY (antidote): Jewel weed, especially if crushed fresh and applied on affected area. Also, Dusty Miller and Aloe Vera.

Internally: 2,000-3,000 mg. vitamin C.

POOR CIRCULATION: Niacin, vitamin E, RNA, folic acid.

PREGNANCY (to prevent toxemia, nausea and edema in pregnancy): Vitamins B_6, B-complex and C, in large doses, preferably natural.

PRICKLY HEAT: Vitamin C, orally, 1,000 mg. or more. Wash with mild soap twice a day, apply apple cider vinegar (1/2 tsp. in glass of water) after bath.

PYORRHEA: Vitamin C-complex, with all the known bioflavonoids, A and B_{12}. Rub the gums morning and evening with vitamin E.

RECTAL ITCH: Hot sitz bath daily (see *Directions: 7*); after bath apply lemon juice or apple cider vinegar with a piece of cotton. Or, rub wheat germ oil on all affected parts after washing and drying.

RED EYES: Vitamin B_2, brewer's yeast.

RING WORM: Apply apple cider vinegar several times a day. Rub with borax. Rub with castor oil or chestnut oil.

SEBORRHEA: Vitamins B-complex, B_2, brewer's yeast, PABA.

SHINGLES: Massive doses of vitamins C, rutin, B-complex, calcium, lecithin, vitamin F. Apple cider vinegar topically, several times a day. Hot baths 2-3 times a week.

SICKLE CELL ANEMIA: Zinc, C, E.

SINUS INFECTION: Garlic, vitamins C and B_6. Herbs: saw palmetto, rose hips, mullein, golden seal, hops, red clover.

SLOW PULSE: Vitamin B_1.

SORES (that do not heal): 1. Topically: Vitamin E, 200 IU a day. 2. Topical application of strong comfrey root and/or leaf tea. Also a dressing of fresh comfrey leaves and root. 3. Dressing: paste made from raw garlic on gauze, for 8 to 10 hours. Orally: C, A, zinc, calcium.

SMELL AND TASTE (depressed): Zinc tablets, orally, 30 to 60 mg.

STERILITY (female): Wheat germ oil, vitamin E, sprouted grains and seeds, raw nuts.

SWELLING (due to edema, arthritis, bruises, sprains, infections, inflammations): *bromelain*, fresh pineapple enzyme, in tablet form, or in the form of fresh pineapple juice.

TEETH, stained or yellow: 1. Brush with fresh strawberries: place a strawberry on the toothbrush and brush as usual. 2. Brush with charcoal powder (obtainable in drug stores).

TENDINITIS: Manganese supplement.

THYROID INSUFFICIENCY (Hypothyroidism): Kelp, granulated or tablets; vitamins C and E; olive oil. Herbs: golden seal, bayberry, myrrh, black cohosh.

VAGINITIS (vaginal yeast infection): B-complex, high potency, orally.

VITILIGO: PABA, pantothenic acid, hydrochloric acid.

PART TWO

HOW TO PROTECT YOURSELF AGAINST COMMON POISONS IN FOOD, WATER, AIR AND ENVIRONMENT

WHAT CAN YOU DO...

HOW TO PROTECT YOURSELF AGAINST COMMON POISONS
IN FOOD, WATER, AIR AND ENVIRONMENT

I don't think I need to waste any ink trying to prove that poisons in our environment are a real threat to our health. Ten years ago – yes. Those of us who warned about danger of environmental poisons were called alarmists and crackpots. Now it is common knowledge that the gradual build-up of disease-producing poisons in air, water, soil and food supplies has reached a critical point.

Many scientists, who have investigated the seriousness of the situation, say that man has already succeeded in destroying and poisoning his own planet – the soil, the air and the water – to the point of no return. They predict that man faces mass extinction through toxic chemicals in the very near future – *unless something drastic is done* . . . and done very fast.

There is no longer any doubt in anybody's mind that poisons in our environment cause all kinds of serious disorders, disease and death – all the way from the vague, subclinical conditions, such as headaches, irritability, chronic mental and physical fatigue and digestive disorders, to our most dreaded killers, heart disease and cancer.

There is much talk today, on every level, *about* the environmental pollution. Even the President of the United States said that "We must clean our environment – or perish!" But if you think that those responsible for our health will take a swift action to clean our air, water and food supplies from disease-producing and killing poisons, you are in for a big surprise. Nothing of decisive value will be done for a long time. You should be prepared to see things get much worse before they get better. Not until real mass tragedies begin to occur, when millions of people will be dropping dead, will any real effective measures be taken. Let's face it: the real powers that run our country are the financial and industrial big boys from the chemical-drug-medical-food processing-auto-oil and other vested interests. They will see to it that nothing is done that can hurt their profits. That all these poisons in air, soil, water and food are making Americans the sickest people in the world, does not bother them. You see, the whole economical structure of American chemical-drug-medical and hospital industry is based on the principle: "The more sickness – the more profit!" The government agencies, which are supposed to protect us from the toxic dangers in our food, drug and other environmental sources, are completely taken over and controlled by these interests.

Therefore, if you want to be protected against ever-increasing amounts of deadly poisons in your environment – in the air you breath, in the water you drink and in the food you eat – *you must do it yourself*, no one else will.

What *can* you do?

I have made a thorough study and research of this question, with the result that I have found many ways and means that you can employ for your protection. The damage to your body by certain common poisons in air, water and food *can* be partially minimized and even prevented by the regular use of certain vitamins, minerals and other food substances. Certain minerals and vitamins neutralize and/or counteract the effect of toxins. Certain foods can help the development and growth of beneficial bacteria in your intestines which can help to detoxify and neutralize certain toxic residues in food. Certain vitamins and food substances can increase your body's tolerance and resistance against toxins. Some other vitamins can help your body to excrete ingested poisons from the system.

Here are some priceless tips that may help to save your health, perhaps even your life, in this poisoned world.

CARBON MONOXIDE

Carbon monoxide is the most health-damaging constituent of polluted air. In interferes with the oxygenation of all the cells of your body by preventing oxygen from being absorbed by your lungs. It can cause respiratory disorders, irritability, loss of memory, headaches, shortness of breath, angina, emphysema, anemia, heart disease and cancer.

Protection

1. **VITAMIN E.** It increases tissue oxygenation and decreases the body's oxygen need, by preventing the undesirable oxidation of lipids in the blood stream.
   Dose: 400 to 600 IU a day. For higher dosage, or if you suffer from high blood pressure or rheumatic heart disease, consult your doctor.

2. **VITAMIN B$_{15}$,** or pangamic acid. It markedly increases your body's tolerance to the oxygen deficiency caused by carbon monoxide.
   Dose: 30 mg. three times a day, or 50 mg. twice a day, morning and evening.
3. **VITAMIN A.** It has a specific protective property against carbon monoxide and other toxins in polluted air, by increasing the permeability of blood capillaries and, thus, facilitating better delivery of oxygen to the cells.
   Dose: 25,000 USP units each day. In severely smoggy conditions, up to 50,000 units each day.

OZONE AND NITROGEN DIOXIDE

These photochemical air pollutants are health-damaging constituents of smog. They can cause many respiratory and other disorders, notably emphysema.

Protection

1. **VITAMIN A.** It protects your mucous membranes, including those of the lungs, against damage by ozone, nitrogen dioxide and other pollutants.
   Dose: 50,000 units per day.
2. **VITAMIN E.** It has been established that vitamin E affords definite protection against toxic effects of ozone and nitrogen dioxide. It also keeps the ozone from destroying vitamin A in the body.
   Dose: up to 1,200 IU a day.

LEAD

Lead is present in air, water and food in increasing amounts. It is one of the most toxic metal contaminants and can be fatal even in small amounts. It comes mostly from leaded gasolines, but also from lead-containing paint, ceramic glazes, and other industrial sources.

Lead is a cumulative poison. Early symptoms of lead poisoning can be hard to diagnose: lack of appetite, fatigue, nervousness. As the poison continues to accumulate, it damages the kidneys, liver, heart and nervous system. Eventually, paralysis of extremities, blindness, mental disturbances, mental retardation and even insanity may develop. Multiple sclerosis is believed by some researchers to be caused by lead poisoning. It can also cause anemia, reproductive disorders, decline in fertility, miscarriages, stillbirths and total sterility. Chronic lead poisoning can also cause sexual impotence in men.

Lead is particularly dangerous to expectant mothers. Children born to lead-poisoned women suffer growth retardation and nervous and mental disorders.

Protection

1. **CALCIUM.** It has both a preventive and curative effect on lead poisoning by helping the body to safely excrete lead from the system.
   Dose: 5 to 10 tablets of bone meal or calcium lactate daily. Calcium gluconate (intravenously) helps to remove pain of acute lead-poisoning colic.
2. **VITAMIN D.** In acute cases of lead poisoning, calcium and vitamin D, injected intravenously, have been successful in speeding the recovery.
3. **VITAMIN C.** A powerful anti-toxin. Helps in neutralizing the toxic effect of lead. Protects muscle tissue from lead damage.
   Dose: 1,000 mg. to 3,000 mg. a day. In acute condition, up to 10,000 mg. (1,000 mg. every hour, preferably intravenously).
4. **VITAMIN B$_1$.** It is of specific value in protecting against damaging effect of lead.
   Dose: 25 mg. to 100 mg., together with one high potency B-complex tablet, each day.
5. **VITAMIN A.** It helps activate enzymes which are involved in detoxifying lead poisons.
   Dose: 25,000 units.
6. **LECITHIN.** Lecithin is a "neutralizer" of poisons in the body. It also protects the myelin sheaths of nerve fibers from being damaged by lead.
   Dose: 1 to 2 tbsp. a day in granular form.
7. **MINERAL AND TRACE ELEMENTS SUPPLEMENT**, in tablet form or natural, like sea water. According to Dr. Henry Schroeder, a mineral-rich diet will help to resist harm caused by heavy metal contamination.
8. **POTASSIUM IODIDE.** Combines with lead in the system and promotes its excretion from the body.
9. **AVOID SMOKING.** Smoking cigarettes can increase your daily intake of lead by 25 percent.
10. **LEGUMES AND BEANS**, used generously in the diet help to excrete lead from the system.
11. **ALGIN** (made from brown Pacific kelp), or sodium alginate, has been shown to help excrete lead from the body. Algin is a chelating agent which moves through the intestinal tract without being absorbed. It attaches to the lead and carries it out as it leaves the body. Powdered algin can be mixed with drinks and foods.

MERCURY

Mercury is one of the most universally present poisons in our environment. It has contaminated our soil, our waters and our food supply.

Mercury is a deadly, cumulative poison. It can damage the brain and central nervous system. It also interferes with enzyme activity, damages kidneys, liver, and causes paralysis and blindness.

Protection

1. **BREWER'S YEAST**. It contains selenium, a trace mineral that acts as an antidote helping to destroy the mercury in the body.
   Dose: 3 to 5 tbsp. a day.
2. Eat only **organically grown foods**. Drink plenty of raw fruit and vegetable juices. Organic foods contain traces of selenium.
3. Do not drink **regular tap water**. Use pure, unpolluted well or spring water, bottled if necessary.
4. Take large doses daily of the following **vitamins** which are known to help you protect against harmful effects of any toxins, including mercury: C, E, A and B-complex.
5. **CALCIUM**. Helps to neutralize mercury and excrete it safely.
   Dose: Up to 1,000 mg. a day.
6. **HYDROCHLORIC ACID**. One tablet after each meal, if you are over 40 and deficient in HCl.
7. **LECITHIN**. Minimizes the toxic effect of mercury.
   Dose: 1 to 2 tbsp. of granules a day.

DDT

DDT is now present everywhere. Although the American government has limited (not banned, as it is commonly believed) its use, it is still *widely* used throughout the world, especially in underdeveloped and "developing" countries. The whole of our planet is contaminated by DDT. If the use of DDT was completely discontinued today, it would take several decades before it would disappear from the environment, as it is an extremely slow decomposing substance.

DDT is a cumulative poison, stored mainly in the fat tissues of the body. Quick-reducing programs, or a rapid loss of weight for any other reason, can, therefore, be dangerous, as poisons will be released from the dissolved fat and can damage the whole system. When fasting is employed for reducing purposes, patients should fast only on juices (see *Directions: 3*), which will minimize the danger of DDT poisoning, and follow the protection program suggested below.

Protection

1. **YOGURT**, and other soured milks. It has been well established that sour milk bacteria neutralizes DDT in the intestines and makes it "safer", that is, minimizes its damaging effect on the body. Use daily.
2. **LECITHIN**. Recent research by the Department of Agricultural Chemistry and Environmental Health Sciences Center at Oregon State University have found that lecithin can bind up DDT and reduce its harmful effect on organism.
   Dose: 2 to 3 tbsp. of granules a day.
3. **WHEY**, powder or tablets. It feeds and encourages the beneficial bacteria in the intestines, which help to neutralize DDT.
4. **VITAMIN C.** Helps to neutralize all poisons, including DDT, and protects body tissues from its harmful effects.

CADMIUM

Although beneficial in minute amounts in natural form, *cadmium*, as an environmental pollutant, is extremely toxic. It is found in smoggy air, coming mostly from automobiles. Many brands of gasoline and lubricating oils contain cadmium. It is also present in commonly used phosphate fertilizers whereby it pollutes the soil, wherefrom it is taken up by vegetables and particularly by cereal grains. Most of our water supplies, especially so-called soft water, are heavily polluted by cadmium.

One of the common causes of slow, chronic cadmium poisoning is the ingestion of water which comes out of the faucet first thing in the morning, as it had picked up dangerous amounts of cadmium by standing in the pipes overnight. Both the galvanized and the newer black plastic pipes contain cadmium, which is dissolved and leached out by acids in the water. Hot water leaches even more than cold water and, therefore, should be never used for cooking or drinking.

Shellfish and animal livers concentrate cadmium and are dangerous to eat for this reason.

Cadmium poisoning can also be caused by the use of enameled utensils and pots. Toxic cadmium is used to achieve the beautiful colors in enamel (the same way as lead is used in ceramics). It is dissolved by acids in food and ends up in our bodies.

Cadmium is even more dangerous to your health than lead. It can cause high blood pressure and heart disease, iron-deficiency anemia, atherosclerosis, emphysema, chronic bronchitis, lung fibrosis, kidney damage and cancer.

Protection

1. **VITAMIN C.** It is a *specific* protector against the toxic and disease-producing effect of cadmium.
   Dose: massive doses up to 3,000 mg. a day. In acute poisoning, even more.
2. Include **zinc-rich foods**, such as pumpkin seeds, sunflower seed and other raw seeds, nuts and whole grains, in your daily diet. Zinc prevents the assimilation of cadmium. Cadmium and zinc are chemical "antagonists." If zinc is present in the diet in abundance, it winds up being stored in our body in place of cadmium.
3. Avoid **white flour** and everything made with it. Seventy-eight percent of the zinc present in whole wheat is removed with bran and wheat germ during the milling process, leaving an abundance of cadmium in white flour.
4. Avoid using **enameled utensils**. Use glass, earthenware or stainless steel utensils.
5. Do not drink regular **tap water**. Use bottled spring water if you live in the city.

STRONTIUM 90

World-wide nuclear tests and explosions have now contaminated the whole globe with toxic Strontium 90. Scientists say that *everyone* has already dangerous amounts of radioactive Strontium 90 in their bones. It stays in the body throughout the lifetime, emitting radioactive rays, like x-rays.

Anemia, leukemia, sarcoma of the bones (bone cancer) and many other cancers are believed to be caused by Strontium 90.

Protection

1. **ALGIN.** Extracted from giant brown Pacific kelp, this non-toxic substance can effectively remove radioactive Strontium 90 from the body. Algin can be used in the daily diet instead of such thickening agents as gelatin or cornstarch, or mixed with milk or other drinks.
2. **PECTIN.** It binds radioactive Strontium in the intestines and reduces its absorption and deposition in the skeleton. Only the pectin derived from sunflowers was found effective. Eat plenty of raw sunflower seeds daily.
3. **CALCIUM AND MAGNESIUM.** Both help your body to pass off Strontium 90. When selecting your mineral supplement, make sure it is not made from American animal bones which contain large amounts of Strontium. The best bonemeal supplements are made from South American bones, which are not so contaminated. Bone

meal with bone-marrow is the best. Deep-mined mineral supplements, such as dolomite and others, are advisable. Dr. Linus Pauling says that heavy calcium supplementation will reduce strontium absorption by 50 percent.

4. **YOGURT** and other soured milks help to neutralize the radioactive chemicals in the intestines and excrete them safety from the body. Up to 1 quart a day of soured milk can be consumed.

5. **B-complex vitamins, or Brewer's yeast.** It has been shown in animal studies that brewer's yeast affords protection against radiation.

6. **KELP.** *Sodium alginate* in kelp reduces absorption of Strontium 90 by 50 to 80 percent. Take 1 to 2 tsp. of granules daily, or 5 to 10 tablets.

7. **LECITHIN.** Lecithin in daily diet can counteract the effects of radiation.

8. The following vitamins can help to guard against radiation toxicity: E, C, and B-complex.

RADIOACTIVE IODINE
(iodine 131)

Radioactive iodine is a dangerous fallout contaminant, like Strontium 90, but can be even more toxic. It is found mostly in milk; therefore, it is particularly harmful to children who drink lots of milk.

Radioactive iodine is readily absorbed by the body, and it concentrates chiefly in one place — the thyroid gland. When the accumulation is sufficiently large, it causes thyroid cancer.

Protection

1. **KELP.** When the diet is amply supplemented with *easily-assimilable organic iodine*, as in kelp, the radioactive iodine is *not* absorbed by the thyroid gland.
   Dose: 1 to 2 tsp. of granules daily, or 5 to 10 tablets.

2. Protective program suggested for Strontium 90.

X-RAYS

X-rays have been used and abused indiscriminately by doctors, hospitals, dentists and chiropractors for decades, ignoring their great potential danger. X-rays are cumulative, so that even small amounts, such as those emitted from a color TV, a wristwatch or an alarm clock, can be dangerous as they add to the total amount received from all sources.

Overexposure can cause leukemia, cancer, birth defects and a later development of leukemia in a child born of a mother who received abdominal x-rays during pregnancy.

Protection

1. **RUTIN.** It strengthens the capillary walls and reduces hemorrhaging caused by x-rays. In animal tests, *rutin* (vitamin P, or bioflavonoid) reduced the death rate caused by excessive x-rays by 800 percent.
   Dose: 100 to 200 mg. a day as protective dose. In case of exposure: 800 mg. or more, a day. It is harmless.
2. **VITAMIN C.** Large doses of vitamin C, taken together with rutin, can strengthen the effect of rutin and help to protect against damaging effect of x-rays.
3. **PANTOTHENIC ACID.** It prevents radiation injuries. In animal studies, the survival rate was increased by 200 percent by giving pantothenic acid prior to exposure.
   Dose: Preventive — 5 mg. to 15 mg. for children; 25 mg. to 50 mg. for adults. A double or triple dose as a therapeutic after exposure. Brewer's yeast is by far the best natural source of pantothenic acid.
4. **BREWER'S YEAST.** It has been established that crude yeast extract provides a definite protection against lethal radiation doses.
5. **VITAMIN F** (essential fatty acids), present in all crude, cold-pressed vegetable oils. Provides protection against the harmful effect of x-rays.
6. **INOSITOL** (present mostly in lecithin, but also available in tablet form). Prevents damage from x-rays and other radiation exposure.
7. **LEMON** or lemon peel concentrate. Experiments in several hospitals show that patients can withstand heavier therapeutic radiation without damage to healthy tissues if given lemon compound (undoubtedly because of bioflavonoids which are present in large amounts in lemon and lemon peel).
8. **LECITHIN,** 2-3 tbsp. a day, will help counteract the effects of radiation.
   NOTE: When x-ray treatment or exposure is anticipated, large doses of the above-mentioned vitamins and special supplements will help you to prevent damage from radiation and permit higher doses of radiation with less harm.

TOXIC EFFECTS OF DRUGS

All chemical drugs are toxic, more or less. All drugs can cause harmful side effects. It is estimated (very conservatively) that at least 10 percent of all patients suffer from drug-caused diseases. Even such an "innocent" drug as aspirin, consumed in the U.S. at the rate of 30 tons a day, has caused many deaths and millions of serious injuries.

Most drugs also interfere with normal enzyme and vitamin action in the body, causing derangement in metabolism and vital body processes.

Drugs destroy vital vitamins and minerals and/or prevent their absorption. Many drugs damage the liver, kidneys and can cause serious diseases, including impotence, infertility, birth defects and cancer. Of course, there are situations in which drugs *are* necessary and can be life-saving. But drugs should be used only in absolute emergencies, and only if ordered by a competent doctor.

Protection

1. When any kind of drugs are taken, increase your intake of the following vitamins:
    *   C — large doses, up to 10,000 mg. a day can be taken when exposed to heavy doses of drugs.
    *   B-complex, high potency. Especially needed after treatment with antibiotics.
    *   LECITHIN — 2 to 3 tbsp. a day.

    These substances will help to protect you against harmful effects of drugs and prevent damage to the liver and other organs caused by a number of drugs.
2. **VITAMINS C AND E** are of specific value as protective agents against damaging side effects of aspirin.
3. **YOGURT AND WHEY.** If antibiotics have been taken, orally or by injection, take yogurt or other soured milks, or acidophilus culture and whey in tablet or powdered form, for a prolonged period after the drug therapy, to help re-establish a new flora of beneficial intestinal bacteria killed by antibiotics.

NITRATES AND NITRITES

Many foods today, particularly all processed meats, are preserved with these toxic chemicals. They are used on fresh meats to enhance the color. Even baby foods contain nitrates. Also, nitrate fertilizers, commonly used today, contaminate the soil and pollute the water supplies.

Nitrosamines, formed in the body from ingested nitrates and secondary amines, are extremely toxic and proven carcinogenic substances. They cause cancer in the liver, stomach, brain, esophagus, bladder, kidneys and several other ograns. They also cause high blood pressure and heart disease.

Nitrates and nitrites interfere with the conversion of carotene into vitamin A in the body, and even destroy the body's own storage of vitamin A.

Protection

1. **VITAMIN C.** Large doses up to 5,000 mg. a day. In acute cases of poisoning, 2,000 mg. every one and one-half hours for one day, then

reduce to 5,000 mg. a day. A recent study conducted at the University of Nebraska's Eppley Institute For Cancer Research, showed that vitamin C can effectively neutralize and destroy nitrites in the stomach, and prevent their conversion into the nitrosamines. Vitamin C should always be taken in large doses when nitrite containing foods have been eaten. It is best to use vitamin C daily as a preventive measure, as these toxins are hard to avoid these days.

2. **VITAMINS B-COMPLEX, A, E AND LECITHIN** are other substances that have been found to be helpful in neutralizing or minimizing the damaging effect of nitrates and nitrites.

GENERAL PROTECTIVE MEASURES
AGAINST TOXIC ENVIRONMENT

The protective measures suggested so far in this section are for *specific* poisons and toxic or harmful substances in your environment. When you know that you are, or will be, subjected to these specific poisons or health-destroying influences, the suggested measures can help you to protect your health against their damaging effect. The information on these specific, harmless vitamin and food substances that you can use to minimize or neutralize the effect of poisons in your environment, can be of great value if you are subjected, or expect to be subjected, to these specific sources of toxic or health-damaging assault.

But the most serious problem, for most of us, *most of the time*, is *not* the isolated poisons but the continuous total toxic assault from all directions. We are all subjected to radioactive substances and hundreds of poisons and toxic chemicals every day of our lives. The air we breath, the foods we eat, the water we drink — even the clothes we wear and the beds we sleep on — all are filled with poisons that none of us can possibly avoid. Even those who most conscientiously and meticulously attempt to live poison-free lives and eat only organically grown foods, are nevertheless subjected to many poisons. Even organically grown foods are grown in polluted air and are watered with polluted, chemicalized water. And the air, just about *anywhere* in the United States, is now seriously contaminated.

We can also be sure that the poisons in our environment are here to stay for a long time. Even if not a speck of new pollutants were added to our soil, air or water beginning from today, the existing pollutants would be here for decades to come, some for centuries.

Therefore, those of us who are aware of the graveness of the situation, should make an everyday effort to do everything there possibly *can* be done to protect us against the killing environmental poisons, which none of us can actually avoid.

Here are some general protective measures which can help our survival in this poisoned world we have created for ourselves:

1. Make every effort to move away from the smoggy cities. Buy a cottage or a little farm outside of the city, and, if necessary, drive one or two hours to work. Then you can also grow most of your own poison-free foods. If you *must* live in a smoggy city, get out to smog-free air, at least a few weeks each year, to give your body, your liver and your lungs a chance to regenerate themselves and build a certain health reserve.

2. Make every effort to eat only organically grown foods. Many health food stores now carry a good supply of them. Or transform your backyard into your own organic garden. Organic foods, or your own backyard vegetables will not be completely poison-free, but they will be *better* than the regular produce you buy at supermarkets.

3. If you are an apartment dweller, get a green thumb by growing wheat grass in boxes on your balcony or kitchen window. Also, everyone can grow his own sprouts.

4. If you must eat supermarket-bought produce, wash all your vegetables and fruits very carefully, with soap and warm water. Just rinsing with water would not do any good. Those fruits and vegetables that cannot be washed should be peeled.

   Here's one method recommended to remove residues of arsenic, DDT and other toxic sprays from vegetables and fruits: Mix 1 ounce of pure hydrochloric acid (sold in drugstores) with 3 quarts of water (use only glass or earthenware utensils). Place vegetables in solution for five minutes, then remove and rinse well with pure water. The solution can be saved and reused many times. Some claim that hydrochloric acid solution much weaker than this can be used.

5. Stop using any and all toxic chemicals in your household: garden sprays, air fresheners, flystrips, cleaning fluids, detergents, bug killers, etc. Use soap as your only cleaning material, even for washing clothes. Avoid dry cleaning of your clothes. If dry cleaning is necessary, ventilate the clothes for several days after the cleaning.

6. Optimum nutrition will help you to better withstand the polluted environment. The Airola Diet of optimum nutrition, as outlined in *Directions: 1* in this book, will assure you of the optimum nutrition and maximum protection against a toxic environment.

7. Fortify your diet with the following vitamins, minerals, special foods and food supplements which have been found in extensive world-wide research to have specific protective, neutralizing and detoxifying properties against poisons in your environment, your air, your water and your food:

- **Yogurt and other soured milks.** It has been found that sour milk bacteria neutralize most poisons, but specifically DDT and Strontium 90, and make them "safer," that is, minimize their damaging effect on the body. One pint to one quart a day.

- **KELP.** An excellent protector against radioactive fallout substances such as Strontium 90 and radioactive iodine. Five to 10 tablets or 1 to 2 tsp. of granules a day.

- **LECITHIN.** Lecithin neutralizes all body poisons. One to 2 tbsp. a day.

- **BREWER'S YEAST.** Best natural protective food against pollution. Helps your liver in its detoxifying work. Use generously: 2, 3 or more tbsp. a day.

- **VITAMIN B-COMPLEX**, high potency. B-vitamins protect you against many toxic residues in foods.

- **VITAMIN B_1.** Specific protector against damaging effect of lead. 25 mg. a day.

- **VITAMIN B_{15}.** Effective protector against air pollution, particularly against dangerous effect of carbon monoxide. 100 mg. a day.

- **PANTOTHENIC ACID.** Protector against radiation injuries, etc. Up to 100 mg. a day. Brewer's yeast is an excellent source.

- **VITAMIN C.** Number one anti-toxin. It will help your body to withstand the toxic assault better and prevent damage. It will protect all your organs and glands. Large doses up to 3,000 mg. a day. In acute cases of poisoning from any source, doses of 1,500 mg. every hour, up to 10,000 mg. a day.

- **VITAMIN E.** Effective protector against poisons in polluted air, especially ozone, nitrogen dioxide and carbon monoxide. Helps liver in its detoxifying work. Protects you against most poison in food, water and air. Up to 600 IU a day. (For higher dosage, or if suffering from rheumatic heart disease, or high blood pressure, consult your doctor.)

- **VITAMIN A.** Improves your body's oxygen economy and, thus, protects you against damaging effect of smog. Up to 25,000 USP units a day.

- **VITAMIN D.** Improves the utilization of calcium, one of the most important anti-toxin minerals. Up to 2,500 USP units a day.

- **CALCIUM AND MAGNESIUM.** Help your body to neutralize and pass off many toxic substances, such as lead, mercury, Strontium 90, radioactive iodine and cadmium. Calcium up to 1,000 mg., magnesium, up to 500 mg. a day. Bone meal tablets (with bone-marrow) and dolomite are good sources of calcium and magnesium.

PART THREE

DIRECTIONS

Description and instructions regarding nutritional, herbal and other biological therapies recommended in PART ONE of this book.

THE AIROLA DIET

**THE OPTIMAL NUTRITIONAL PROGRAM FOR CORRECTING
DISEASE AND RESTORING, BUILDING
AND MAINTAINING HEALTH.**

In *Part One* of this book we often refer to the *Airola Diet* as one of the most effective therapeutic ways to treat the majority of man's ills, correct disease and restore, build and maintain health. What is the Airola Diet?

First, let me say a few words regarding the name. Throughout my several decades of teaching, lecturing and writing, I have made references to an ideal diet which has the greatest potential for the prevention of disease and the maintenance of health. I have described such a diet in detail, as in my book "Are You Confused?", with instructions, menus and recipes – but never gave it a specific *name*. Sometimes, in my writings I refer to this diet as the Optimum Diet or the Modern Macrobiotic Diet. But during the last several years I have noticed that thousands of my readers, students and those who hear my lectures, insist on referring to the diet I recommend as "your diet" or the "Airola Diet". In fact, "the Airola Diet" became a firmly established referential concept of a lacto-vegetarian diet, with emphasis on the three basic foods: (1) Seeds, grains and nuts, (2) vegetables, and (3) fruits (in this order of importance), supplemented with milk and milk products, fermented lactic acid foods, cold-pressed vegetable oils, honey, brewer's yeast and a long list of vitamins and mineral supplements. Because of such massive insistance of referring to the diet I recommend as "The Airola Diet" I finally capitulated and, with the publication of this book, decided to make it "official". Perhaps I should point out that this nutritional program is the result of my life-time studies, research and personal and clinical experience, and that it differs essentially on many vital points from other well-known lacto-vegetarian diets, such as the Waerland Diet or the Bircher-Benner Diet, both of which were formulated several decades ago, or before most vitamins were discovered and before man was subjected to universal pollution. The Airola Diet combines the knowledge of Waerland and Bircher-Benner with the newest nutritional discoveries and the ecological and environmental requirements of the Seventies. It is an Optimum Diet for optimum health, prevention of disease, and long life adopted to the modern age with its growing amounts of health-destroying environmental factors.

Although the majority of American orthodox doctors generally dismiss nutrition as an important factor in health and disease, all responsible nutritionists and a few biologically and nutritionally oriented doctors agree that proper nutrition *is* a number one factor affecting one's health. Disagreement among nutritionists starts when they attempt to determine *WHAT IS PROPER NUTRITION, or What constitutes an Optimum Diet for Optimum Health.*

There are those who believe that the so-called "Basic Four" food groups will assure optimum nutrition. There are those who advocate a high animal protein diet, with lots of meat. There are those who condemn all seeds and grains ("seeds are for the birds") and those who would eat seeds, but not grains. There are those who advocate eating only raw foods, and those who consider the discovery of the fire the greatest boon to man's nutrition. There are those who eat only vegetables that grow above the ground, and again those who consider tomatoes and onions to be poisonous. Then there are nutritionists and health writers who wish to please everyone (just like the politicians – it's good business you know) and advise eating anything that you like, or "what agrees with you", as long as it is natural and unprocessed. There are those who feel that you should supplement your diet with added vitamins – and there are those who claim that all added vitamins are harmful, and that you should get your vitamins from the foods you eat.

Who is right and whom can you believe?

The Airola Diet, presented below is not based on my own personal, subjective beliefs or wishful thinking, but is based on reliable scientific sources and corroborated by overwhelming empirical evidence and my own life-long research. This diet has not only the greatest potential for building health, preventing disease and maintaining health, but also is the most effective diet for restoring health where health has been lost.

Here are, then, in a nutshell, the

TEN BASIC PRINCIPLES OF THE
OPTIMUM NUTRITION

The Airola Diet for Optimum Health, Youthful Vitality and Long Life.

1. YOUR OPTIMUM DIET SHOULD BE MADE UP FROM THESE THREE BASIC FOOD GROUPS

(In this order of importance):
A. Seeds, nuts and grains
B. Vegetables
C. Fruits

A. *SEEDS, NUTS AND GRAINS* are the most important and the most potent foods of all. Their nutritional value is unsurpassed by any other food. Eaten mostly raw and sprouted, but also cooked, they contain *all* the important nutrients essential for human growth, sustenance of health and prevention of disease in the most perfect combination and balance. In addition, they contain *the secret of life itself, the germ*, the reproductive power that assures the perpetuation of species. This reproductive power, the spark of life in the seeds, is of extreme importance for the life of man, his health, and his own reproductive capacity and power.

All seeds and grains are useful and beneficial, but you should eat predominantly those that are grown in your own environment. Millet, buckwheat, wheat, oats, barley, brown rice, sesame seeds, beans, peas – all are wonderful health foods. Wheat, mung beans, alfalfa seeds and soybeans make excellent sprouts. Sprouting increases their nutritional value tremendously. Sunflower seeds, pumpkin seeds, almonds, peanuts, sesame seeds, buckwheat and soybeans – all contain complete proteins of highest biological value. Those seeds and grains that do not contain complete proteins (or all the essential amino acids), will become complete protein foods if eaten together (like corn tortillas and beans; or buckwheat and wheat), or if eaten with vegetables or milk.

Seeds, nuts and grains are not only excellent sources of proteins but also the best natural sources of essential *unsaturated fatty acids* without which health cannot be sustained. They are also nature's best source of *lecithin* and most of the *B-complex vitamins.* Sprouted seeds are a good source of *vitamins C and A.*

Perhaps the most important vitamin for preservation of health and prevention of premature aging is *vitamin E.* Whole seeds, grains and nuts are, by far, the best natural sources of this vital vitamin.

Seeds, grains and nuts are also goldmines of *minerals* and *pacifarins*, an antibiotic resistance factor that increases man's natural resistance to disease. They also contain *auxones*, natural substances that help produce vitamins in the body and play a part in the rejuvenation of cells, preventing premature aging. Whole grains, seeds and nuts will also supply the necessary bulk in the diet. The bran of the grains and seeds is vital for the normal function of the digestive organs and for the prevention of such diseases as appendicitis, diverticulitis and cancer of the colon, as shown by recent studies by Dr. Dennis P. Burkitt.

All seeds and nuts should be eaten raw. Those that can be sprouted, should be used in sprouted form. Some grains, such as rice, buckwheat, millet, rye and barley, can be cooked in the form of cereals or bread (see *Recipes* for sprouting or making breads and cereals). Particularly, sourdough bread is extremely beneficial. During the natural souring process, due to the enzymatic action on the grain, valuable lactic acid develops, which is a health-promoting and disease preventing factor, as demonstrated by Dr. Johannes Kuhl and others. Also the fermentation makes certain nutrients in grains more easily available for assimilation in the intestinal tract. This is particularly true in regard to zinc, manganese and other trace minerals. Rye is the most suitable grain to make sourdough bread. Millet and buckwheat cereals are most delicious and nutritious foods. Beans and peas can be cooked, and should be used often.

B. The next in importance from "the basic three" are **VEGETABLES.**

Vegetables are extremely important sources of minerals, enzymes and vitamins. Most green vegetables also contain complete proteins of highest quality; in fact often of better biological value than proteins of animal sources — proteins of potatoes and green leafy vegetables are complete proteins of highest biological value.

Most vegetables should be eaten raw in form of raw salads. Some vegetables, such as potatoes, yams, squashes or green beans can also be cooked, baked or steamed.

Generous use of garlic, onions and numerous herbs and natural spices will improve your health and turn dull vegetable dishes into gourmet food.

Food is your best medicine — and vegetables (herbs) are your best medicinal foods.

C. The third most important food group in your Airola Diet are **FRUITS.**

Like vegetables, fruits are excellent sources of minerals, vitamins and enzymes. Fruits are a cleansing food. They are easily digested and exert a cleansing effect on the blood and the digestive tract.

In addition to all available fresh fruits, in season, the Airola Diet can include dry fruits, particularly when fresh fruits are not available. Unsulfured, organically grown raisins, prunes, dried apricots and figs are available from health food stores.

Fruits are best eaten for breakfast in the morning or as a snack between meals. Roughly, each food group should supply the bulk of one of the three meals: Fruits for breakfast, seeds, nuts or cereal for lunch, and vegetables for dinner; although this order can be interchanged, of course. See the suggested *HEALTH MENU* at the end of this section.

2. EAT MOSTLY RAW, LIVING FOODS

At least 75% to 80% of your diet should consist of foods in their natural uncooked state. There are numerous studies which demonstrate superiority of raw, living foods, both for maintenance of health and prevention of disease, as well as for the healing of disease. Cooking destroys much of the nutritional value of most foods. Many vitamins are partly destroyed, minerals are leached (if boiled in water) and all enzymes are destroyed by temperatures over 120°F.

Cooking also changes the biochemical structure of amino acids (proteins) and fatty acids, and makes them only partially digestible. For example, it has been demonstrated recently at the Max Planck Institute For Nutritional Research that you need only one-half the amount of protein in your diet *if you eat protein foods raw* instead of cooked.

Sprouting is an excellent way to eat seeds, beans and grains in raw form. Sprouting increases nutritional value of foods; many new vitamins are created or multiplied in seeds during sprouting. Sprouting also improves the protein quality in seeds and grains. Some grains and legumes, which do not contain complete proteins, become complete protein foods after they are sprouted. (See *Recipes* for instructions on sprouting.)

Another excellent way to increase the amount of raw food in your diet is to eat lots of fermented lactic acid foods, such as homemade sauerkraut, pickles or lactic acid vegetables (see *Recipes*). Especially for those who live in cold, northern regions, fermenting foods is an excellent way to preserve vegetables for winter use, and not only preserve, but increase their nutritive value — without cooking!

It would be ideal, of course, to eat a 100% raw food diet. This is possible to do if you live in an ideal tropical or subtropical climate, man's natural habitat, where fresh, natural foods are available year round. In colder, northern regions of the United States, Canada and Europe, a 100% raw food diet would be difficult for most people to maintain indefinitely, although a few nutritionally-well-educated raw foodists are able to do this. A good practical solution, therefore, would be to eat *most* of your food, perhaps 80%, in the raw, uncooked state. Practically all fruits, vegetables and seeds can be eaten raw. A few vegetables such as potatoes and yams, dried beans and peas, and some grains such as rye, rice, buckwheat and millet, can be used in cooked form; however, cooked foods should not comprise more than 20% of the total caloric intake.

When the Airola Diet is used as part of a therapeutic program in treating disease, usually a 100% raw food diet is advisable, unless it is contraindicated for some conditions (see *Part One*).

3. EAT ONLY NATURAL FOODS

Your foods should be whole, unprocessed and unrefined, and be organically grown in fertile soil. They should be preferably grown in *your own environment*, and eaten in *their season.*

That your health and longevity are in a direct relationship to the *naturalness* of the foods you eat is a well-established scientific fact. Where natives eat a diet of natural, whole, unprocessed and unrefined foods, they enjoy perfect health, absence of disease and long life. When denatured, refined, processed, man-made foods, such as white sugar and white flour, and canned and processed foods enter into their lives, disease becomes rampant among them.

Natural foods are foods that are grown in fertile soils without chemical fertilizers and sprays and are consumed in their *natural* state, with all the nutrients nature put in them intact, *nothing removed and nothing added.* White bread is, for example, a denatured food, from which most vital nutrients have been removed; the so-called "enrichment" is a hoax – only 4 nutrients are returned, while over 20 vital nutrients are removed in refining the flour. Breakfast cereals are all denatured foods with some "added features" – toxic preservatives and health-destroying white sugar. Supermarket quality eggs are not natural food; they are produced by cooped-up chickens, without a rooster (thus infertile), which are fed chemicalized commercial mash. Such eggs have a lower nutritional value, less vitamins and more cholesterol than natural eggs.

Organically grown fruits and vegetables contain more vitamins and minerals, as has been shown in many tests. They also contain more enzymes than the produce grown on depleted, chemically fertilized soils. Such foods have greater a health-building and disease-preventive potential. Researches reported recently that "Anti-malignancy factors are apparently present in organically grown foods".

These are only a few examples to show that only natural foods can produce optimum health and prevent disease. Synthetic, denatured and devitalized foods will not sustain health, but will inevitably bring about a gradual degeneration of normal body functions and, ultimately, disease.

It is of specific importance to see that all foods are natural when planning a therapeutic diet for treatment of disease. Only natural, whole, unprocessed and organically grown foods possess therapeutic value.

4. EAT ONLY POISON-FREE FOODS

Your food should be grown without the aid of chemical fertilizers and should contain no residues of toxic insecticides, chemical additives or preservatives.

Almost all food sold at supermarkets today contains some chemicals, either used in food producing or added during food processing or packing. Many of the poisons in fruits or vegetables are systemic, that is, they cannot be washed out or peeled out, as they penetrate the whole fruit. The only solution seems to be to grow your own food, or buy the certified organically grown food. And, of course, to avoid eating all processed and packaged foods, which contain the most chemicals.

Since it is unlikely that in this poisoned world any of us can escape getting some poisons into our systems, it would be wise to follow the advice given in *Part Two* of this book: "How to Protect Yourself Against Common Poisons In Food, Water, Air and Environment".

5. COMPLEMENT YOUR THREE BASIC HEALTH-BUILDING FOODS WITH THE FOLLOWING:

A. **MILK**. The value of milk in human nutrition has been highly disputed in the United States. Some authorities claim that milk is an excellent and indispensible food for man — others insist that milk is food for calves and poison for man, that man cannot digest milk properly, that milk causes mucus, allergies, etc.

The answer to the milk controversy is simple: both sides are right! *Milk is an excellent food for those who are milk-tolerant, and poison for those who are not.*

Who is tolerant and who is not? Simple again, as so ably explained by Dr. Robert D. Mc Cracken, anthropologist at the University of California School of Public Health. Descendants of the countries and the ancestors who historically herded dairy animals and traditionally lived on a lactose-rich diet (milk, cheese, etc.) are usually *tolerant to milk*. Their intestines contain plenty of the enzyme, *lactase*, that breaks down milk sugar, *lactose*, into a form that the body can use. Thus, milk for them will be an excellent health food. Conversely, those whose ancestors never or seldom used milk as a major element of the diet, are usually *intolerant to milk*, because their intestines do not contain sufficient lactase.

So, if your ancestors come from Europe, or the Middle East, your body is genetically programmed to use milk and digest it effectively. If your ancestors are from Africa (except the East African Nilotic Negroes), China, the Philippines, or New Guinea, or if your heritage is that of American Indians, Australian Aborigines, or Eskimos, your body is *not programmed* to digest milk properly.

Thus, 75% of American Blacks have been found to be intolerant of milk, while over 95% of white Americans have no problem in digesting milk. As simple as that! *

Needless to say, when I recommend supplementing the diet with milk, I mean *only the highest quality, uncontaminated, raw milk from healthy animals.* Today's pasteurized supermarket-sold milk is loaded with toxic and dangerous drugs, chemicals and residues of pesticides, herbicides and detergents — such milk is not suitable for human consumption. If you are fortunate enough to get *real* milk, fresh, raw, "farmer" milk from healthy cows fed organic food, then you can add milk to your diet. Note that the people we always associate with remarkable health — Scandinavians, Bulgarians, Russians — are traditionally heavy milk drinkers.

The best way to take milk is in its soured form: as yogurt, kefir, acidophilus milk or regular clabbered milk. Homemade cottage cheese can be made from any of these soured milks (see *Recipes*). Soured milks are superior to sweet milk, as they are in *predigested* form and very easily assimilated. They also help to maintain a healthy intestinal flora and prevent intestinal putrefaction and constipation.

Goat's milk is better than cow's milk as human food. While cow's milk is not recommended in the dietary program for arthritis, rheumatic diseases or cancer, goat milk contains both anti-arthritic and anti-cancer factors and is recommended for these conditions.

B. COLD-PRESSED VEGETABLE OILS. High quality fresh, cold-pressed, crude and unrefined vegetable oils are recommended as an addition to the diet. The average daily amount should not exceed 2 tbsp.

Vegetable oils are rich in unsaturated fatty acids, vitamins F and E, and lecithin.

Make sure that oils are *not rancid* (you can taste rancidity) and that they are *actually cold-pressed.* Most oils so marked, are *not* cold-pressed, but chemically extracted or heat extracted. Since there is no law against

---

* By the way, you *cannot* change this genetic programming in just a few generations — it would take thousands of years to accomplish this.

it, manufacturers deceive the public. The only oils that would likely to be the real cold-pressed oils which you could find in the United States would be olive oil, sesame seed oil or sunflower seed oil sold in health food stores, or olive oil imported from Italy or Spain and sold in tin cans in most Italian delicatessens.

C. **HONEY**. Natural, raw, unheated, unfiltered and unprocessed honey is the only sweetener used in the Airola Diet, particularly in the diet of older people and children — 1 or 2 tbsp. a day is recommended. Honey possesses miraculous nutritional and medicinal properties and has been used for healing purposes since early history. It has been found that most centenarians in Russia and Bulgaria use honey liberally in their diets.

Better than any other food, honey fulfills Hippocrates' requirement for an ideal food: "Our food should be our medicine — our medicine should be our food". Honey increases calcium retention in the system, prevents nutritional anemia, is beneficial in kidney and liver disorders, colds, poor circulation and complexion problems.

D. **SPECIAL PROTECTIVE FOODS**: Brewer's yeast, kelp, wheat germ (only if available fresh, not more than one week old after it is *made*) and fish liver oils (only in colder climates during dark winter months).

The above foods are truly "wonder" foods. They are storehouses of important nutrients.

Brewer's yeast is real super food and should form an essential part of every diet. It contains 40% highest quality protein; it is a superior source of the B-complex vitamins; it is one of the richest sources of organic iron and an excellent source of most minerals and trace elements. It has been recently shown in scientific studies that generous addition of brewer's yeast in the diet can prevent cancer development.

Kelp is another miracle food. It contains a valuable iodine and most other minerals and trace elements. It also contains complete proteins and vitamins C, K, A, E, D and B_{12} (which is otherwise seldom found in vegetable foods).

Wheat germ is a super food loaded with complete proteins, essential fatty acids, B-complex vitamins and vitamin E. Wheat germ would make an excellent addition to the Airola Diet, *if you would be able to find it fresh enough.* It is extremely perishable and becomes inedible (rancid) in one week. Make sure the one you eat is *not* rancid. Rancid foods are extremely harmful and carcinogenic!

Finally, fish liver oil supplies important vitamins. Most people, particularly those living in northern countries, are deficient in vitamins A and D. Make sure that you get oil which is *not fortified* with synthetic vitamins — just plain natural cod or halibut liver oil. It is also available in capsule form. Fish liver oil should be used particularly during winter months, and especially in the diet of very young and very old.

E. **NATURAL VITAMIN AND MINERAL SUPPLEMENTS,** as an effective assurance against nutritional deficiencies and protection against harmful effects of our increasingly toxic environment and toxic residues and additives in foods. See *PART TWO* and *Directions: 2* for practical instructions on how to use vitamins and mineral supplements in your diet.

6. AVOID AN EXCESS OF PROTEIN IN YOUR DIET

The Airola Optimum Diet of three basic foods — seeds, nuts and grains; vegetables; and fruits — supplemented with the special super-foods and food supplements named above, will assure you a complete and adequate supply of all required nutrients for optimum health, *including sufficient amounts of complete high quality proteins.* A moderate amount of eggs, fish or meat may be added to this basic diet, if desired (particularly the fish in coastal areas or meat in far northern regions with long winters), *but their inclusion is not necessary.* In temperate, subtropical and tropical climates, the highest level of health and extended longevity can be best achieved and maintained without meat.

Furthermore, when diet is used therapeutically, that is as a part of an overall program in healing disease, the pure vegetarian or lacto-vegetarian diet is always preferable. Animal proteins, especially meat, always have a detrimental effect on the healing processes.

But even in a diet aimed at preventive or prophylactic purposes, an excessive consumption of animal proteins should be avoided. A high animal protein diet is definitely detrimental to health and may cause or contribute to many of our most common diseases.

In this era of "high protein cult" you have been brought to believe that a high protein diet is a must if you wish to attain a high level of health and prevent disease. Health writers and "experts" who advocated high protein diet were misled by slanted research, which was financed by dairy or meat industries, or by insufficient and outdated information. Most recent research, worldwide, both scientific and empirical, shows more and more convincingly *that our past beliefs in regard to high requirement of protein are outdated and incorrect, and that the actual daily need for protein in human nutrition is far below that which has long been considered necessary.* Researchers, working independently in many parts of the world, arrived at the conclusion that our actual daily need of protein is only 25 to 35 grams — *even less if raw proteins from milk and vegetable sources are used* (raw proteins being utilized twice as well as cooked). Independent researchers, not associated with or paid by dairy or meat industries, also point out that, contrary to past beliefs, proteins from many vegetable sources are superior or equal to animal proteins in their biological value — not inferior, as some meat cultists claim. Almonds, sesame seeds, soybeans, buckwheat, peanuts, sunflower seed, pumpkin seeds, potatoes, and all leafy green vegetables contain *complete proteins*, which are comparable in quality to animal proteins. This revealing information comes from the most reliable and respected nutrition research organization in the world, the Max Planck Institute for Nutritional Research, in Germany.

But, what is even more important, the worldwide research brings almost daily confirmation of the scientific premise which I first presented in the United States six years ago in my book "There *IS* A Cure For Arthritis", and which shocked high-protein-brainwashed Americans — *that proteins, essential and important as they are,* CAN BE EXTREMELY HARMFUL WHEN CONSUMED IN EXCESS OF YOUR ACTUAL NEED. Especially an excess of *cooked* animal protein can cause serious health disorders.

The metabolism of proteins consumed in excess of the actual need leaves toxic residues of metabolic wastes in tissues, causes autotoxemia, over-acidity and nutritional deficiencies, accumulation of uric acid and purines in the tissues, intestinal putrefaction, and contributes to the development of many of our most common and serious diseases, such as arthritis, kidney damage, pyorrhea, schizophrenia, osteoporosis, athero-sclerosis, heart disease and cancer. A high protein diet also causes premature aging and lowers life expectancy.

All the above mentioned results of a high-animal-protein diet are well documented by reliable scientific research.

A recent American research done under the direction of Dr. Lennart Krook, shows that overindulgence in meat leads to a mineral imbalance in the system — too much phosphorus and too little calcium (meat has 20 times more phosphorus than calcium) which leads to severe calcium deficiency and resultant loss of teeth or pyorrhea.

A recent study, made at the U.S. Army Medical Research and Nutrition Laboratory in Denver, Colorado, demonstrated that the more meat you eat, the more deficient in vitamin B_6 you become. A high protein diet causes severe deficiencies of B_6, magnesium, calcium and niacin, or vitamin B_3. Mental illness and schizophrenia are often caused by niacin deficiency and have been recently successfully treated with high doses of niacin. Russian researcher, Dr. Uri Nikolayev, has been extremely successful in treating schizophrenia patients with a low protein diet.

Extensive studies made in England showed a clear connection between a high protein diet and osteoporosis. And doctors at the Vascular Research Laboratory in Brooklyn conducted research which indicates that excessive meat-eating can be a cause of widespread arteriosclerosis and heart disease. To the same conclusion, came researcher Dr. C. D. Langen, from Holland, and Dr. A. Hoygaard, from Denmark.

Dr. Ph. Schwarz, of Frankfort University, in Germany, and Dr. Ralph Bircher, a famous biochemist from Zurich, Switzerland, report that the aging process is triggered by *amyloid*, a by-product of protein metabolism, which is deposited in all the connective tissues and causes tissue and organ degeneration — thus leading to premature aging. This explains why people who traditionally eat low protein diets — Hunzakuts, in Pakistan, Bulgarians, Russian Caucasians, Yucatan Indians, East Indian Todas — also have the highest average life expectancy in the world, 90 to 100 years! And,why the people who live on high animal protein diets, such as Eskimos, Greenlanders, Lapplanders, Russian Kurgis-tribes, etc. have the lowest life expectancy in the world — 30 to 40 years. Americans lead the industrialized world in per capita meat consumption — and they also are in 21st place in life expectancy among industrialized nations!

Recently, Dr. Willard J. Visek, of Cornell University, implicated a high protein diet in the development of cancer. *Ammonia*, which is produced in great amounts as the by-product of meat metabolism, is highly carcinogenic and can cause cancer development. A high protein diet also breaks down the pancreas and lowers resistance to cancer, as well as contributes to the development of diabetes.

These are just a few examples of recent research and overwhelming scientific evidence which show that a high animal protein diet is *a very dangerous course to follow.*

Not only animal proteins but *all* proteins should be consumed in moderation. Excessive protein consumption, even if from such sources as milk or concentrated protein powders of vegetable origin, can be dangerous.

A good rule regarding proteins should be: *Enough, but not too much.* By eating the three basic foods of the Airola Diet — seeds, nuts and grains; vegetables; and fruits — supplemented with milk and brewer's yeast, 80% of which are consumed in their natural uncooked state, you can be assured of obtaining *all* the vital nutrients you need for vigorous and vibrant health and prevention of disease, *including adequate amounts of complete proteins*, in a natural balance and in proper combination with all the other vital nutrients.

7. DRINK PURE, NATURAL WATER

Drinking pure, uncontaminated, natural spring, river or well water is an important part of the Optimum Airola Diet for optimum health.

Avoid prolonged drinking of distilled water, which has become a fad recently, motivated by the universal water contamination. Distilled water is totally void of all minerals, and prolonged use of it may leach out the body's own mineral reserves and lead to severe mineral deficiencies and such diseases as osteoporosis, diabetes, tooth decay and heart disease. It has been proven by extensive world-wide studies that where people drink naturally "hard" or heavily mineralized water, there is a lesser incidence of the above-mentioned diseases. Minerals, as they are naturally present in drinking water, have been an essential part of man's mineral nutrition since the beginning of man's life on this planet.

Contrary to what some "experts" claim, inorganic minerals in natural waters *are* effectively absorbed and well utilized in human metabolism. And they do *not* cause hardening of arteries, kidney stones or other supposed diseases. Quite to the contrary! *We need* both *inorganic* and *organic* minerals for optimum health. Hunzakuts, considered the healthiest people in the world, who never had any hardening of the arteries, kidney stones, tooth decay, arthritis, osteoporosis or heart disease, have for 2,000 years been drinking water so heavily mineralized with lime and other inorganic minerals that it is milky in appearance. This is perhaps better evidence than any quasi-scientific reasoning.

Unfortunately, it is becoming more and more difficult to obtain uncontaminated pure natural water in this poisoned world of ours. Most places now sell bottled spring or purified waters. See that natural minerals are left intact in the purification process. If you are forced to drink distilled water, add natural minerals to it, such as pure sea water — 2-3 tsp. of sea water to a quart will do. But, *if you can get it*, we recommend using pure, uncontaminated, naturally mineralized spring water.

8. CLEANSE YOUR SYSTEM PERIODICALLY WITH JUICE FASTING

Continuous over-abundance and over-indulgence in food is a relatively recent phenomenon in man's history. Historically and traditionally our genetic code is programmed for a periodic abstinence from food, which was necessitated by the periodic unavailability of food, particularly during famines and during winter and early spring, when the storage supply of food was exhausted and the new crops were still unripe. In Hunza, and many other parts of the world, such spring starvation is a common occurrence even today. Every spring there is a period of 4 to 6 weeks when people must tighten their belts and go through a natural, unintentional fast, because there is not much food left from winter supplies.

Although the primitive populace, who were forced to starve (fast), did not, of course, understand or appreciate the health benefits they derived thereby, the fact remains that periodic abstinence from food had a far-reaching beneficial effect on their health. Our ancestor's bodies used these periods to cleanse themselves from the toxic wastes accumulated during the periods of over-indulgence. These periodic fasts also helped to repair and heal any health disorders, give digestive and elimination organs a rest, and to restore and normalize the functions of all glands and organs. They enjoyed better health, their resistance against disease was increased, and they lived longer, because of these involuntary fasts. We are able to say this now because modern scientific research has shown that *systematic undereating and periodic fasting are the two most important health and longevity factors.*

What our ancestors did against their will, forced to it by the unfavorable environmental conditions and circumstances beyond their control, *we must do now intentionally.* A periodic cleansing fast, perhaps once a year every spring, for a couple of weeks, would help tremendously to improve our health, prevent disease, and increase life span. Because of our sedentary life, lack of exercise and tendency to overeat, our body mechanisms need such spring cleaning to keep in good working order.

Juice fasting has been shown to be the safest and most effective way to restore health, as a part of the overall biological therapeutic program. But juice fasting has also a tremendous preventive potential. Periodic juice fasting will speed up the process of elimination of toxic waste matter and the dead cells from the body and accelerate and stimulate the building of new cells. It will also normalize all metabolic and nervous functions and increase cell oxygenation. After fasting, the digestion of food and utilization of nutrients is greatly improved and sluggishness and further water retention are prevented. All this will have a far reaching effect on the body's ability to withstand stress and prevent disease.

(See *Directions: 3* and *Directions: 5* for more details about juice fasting: Why, when, how, etc.).

9. CULTIVATE THE FOLLOWING HEALTH-PROMOTING EATING HABITS

1. Eat only when really hungry.

There are all kinds of *theories* regarding eating and drinking — when you should or shouldn't eat or drink — *theories invented by scientists.*

They tell you that you should eat a large, heavy protein breakfast, with meat, liver, eggs, etc., the first thing in the morning. They tell you when to eat heavy meals and when to eat lightly. They tell you when and how much to drink. Etc., etc. All these are unsubstantiated pseudo-scientific theories. You don't need any scientists or their theories to tell you when and how much to eat. *Nature* has provided a built-in mechanism within your brain which will tell you unmistakably *when* you should eat or drink. You should eat *when you are hungry*, and drink *when you are thirsty*. Contrarywise, you should *never* eat when you are *not* hungry (very few people are hungry in early morning, for example, no matter what "experts" tell you) and you should never drink when you are *not* thirsty. This is the *only* sure and safe way to solve this controversial question *for you*. Your requirements for food and drink are *unique*, different from those of everybody else. But you can never go wrong if you follow your hunger and thirst signals.

Food eaten without appetite will do you no good. It will, in fact harm you by overburdening the digestive organs with unwanted material and create indigestion, gas and other disturbances.

2. Eat slowly in a relaxed unhurried atmosphere.

Slow eating and thorough mastication are essential for good digestion. Good chewing increases the assimilation of nutrients and makes you feel satisfied with a smaller amount of food. "Fletcherize" your food — chew every mouthful at least 40 times! Saliva contains digestive enzymes. Therefore, well chewed and generously salivated food is practically half-digested before it enters the stomach.

Also, food should be eaten in a relaxed atmosphere and *enjoyed*. Biologically, only the foods eaten with genuine pleasure will do you any good. A peaceful, unhurried and happy atmosphere around the table will pay good dividends in improved digestion and assimilation of food — and, hence, in better health.

3. Eat several small meals during the day in preference to a few large meals.

In my lifelong study of nutrition I could find no scientific support for the idea of eating a few large meals a day. In my travels and studies of eating habits of various natives known for their excellent health, I have found that they always eat several small meals a day. In addition to 2 or 3 main meals, they have some snacks in between as they go about their usual work. Watching peasants work in the field in Russia and Ukraina, I noticed that they interrupt their work every two hours or so to eat and drink a little something: a fruit, a glass of cool sour milk, a watermelon, a plate of cold summer borsch, or whole fresh vegetables, such as cucumber, tomato, carrot — or just a slice of sour bread with onions! When a Mexican laborer goes to work, he takes with him several oranges, mangoes, ever-present limes or a large jicama, and has a snack of something every now and then.

It is better to eat 4, 5 or 6 small meals a day than 2 or 3 large meals. Such eating habits would also solve 99% of all hypoglycemia, or low blood sugar, problems. Also, if you have a tendency toward obesity, you should know that while 2,000 calories eaten at two meals will result in a new fat accumulation, the same 2,000 calories eaten in 6 small meals, with 2 or 3 hour intervals, will not only fail to add weight but may actually help you to reduce!

4. Do not mix too many foods at the same meal.

There is much evidence to the effect that the fewer foods you mix at the same meal, the better your digestion and assimilation will be. Every food — every fruit or vegetable — requires a different enzyme system and (too many at one time) results in less effective digestion.

5. Do not mix raw fruits and raw vegetables at the same meal.

Raw vegetables and raw fruits require totally different enzyme combinations for their effective digestion, and, therefore, they should never be eaten at the same meal. Such combination will only result in poor digestion and gas. Fruit and vegetable juices should never be mixed either.

It would be advisable to make one meal of the day a *fruit meal*, where any available fruits are eaten, possibly with yogurt and raw seeds and nuts; and the other meal a vegetable meal. The third meal can be a cereal meal.

The exceptions to the above rule (it seems there are always exceptions to every rule!): lemon and papaya. Both can be used with any foods. Another exception: avocado (which is a fruit) can be eaten with vegetables.

6. When protein-rich foods are eaten with other foods — eat the protein-rich foods first!

Proteins require a generous amount of hydrochloric acid in your stomach in order to be properly digested. When you eat carbohydrate-rich foods such as vegetables, you stomach does not secrete much hydrochloric acid, because it is not needed for the digestion of carbohydrates. If you first fill your stomach with predominantly carbohydrate foods (as you do when you start your meal with a large, raw vegetable salad, as "experts" tell you to do) and then finish your meal with a protein food, *the protein will remain largely undigested* because of an insufficient amount of hydrochloric acid in the stomach.

Therefore, it is best to eat protein foods first, on an empty stomach, when the hydrochloric acid secretion will be generous; then continue with carbohydrate foods. In practical terms that would mean: *steak first and then salad*! Or beans & tortillas first and then the salad. Or, if you wish, eat your salad *with* protein food, but not before. Now, this is contrary to what you have been told by "experts", isn't it? But the proof of the pudding is in the eating — it works! Try and see for yourself how your digestion will improve and how even beans will cease to be a "musical food".

7. Finally, practice systematic undereating.

Systematic undereating is the *NUMBER ONE* health ahd longevity secret. Overeating, on the other hand, *even of health foods*, is one of the main causes of disease and premature aging.

Studies of centenarians around the world show that all of them are moderate eaters throughout their lives. You never see an obese centenarian.

Scientific studies made in Russia and the United States show that overeating is one of the prime causes of most degenerative diseases. Food eaten in excess of actual body need acts in the system as a poison. It interferes with proper digestion, causes internal sluggishness, gas, incomplete assimilation of nutrients (thus even nutritional deficiencies), putrefaction in bowels, and actually poisons the whole system. Overindulgence in protein is particularly harmful. Overeating is especially dangerous for older people, who are less active and have a slowed down metabolism.

The unbelievable truth is that *the less you eat, the less hungry you feel*, because the food will be more efficiently digested and better utilized.

10. AVOID THE FOLLOWING HEALTH DESTROYERS:

The following is the list of *do nots*, the health destroyers that you *must* avoid if you wish to achieve optimum health. All these factors are scientifically well-proven as potent health-destroyers. My files are bulging with overwhelming research and incriminating evidence on each item.

- Tobacco, including cigars.
- Coffee, tea, chocolate, cola drinks and soft drinks.
- Excessive use of salt.
- Excessive consumption of alcohol
- Harmful spices, mustard, black and white pepper, white vinegar.
- Refined white sugar and white flour and everything made with them: bread, pastry, packaged cereals, pies, donuts, ice cream, candy, cookies, gum, etc., etc.

- All processed, refined, canned or factory-made foods.
- All rancid foods, even such health foods as wheat germ, seeds and vegetable oils, if they are not absolutely fresh.
- All chemical drugs, except in absolute emergency, ordered by a doctor.
- All household and environmental toxic chemicals: garden sprays, air fresheners, household chemicals and cleaners, detergents (use soap flakes), hair sprays, chemically cleaned or treated clothes, beds or wallpaper, bug and fly killers, etc.
- Avoid a sedentary life and lack of sufficient exercise and relaxation.

All the above points and factors are self explanatory and the average reader is well aware of their potential health danger. The last point I would like to elaborate upon a bit.

Today's soft, sedentary living is one of the main causes of our physical degeneration. Since I am a nutritionist, most of my writings deal with nutrition as it is related to health and disease. This does not mean, however, that I minimize the importance of other vital factors, such as fresh air, sufficient exercise, adequate relaxation and peace of mind. These are all extremely important health building and disease-preventive factors.

Medical evidence to the effect that ample regular exercise is imperative for optimum health is overwhelming. Lack of sufficient exercise contributes to many of our most killing diseases and is one of the main causes of one million deaths from heart attacks yearly in the United States.

Sufficient exercise is imperative for good health for two reasons. *One*, it will tone up your muscles, improve digestion and general metabolism, keep your eliminative organs doing their work effectively — and in general, contribute to the better circulation and better function of all your organs and glands. *Two*, it will increase and improve your *tissue oxygenation*. The ultimate cause of all disease and premature aging is a lack of oxygen in your cells. Vigorous daily exercise will keep all your cells and tissues well oxygenated and in the peak of their efficiency.

Relaxation and peace of mind — these are two other vital health factors that are missing in modern man's life. Emotional and mental stress can tear your health down faster than inadequate nutrition can. And this is quite a statement to come from a dedicated nutritionist.

It has been scientifically established that emotional and mental stresses, such as fears, anxiety, worries, tensions, depression, hate, jealousy, unhappiness, depreviation of love, and loneliness, can cause practically every disease in the medical dictionary including arthritis, ulcers, constipation, asthma, strokes, diabetes, high or low blood pressure, angina, glandular disturbances, heart disease and cancer.

Relaxation, peace of mind, a positive outlook on life, a contented spirit, an absence of envy and jealousy, cheerful disposition, love of mankind and faith in God — these are all powerful health-promoting factors without which optimum health cannot be achieved. When health is lost, it cannot be restored *unless* all the above mentioned underlying emotional and mental stress factors are eliminated, and an adequate nutritional and biological program is "supplemented" with a good dose of "vitamin X": relaxation, peace of mind, positive and happy disposition and faith that Nature and God will do *their part* in helping to restore our health, if we do *our part*.

Here you have it, in a nutshell, *the Airola Diet* — a scientifically and empirically proven nutritional system that has produced superior health for millions of people around the globe during the thousands of years of actual application. This Optimum Nutrition program will assure you the highest level of health, greater resistance against disease, bouyant, dynamic strength and more endurance, better mental efficiency, greater virility, and longer life in youthful vitality.

YOUR HEALTH MENU

Based on the material and information presented in this section, your daily menu of health-building and vitalizing Airola Diet should look something like this:

UPON ARISING: Glass of pure water, plain, or with freshly squeezed citrus juice: ½ lime, or ¼ lemon, or ½ grapefruit, or one orange to a glass of water.

OR: Large cup of warm herb tea sweetened with honey. Choice of rose hips, peppermint, camomile, or any of your favorite herbs (see *Directions: 6*).

OR: Glass of freshly made fruit juice from any available fruits or berries in season: apple, pineapple, orange, cherry, pear, etc. The juice should be diluted with water, half and half. No canned or frozen juices — the juice must be freshly made on your own juicer just before drinking, or squeezed from the fruit.

After this morning drink you should walk for one hour in the fresh air, combining your walk with deep-breathing exercises and all the calisthenics you can manage to squeeze in. If you have a garden, or if you live on the farm, you should get in a couple of hours of hard physical labor.

Upon returning from your long walk, or garden work, and after a cold shower to wash the prespiration away, you are now, *but not before*, ready for your breakfast.

BREAKFAST: Fresh fruits: apple, orange, banana, grapes, grapefruit, or any available berries and fruits *in season*. All fruits preferably organically grown in your own locality and environment.

Cup of yogurt, kefir, or homemade soured milk, preferably goat's milk (see *Recipes*).

Handful of raw nuts, such as almonds, cashews, peanuts, or a couple of tablespoons of sunflower seeds, pumpkin seeds or sesame seeds. Nuts and seeds can be crushed or ground in your own seed grinder (sold in health food stores) and sprinkled over yogurt.

½ cup of homemade cottage cheese (see *Recipes*).

OR: Large bowl of fresh Fruit Salad á Lá Airola (see *Recipes*).

OR: Bowl of rolled oats, uncooked, with 4-6 soaked prunes, or 2-3 figs, and a handful of unsulfured raisins.

Glass of raw, unpasteurized milk, preferably goat's milk, or yogurt.

OR: Bowl of sprouted wheat or other sprouted seeds with yogurt and/or available fresh fruits.

MIDMORNING SNACK: One apple, banana, or other fruit.

LUNCH: Bowl of whole-grain cereal, such as millet cereal, buckwheat cereal or Kruska (see *Recipes*). Any other available whole-grain cereals can be used, such as oats, barley, rice, corn, etc. Dry milk powder (non-instant kind) can be added to the water when cereals are cooked.

Large glass of raw milk, preferably goat's milk.

One tablespoon of cold-pressed vegetable oil, and/or one tablespoon of honey can be used on cereal.

OR: Large bowl of fresh Fruit Salad á Lá Airola (if not eaten for breakfast).

OR: Bowl of freshly prepared vegetable, pea or bean soup, or any other cooked vegetable dish, such as potatoes, squash, beans and corn tortillas, yams, etc. Kelp, sea salt, cold-pressed vegetable oil and fresh butter can be used for seasoning.

Glass of yogurt or other soured milk.

1-2 slices of whole-grain bread, preferably sourdough rye bread (see *Recipes*), 1 or 2 slices natural cheese, available at health food stores. Never use processed cheeses.

MID AFTERNOON: Glass of fresh fruit or vegetable juice.

OR: Cup of your favorite herb tea, sweetened with honey.

OR: One apple, or other available fruit.

DINNER: Large bowl of fresh, green vegetable salad. Use any and all available vegetables, preferably those *in season*, including tomatoes, avocadoes and all available sprouts, such as alfalfa seed sprouts, mung bean sprouts, etc. Carrots, shredded red beets and onions should be staples with every salad. Garlic, if your social life permits. Salad should be attractively prepared and served with homemade dressing of lemon juice (or apple cider vinegar) and cold-pressed vegetable oil, seasoned with herbs, garlic powder, a little sea salt, cayenne pepper, etc. But all vegetables can be also placed attractively on the plate without mixing them into salad and eaten one at a time — this is, by far, the superior way of eating vegetables.

2 or 3 middle sized boiled or baked potatoes in jackets. Prepared cooked vegetable course, if desired: eggplant, artichoke, sweet potatoes, yams, squash or other vegetables. Use kelp powder or sea salt sparingly for seasoning, also any or all of the usual garden herbs.

Fresh homemade cottage cheese, or 1-2 slices of natural cheese.

Fresh butter or 1 tbsp. of cold-pressed vegetable oil (can be used on salad, soup or potatoes).

Glass of yogurt or other soured milk.

OR: Any of the recommended lunch choices, if fresh vegetable salad is eaten at lunch.

BEDTIME SNACK: Glass of fresh milk, or nut-milk, or seed-milk (made in electric liquifier from raw seeds or raw

nuts and water and milk or without milk) with a
tablespoon of honey.

OR: Glass of yogurt with brewer's yeast.

OR: Cup of your favorite herb tea with a slice of
whole grain bread with butter and a slice of
natural cheese.

OR: One apple.

Vital points to remember

1. The above menu is only a very general outline, a skeleton, around which an individual diet for optimum nutrition should be built. It can be followed as it is, of course. I know of thousands of people who live on such a diet and enjoy extraordinary health. But it also can be modified and changed to adapt to your specific requirements and conditions, your country's customs, your climate, the availability of foods, your health conditon, your preferences, etc.

2. Whatever changes you make, keep in mind, however, that the bulk of your diet should consist of seeds, nuts and grains, and fresh vegetables and fruits, preferably organically grown, and up to 80% of them eaten raw. Eat as great a variety of available foods as possible, but not in the same meal, of course. Do not shun potatoes and avocados and bananas because you think they are fattening – they are not!

3. The menu for lunch and dinner is interchangeable. One big vegetable meal should be eaten at least once a day. If it is eaten for lunch some of the lunch suggestions can be eaten for dinner.

4. Remember, when you eat protein-rich foods (cottage cheese, nuts, beans, etc.) together with carbohydrate-rich foods (salads, fruits, etc.) – eat the protein-rich foods *first*, or *together with* carbohydrate-rich foods, but not *after*.

5. Do not drink liquids with meals. If thirsty, drink between meals or 15 minutes before meals. Milk or yogurt are foods.

6. If you are taking vitamins and other food supplements, take them *with* meals. See *Directions: 2* for information on what supplements I recommend and how to take them.

7. One or two tbsp. of brewer's yeast should be taken either with breakfast or lunch, or between meals with fruit juice or yogurt.

8. Finally, follow this Health Menu *every day of your life* and you will live a long life and enjoy the highest possible level of health. And be assured that this Airola Optimum Diet will supply you not only with *all* the vitamins, minerals, essential fatty acids, trace elements, enzymes and the other identified and unidentified nutritive substances, but also with adequate amount of the highest quality proteins you need for optimum health!

WHY AND HOW TO USE VITAMINS AND FOOD SUPPLEMENTS

Ideally, all vitamins, minerals, and other nutrients should be obtained from foods, without the addition of concentrated vitamins in pill or tablet form. This was also possible 100 or even 50 years ago, when all foods were grown on fertile soils, were unrefined and unprocessed, and contained all the nutrients nature intended them to contain. But today, when soils are depleted, when foods are loaded with residues of hundreds of toxic insecticides and other chemicals, and when the nutritional value of virtually all foods is drastically lowered by vitamin-, protein- and enzyme-destroying food-producing and food-processing practices (such as the tendency to harvest the produce before it is ripened, for example), the addition of vitamins and food supplements to the diet is of vital importance. Nutritionally inferior and poisoned foods of today cause many nutritional deficiencies, derangement in body chemistry and lowered resistance to disease.

The prime purpose of food supplementation is to fill in the nutritional gaps produced by faulty eating habits and by nutritionally inferior foods.

Since in this book we are primarily concerned with the healing of disease, vitamins and food supplements, used therapeutically, can be of tremendous help in fighting disease and speeding recovery.

Vitamins can be used in two distinctly different ways:

1) *Correcting deficiencies.* When a specific vitamin or mineral deficiency is indicated, the prescribed vitamins or minerals can correct the deficiency and cure the condition caused by the nutritional deficiencies.

2) *As Drugs.* Many avant-garde practitioners around the world are now using vitamins in massive doses, *doses that are far above the actual nutritional needs*, in the treatment of all kinds of conditions of ill health. It has been found that in large doses many vitamins have a miraculous healing, stimulating and/or protective effect on a variety of body functions — an effect that is totally different from the usual vitamin activity as nutritional and metabolic catalysts.

Here are a few examples:

Vitamin C. You need 100 mg. to 200 mg. of vitamin C a day for the maintenance of normal, healthy functions of your body. But when you take the same vitamin in huge doses, we'll say 5,000 to 10,000 mg. a day, it will assume totally different functions and can perform such miracles as:

- Killing pathogenic bacteria, acting as a harmless antibiotic.
- Preventing and curing colds and infections, having a natural antihistamine activity.
- Effectively neutralizing various toxins in the system, being a most potent antitoxin.
- Speeding healing processes in virtually every case of ill health.
- Increasing sexual virility.
- Preventing premature aging by strengthening the collagen, and preventing the degenerative processes.

Vitamin E. For normal, healthy functions of all your organs and glands you need, perhaps, 100 IU of vitamin E a day (the official estimation is only 45 IU). But when you take large doses of vitamin E, such as 600 to 1,600 IU or even more, it assumes a drug-like role and can perform the following activity.

- It markedly decreases the body's need for oxygen.
- It protects against the damaging effect of many environmental poison in air, water and food.
- It saves lives in cases of atherosclerotic heart disease by dilating blood vessels and acting as an effective anti-thrombin.
- It prevents scar tissue formation in burns, sores and post-operative healing.
- It has a dramatic effect on the reproductive organs: prevents miscarriage, increases male and female fertility and helps to restore male potency.

Vitamin A. The official recommended daily allowance is set at 4,000 U.S.P. Units. But when taken in such large doses as 100,000 U.S.P. Units per day, vitamin A has been known to:

- Cure many stubborn skin disorders.
- Cure chronic infections and eye diseases.
- Increase the body's tolerance against poisons.
- Prevent premature aging, particularly the aging processes of the skin.

Niacin. The official recommended allowance is set at 10 mg., but many doctors around the world have been using large doses of niacin (up to 25,000 mg.) to treat schizophrenia, actually achieving dramatic cures with this so-called mega-vitamin therapy.

These few examples show that vitamins can be used successfully in large doses *instead* of many commonly used drugs. While drugs are always toxic and have many undesirable side effects, vitamins are, as a rule, completely non-toxic and 100% safe.

In *Part One* of this book we specified vitamins and food supplements that can be successfully used in treatment of various diseases (see *Introduction*: "How to Use This Book," sections 5 and 6, on how to use vitamins therapeutically).

Where no specific disease is present, but a person needs a strengthening, health-building diet to achieve *optimum* health, more vitality and greater resistance against disease, we recommend the AIROLA DIET (see *Directions: 1*) supplemented with the following food supplements and vitamins. This supplementation is also advised for all those who are recuperating from disease and wish to restore health and vitality as fast as possible.

1) **Vitamin C** — preferably in natural form from rose hip concentrate, or other natural sources: 1,500 to 3,000 mg. a day; even more in all acute conditions of ill health. Vitamin C is completely non-toxic even in large amounts.

2) **Vitamin A** — natural, from fish liver oil, or lemon grass: 25,000 U.S.P. units a day. Under doctor's supervision it can be taken in doses up to 100,000 units a day for shorter periods.

3) **Vitamin E** — natural d-alpha tocopherol from vegetable oil: 600 IU a day. If you have not used vitamin E before, start with 100 IU and increase by 100 IU each week. If suffering from high blood pressure or rheumatic heart disease, consult your doctor on the proper dosage for your particular condition.

4) **Vitamin B-complex, with B_{12}** — natural, from yeast concentrate, highest potency: 1 to 3 tablets or capsules a day. (The usual strength of *natural* B-complex does not exceed 10 mg. for B_1, B_2 and B_6.)

5) **Brewer's yeast** — or primary grown food yeast: 1 to 3 tbsp. a day.

6) **Kelp**: 1 to 2 tsp. of granules a day, or 3 tablets.

7) **Fish liver oil** — unfortified, for vitamin D and A: 1 tsp. a day.

8) **Lecithin**: 1 to 2 tsp. of granules a day.

9) **Mineral supplement** — bone meal or calcium lactate: 1 tsp. of powder or 3 tablets a day.

A few tips on how to take vitamins and supplements

1) As a general rule, all vitamins and food supplements should be taken with meals, or immediately after the meals. They are better utilized with foods.

2) Divide all the suggested daily amounts equally between three meals.

3) Take *all* vitamins and food supplements *continuously*, with the exception of high potency B-complex vitamins, large doses of synthetic isolated B-vitamins, and large doses of vitamins A and D — these should be taken for one month, then after a one-month interval, taken for another month, and so on. The reason for this is that the above-mentioned vitamins are cumulative and may cause vitamin imbalances in the system if taken in large doses over a prolonged period of time. Also, the continuous ingestion of certain isolated B-vitamins in large doses may cause deficiencies of other B-vitamins, and/or interfere with the body's own synthesis of these vitamins in the intestines. Naturally, brewer's yeast (B-complex) and plain fish liver oils (A & D) can be taken continuously.

4) In *Part One* of this book, special medicinal supplements, such as digestive enzymes, hydrochloric acid, special vitamins and minerals *in massive doses*, etc., are recommended. These should be taken only during the treatment, or for about one to three months, *then discontinued.* After a one to three month interval, treatment can be repeated if needed. Between treatment periods, vitamin and mineral-rich natural food supplements should be used, such as brewer's yeast, bone meal, lecithin, fish liver oils, rose hips, etc. Vitamin C can be used continuously in reduced dosage. When vitamin E is used for a heart condition it also should be used continuously.

5) Although vitamin E in the form of mixed tocopherols is perfectly safe to take by a healthy person who takes vitamins for preventive purposes, those who take vitamin E for therapeutic purposes or for treatment of specific conditions, should take only the *pure d-alpha tocopherol capsules* (possibly supplemented by mixed tocopherols). Only the alpha-tocopherol fraction of E vitamin complex is known presently to be effective in treatment of disease.

6) As a rule, all vitamins and food supplements should be taken *together*; being synergistic in action, they work best that way and complement each other. There is, however, a notable exception to this rule. Vitamin E and iron supplements are *antagonists.* Iron tablets have an adverse effect on the utilization of vitamin E. Therefore, when iron tablets are taken, as for example in anemia, they should be taken 8 to 12 hours *after* or *before* taking vitamin E. For example, take the total daily dose of vitamin E

for breakfast and iron tablet at dinnertime. Natural iron-rich *foods*, however, have no adverse effect on vitamin E utilization.

7) We must stress again, as we did in the *Introduction*, that although in *Part One* of this book we list specific vitamins for the biological treatment of most ailments, and, in most cases, list the commonly used therapeutic doses, *there is no such thing as a common or an average person or patient.* As Dr. Roger J. Williams stressed so expertly, "Individual human beings have great diversity in human nutritional needs." There is also a great difference in every patient's *response* to vitamins and other therapeutic substances, depending on his health condition, nutritional stature, the quality of the foods he eats, his ability to assimilate nutrients, the mineral content of the water he drinks, the toxicity degree of his environment, his emotional health, etc. Due to many physical and mental disorders, vitamins may not be utilized properly. Poor teeth, diarrhea, the lack of digestive juices, intestinal parasites, infections, colitis, gall bladder or liver disorders, mental stresses — these are just a few of the conditions which interfere with vitamin utilization. Then there are countless vitamin antagonists which destroy or interfere with ingested vitamins, such as smoking (vitamin C), aspirin and other drugs (vitamin C), alcohol (Vitamin B), rancid foods (vitamin E), chlorinated water (vitamin E), laxatives (vitamins C & B), etc., etc.

Therefore, *please understand* that suggested daily doses of vitamins and other supplements, as given in *Part One* of this book, are given only for a *very general guidance*, referring generally to maximum doses used by most practitioners who specialize in vitamin therapy. These doses are *not* recommended for *every* individual, *as every individual's needs are different.* Your doctor, upon a careful examination and nutritional and metabolic evaluation of your condition must determine the *exact dosage* and the *duration* of the vitamin therapy *FOR YOU.*

8) When possible, all vitamins should be *natural*, not *synthetic.* See the following section for the difference between the two, and how you can know which is which.

NATURAL VS. SYNTHETIC VITAMINS

Most drugstore-quality vitamins are made from synthetic chemicals — they are not derivatives of natural food substances. Although this is also true of some brands sold in health food stores, most vitamins sold in health food stores are concentrations of nutrients from such natural sources as rose hips, green peppers and acerola berries (vitamin C); brewer's yeast, liver or rice polishings (vitamin B); fish liver oil, or lemon grass (vitamins A and D); vegetable oils (vitamin E); kelp (iodine); bone meal, egg shells and milk (minerals); etc.

There is a great deal of controversy regarding the difference and the usefulness of synthetic vs. natural vitamins. Natural health authorities usually claim that synthetic vitamins are useless, ineffective and extremely harmful. Most orthodox doctors and nutritionists claim that synthetic vitamins have a molecular chemical structure identical to the so-called natural vitamins, and that they are just as effective. Who is right?

I have made studies of world-wide vitamin research to find an intelligent answer to this question.

In Sweden, two groups of silver foxes were fed identical diets, but one group received a food supplement in the form of all the known synthetic B-vitamins; the control group received vitamins in the form of brewer's yeast and liver. The synthetically fed animals failed to grow, had bad fur and acquired many diseases. Animals fed the natural vitamins grew normally, developed beautiful fur and enjoyed good health. Approximately similar results were demonstrated in other animal studies in various countries.

"On the whole, we can trust nature further than the chemist and his synthetic vitamins", explained Dr. A. J. Carlson, of Chicago University.

We must keep in mind that in nature vitamins are never isolated. They are always present in the form of vitamin complexes. There are 24 known factors in vitamin C-complex. There are 22 known B-vitamin factors. E vitamin, as we know it, is composed of at least 9 natural tocopherols. And so on. When you take natural vitamins, as for instance in form of rose hips, brewer's yeast or vegetable oil, you are getting *all* the vitamins and vitamin-like factors that naturally occur in these foods — that is, all those that are already discovered as well as those that are not discovered yet. Our knowledge of vitamins is not complete. New vitamins are discovered frequently. For example, it has been clinically demonstrated that foods which are naturally rich in B-vitamins, such as brewer's yeast and liver, contain some potent, *but as yet unidentified or isolated*, B-vitamin factors. When you take your vitamins in the form of vitamin-rich supplements or in the form of "complexes", you are getting the benefit of all the known as well as unknown vitamins.

Does this mean that synthetic vitamins are useless? Not necessarily. *The rightful place of synthetic vitamins is in their therapeutic use where extremely large doses of easily-soluble and fast-acting vitamins are necessary.* For example, Dr. W. J. McCormick, the world-famous authority on the therapeutic uses of vitamin C, has successfully used huge doses of ascorbic acid (vitamin C) in acute cases of poisoning or infection, preferably *intravenuously*. His treatments brought spectacular results and often saved lives. You cannot very well inject rose hips intravenously and get such results. Dr. Linus Pauling had used synthetic ascorbic acid to successfully prevent or cure the common cold. In huge doses, synthetic vitamins perform as fast-acting drugs. Their action is often more rapid than the action of natural vitamins. This fact can be invaluable in acute conditions of poisoning or ill health.

Vitamin E is a good example. Proponents of natural vitamins advise taking vitamin E-rich vegetable oils, particularly wheat germ oil instead of isolated vitamin E capsules. Or, if capsules are used, they advise taking vitamin E in the form of *mixed* tocopherols, as it occurs in nature. But, Drs. Evan and Wilfred Shute, the world's foremost authorities on therapeutic uses of vitamin E, use only an isolated alpha-tocopherol in their successful practice and research work. They contend that alpha-tocopherol is *the only* active part of the vitamin E complex and that the other tocopherols are not necessary in therapeutic use.

I know personally of a few cases where health food-minded patients, suffering from a heart condition, tried to protect their hearts and avoid a heart attack by taking vitamin E in the form of mixed tocopherols. Some of them paid with their lives for their experiment. You see, Dr. Wilfred Shute recommends up to 1,600 IU of vitamin E for heart cases. If a heart patient is taking 1,600 IU of vitamin E in the form of mixed tocopherols he may be getting only 400 IU or less of the active alpha-tocopherol a day — and, thus, actually endangering his life.

The intelligent solution to the controversy *synthetic vs. natural* vitamins seems to be as follows:

The isolated and synthetic vitamins and minerals in large doses have their rightful and indispensible place in the short term treatment of acute conditions or severe dificiency diseases, or where only the isolated fractions of a vitamin complex are needed for specific therapeutic purposes. But those who do not suffer from any specific disease or deficiency, but are interested in food supplements and vitamins mainly for preventive purposes — that is, to protect their health and to prevent disease and premature aging — should use natural vitamins in form of food supplements, such as brewer's yeast, rose hip concentrate, kelp, bone meal, fish liver oil, vegetable oils, etc. In these supplements all the vitamins and other nutritional substances are present in their natural, balanced combinations which is essential for better assimilation, synergistic action and maximum biological effect.

For those who are confused as to which vitamins are synthetic and which are natural (as even most health food stores carry and sell both) we advise reading the labels. As a rule, if the formula on the bottle does not say that vitamin is natural or is derived from natural source, it is synthetic. Manufacturers of natural products are always eager to advertise their natural source. We must note, however, a disgraceful fact that there is a growing number of vitamin companies who sell their products in health food stores and use 100% synthetic vitamins, but have words "natural" and/or "organic" on their labels. Actually, there are only a very few B-complex products available that are made completely from natural sources. Often, fancy chemical names are used which the consumer doesn't understand, and, thus, cannot make an intelligent choice. Also, some manufacturers try to mislead you by clever wording, or even by colorful pictures of fruit or berries, to make you believe that theirs is 100% natural product, when it is actually not. For example, if the label reads "Vitamin C — Rose hips", it does not necessarily mean that the product is made *from* rose hips, it only may mean that ascorbic acid has an added rose hip concentrate with it, perhaps 95% ascorbic acid and 5% rose hips. You have to be expert label reader, even in a health food store!

To help you to orient yourself as you look through long shelves of many vitamin bottles, here is a helpful chart on the most commonly used vitamins:

SYNTHETIC AND NATURAL VITAMINS

Vitamin:	If the source given is only:	It is:
Vitamin C	Rose hips, acerola, citrus fruits, green peppers	Natural
Vitamin C	Ascorbic acid, or if source not given	Synthetic
Vitamin B-complex	Brewer's yeast	Natural
Vitamin B-complex	If source not given	Synthetic
Vitamin B_1	Yeast or rice bran	Natural
Vitamin B_1	Thiamine Hydrochloride or Thiamine Chloride	Synthetic
Vitamin B_1	Thiamine Mononitrate	Synthetic
Vitamin B_2	Yeast or rice bran	Natural
Vitamin B_2	Riboflavin	Synthetic
Vitamin B_6	Yeast or rice bran	Natural
Vitamin B_6	Pyridoxine Hydrochloride	Synthetic
Niacin (B_3)	Yeast or rice bran	Natural
Niacin or Niacinamide	If source not given	Synthetic
Vitamin B_{12}	Yeast, liver or fermentation concentrate	Natural

Vitamin B_{12}	Cobalamin or Cyanocobalamin	Natural fermentation product
PABA	Yeast	Natural
PABA	If source not given	Synthetic
Folic acid	Yeast	Natural
Folic acid	Pteroylglutamic acid, or if source not given	Synthetic
Pantothenic acid	Yeast	Natural
Pantothenic acid	Calcium Pantothenate	Synthetic
Inositol	Soy beans, corn or yeast	Natural
Choline	Soy beans or yeast	Natural
Choline	Choline Bitartrate	Synthetic
Biotin	Yeast	Natural
Biotin	d-biotin	Synthetic
Vitamin A	Fish oils or lemon grass	Natural
Vitamin A	Acetate or Palmitate	Synthetic
Vitamin D or D_3	Fish oils	Natural
Vitamin D or D_2	Irradiated Ergosterol or Calciferol	Synthetic
Vitamin E	Vegetable oils, wheat germ, mixed tocopherols	Natural
Vitamin E	d-alpha tocopherol or tocopheryl acetate	Natural
Vitamin E	Alpha tocopherol acetate or dl-alpha tocopherol (or tocopheryl) acetate	Synthetic
Vitamin E	Succinate	Can be natural or synthetic
Vitamin K	Alfalfa	Natural
Vitamin K	Menadione	Synthetic
Vitamin P or Bioflavonoids	Citrus Bioflavonoids, rutin, hesperidin, citrin	Natural

JUICE FASTING - - ROYAL ROAD TO HEALTH AND LONG LIFE

The main causes of disease and aging are to be found in biochemical suffocation, the systematic disorder that interferes with the normal processes of cell metabolism and cell regeneration. As the famous Canadian "stress doctor" Hans Selye, said, "Life, the biological chain that holds our parts together, is only as strong as the weakest vital link," the cell. You are as healthy and as young as your smallest links, the cells, are. Disease and aging begins when the normal process of cell regeneration and rebuilding slows down. This slowdown is caused by the accumulation of waste products in the tissues which interferes with the nourishment and oxygenation of cells.

Each cell of your body is a complete living entity with its own metabolish. It needs a constant supply of oxygen and adequate nourishment in the form of all the known nutritive substances, such as proteins, minerals, fatty acids, trace elements, etc. When nutritional deficiencies, sluggish metabolish, sedentary life, lack of fresh air and water, overeating and consequent poor digestion and assimilation of food cause our cells to be deprived of the nourishment they need, they start to degenerate and break down. The normal process of cell replacement and rebuilding slows down and your body starts to grow old. Its resistance to diseases will diminish and various ills will start to appear. This may happen at any age.

Only about half of all your cells are in the peak of development and working condition. One fourth are usually in the process of growth and the other fourth in the process of dying and replacement. It is of vital importance that the dying cells are decomposed and eliminated from the system as efficiently as possible. Quick and effective elimination of dead cells stimulates the building and growth of new cells.

Here's where juice fasting comes in as the most effective way to restore health and rejuvenate the body. During the juice fast, the process of elimination of the dead and dying cells is speeded up, and the new-building of cells is accelerated and stimulated. At the same time, the toxic waste products that interfere with the nourishment of the cells are effectively elminiated and the normal metabolic rate and cell oxygenation are restored.

Why fasting is so effective?

Here's why:

1. During a prolonged fast (after the first three days), your body will live on its own substance. When it is deprived of needed nutrition, particularly of proteins and fats, it will burn and digest its own tissues by the process of *autolysis*, or self-digestion. But your body will not do it indiscriminately! In its wisdom — and here lies the secret of the extraordinary effectiveness of fasting as curative and rejuvenative therapy! — your body will *first* decompose and burn those cells and tissues which are diseased, damaged, aged or dead. In fasting, your body feeds itself on the most impure and inferior materials, such as dead cells and morbid accumulations, tumors, abcesses, fat deposits, etc. Dr. Otto Buchinger, M.D., perhaps the greatest fasting authority in the world (and, I am proud to say, one of my fasting teachers), calls fasting — very pertinently — a "refuse disposal", a "burning of rubbish." The essential tissues and vital organs, the glands, the nervous system and the brain are not damaged or digested in fasting.

2. During fasting, while the old cells and diseased tissues are decomposed and burned, the building of new, healthy cells is speeded up. This may seem unbelievable, since no nourishment, or only a limited amount of nourishment during a juice fast, is supplied. But this is nevertheless a physiological fact. During the famous Swedish fast marches, when first 11 and then 19 men walked from Gothenburg to Stockholm, a distance of over 325 miles, in 10 days *while on a total fast*, it was observed that the protein level of the blood (serum albumin reading) of the fasting people remained *constant* and *normal (blood sugar levels also remained normal!)* throughout the fasting period, in spite of the fact that no protein was consumed. The reason for this is that proteins in your body are in the so-called *dynamic state*, being constantly decomposed and resynthesized and re-used for various needs within the body. When old or diseased cells are decomposed, the amino acids are not wasted, but are released and used again in the process of new-building of young, vital cells.

3. During a juice fast, the eliminative and cleansing capacity of the eliminative organs — lungs, liver, kidneys and the skin — is greatly increased, and masses of accumulated metabolic wastes and toxins are quickly expelled. For example, during fasting, the concentration of toxins in the urine can be ten times higher than normal. This is due to the fact that the alimentary canal, liver and kidney are relieved from the usual burden of digesting foods and eliminating the resultant wastes, and can concentrate on the cleansing of old accumulated wastes and toxins, such as uric acid, purines, etc., from the tissues. This eliminative process

is evidenced by the following typical symptoms of fasting: offensive breath, dark urine, continuous and generous discharge from the colon with enema, skin eruptions, excessive perspiration, and catarrhal elimination of mucus.

4. Fasting affords a physiological rest to the digestive, assimilative and protective organs. After fasting, the digestion of food and the utilization of nutrients is greatly improved, and sluggishness and further waste retention are prevented.

5. Finally, the fast exerts a normalizing, stabilizing and rejuvenative effect on all the vital physiological, nervous and mental functions. The nervous system is rejuvenated; mental powers are improved; glandular chemistry and hormonal secretions are stimulated and increased; the biochemical and mineral balance of the tissues is normalized.

It is easy to see from the above why fasting is such an effective health-restoring and rejuvenative measure.

Medical science re-discovers fasting

Fasting is the oldest therapeutic method known to man. Even before the advent of the healing arts, man instinctively stopped eating when feeling ill and abstained from food until his health was restored. Perhaps he learned this from animals, which always fast when not feeling well.

Throughout medical history, fasting has been regarded as one of the most dependable curative methods. Hippocrates, Galen, Paracelsus and many other "greats" of medicine prescribed fasting.

But with the advent of modern, drug-oriented medicine, fasting has fallen into disregard in the eyes of the orthodox practitioners. All kinds of reducing diets — yes; but the total abstinence from food — the best form of reducing as well as healing — is seldom tried.

Happily, things are beginning to change. Many scientific studies are now being made around the world, particularly in Europe, to determine the prophylactic, therapeutic and rejuvenative effects of fasting.

The Karolinska Institute in Stockholm, a world famous medical research institution, has made clinical studies of fasting up to 55 days under Drs. P. Reizenstein and J. Kellberg. Studies demonstrated that fasting is not only a perfectly safe measure, but that it also has a definite beneficial healing effect.

The famous Swedish fast marches, led by Dr. Lennart Edrén, proved to the world the great potential of fasting as well as its safety. Although the fasting participants were under an extremely severe stress walking 33 miles a day for 10 days, their health condition only *improved* and "they felt stronger and had more vigor and vitality after the fast than before it", as expressed by Dr. Karl-Otto Aly, M.D., one of the participants of the fast march.

In Germany, fasting is now used in hundreds of biological clinics operated by medical doctors. One doctor, Otto Buchinger, Jr., has supervised over 90,000 successful fasts. In German and Swedish clinics fasting is now routinely used to treat virtually every disease — rheumatic conditions, digestive disorders, skin conditions, cardio-vascular disorders, etc.

In Russia, doctors have used fasting experimentally for 23 years and report excellent results. The latest report from Russia shows that controlled fasting was found to be the most effective treatment for schizophrenia — 64% of the patients had improved mentally after 20-30 days of controlled fasting.

Some recent animal studies in the United States have shown that periodic fasting can increase the life span considerably. In one study, fasting worms periodically — every other day — caused them to live 50 times as long as usual! Larger animals or man may not do as well, but the Cornell University sutides with rats showed that keeping them from overeating and starving them systematically increased their life span 2½ times!

How safe is fasting

This actually happened in England. A broken-hearted 50 year-old man, whose wife left him for a younger lover, decided to end it all by starving himself to death. He ran away into high mountains, abstained from all eating, contemplating his broken marriage and occasionally sipping fresh water from the mountain springs. He expected to expire in a few days. But to his surprise, the desired death would just not come. In fact, he noticed with dismay, that as the days went by, he felt better and stronger.

The end of the story is that in due time — after 74 days in the wilderness without food — the man finally changed his mind (fasting does improve mental capacity and contributes to a logical and clear thinking!), feeling that she wasn't worth killing himself for, after all, that certainly there must be other women in this world. He returned to civilization and lived happily for another 30 years — with a new wife!

I know personally of a young man of 27 in Sweden who fasted 143 days. No, it wasn't an anti-Vietnam demonstration, but to "cleanse, regenerate and rejuvenate his body and mind" (as many great philosophers, including Plato and Socrates, did in the past). And he lived to tell about his experience in a book called "Man Who Ate His Muscles."

One 54-year old Scottish woman fasted 249 days on juices and not only did she not harm herself, but she lost 74 pounds and got rid of her painful arthritis, as a pleasant side effect!

I have supervised hundreds of fasts in Europe, the U.S., Canada and Mexico and have seen most remarkable results in recovery from a great variety of ills. Many of my patients fasted up to 40 days and, almost without exception, all have told me that they felt stronger and had more vitality after the fast than before it — in addition to the fact that most of their symptoms of ill health had completely vanished during the fast.

Miss B.B. fasted for her heart condition and many vague but persistent symptoms of aging — she was well over 70. She amazed the whole Spa by increasing her daily walking distance, until at the end of her 40-day fast (she called it "40 days and 40 nights") she walked 5 miles a day. Although she did experience a few so-called fasting crises during her long fast (caused by accelerated elimination of accumulated wastes from her body) she felt healthier and stronger on the 40th day than she did on the 1st day of fasting. And you should have heard the ovation she received from the Spa guests when she finally broke her fast.

I could fill a book with actual cases of successful fasts which I supervised. Those who are interested in studying fasting in more detail, reading of many actual cases and perhaps trying to fast for themselves, should read my book, *HOW TO KEEP SLIM, HEALTHY AND YOUNG WITH JUICE FASTING.* *

So, to answer the question "Is fasting safe," I can truthfully say — after studying fasting for 30 years with some of the greatest fasting specialists in the world (Dr. Are Waerland, Dr. Ragnar Berg, Dr. Otto Buchinger, Jr., etc.) and evaluating their results as well as my own experience with hundreds of patients — that fasting is not only the most effective healing method known to man, *but also the safest.*

The best way to fast

The best, safest and most effective method of fasting is *juice fasting.* Although the old, classic form of fasting was a pure water fast, all the leading fasting authorities today agree that juice fasting is far superior to a water fast. Perhaps, if the effective way of making raw vegetable and fruit juices was known before, the healers of the past would have used them, too. I have supervised both types of fasting and I agree with Dr. Otto Buchinger, Jr., who has supervised more fasts than any other doctor, that fasting on fresh raw juices of fruits and vegetables, plus vegetable broths and herb teas, results *in much faster recovery from disease* and more effective cleansing and rejuvenation of the tissues than

---

* Paavo O. Airola, *HOW TO KEEP SLIM, HEALTHY AND YOUNG WITH JUICE FASTING,* HEALTH PLUS Publishers, P.O. Box 22001, Phoenix, Arizona 85028.

does the traditional water fast. It is too bad that some old American practitioners are still using the antiquated water fast method. The water fast exerts severe physical and emotional stress on the patient and therefore results are often unsuccessful. Perhaps this is the reason why fasting is hardly ever used any more in the United States, while in Europe it is practiced on a grand scale. There are hundreds of clinics in Germany alone where fasting is a number one method of healing. And all of them use juice fasting exclusively.

Here's what Dr. Ragnar Berg, world-famous authority on nutrition and biochemistry, says about the superiority of juice fasting to water fasting:

"During fasting the body burns up and excretes huge amounts of accumulated wastes. We can help this cleansing process by drinking alkaline juices instead of water while fasting. I have supervised many fasts and made extensive examinations and tests of fasting patients, and I am convinced that drinking alkali-forming fruit and vegetable juices, instead of water, during fasting will increase the healing effect of fasting. Elimination of uric acid and other inorganic acids will be accelerated. And sugars in juices will strengthen the heart ... Juice fasting is, therefore, the best form of fasting."

Vitamins, minerals, enzymes, trace elements and natural colorings of fresh, raw vegetable and fruit juices are extremely beneficial in normalizing all the body processes, supplying needed elements for the body's own healing activity and cell regeneration, and, thus, speeding the recovery. These juices require no digestion and are easily assimilated directly into the bloodstream — thus, they do not disrupt the healing and rejuvenating process of autolysis, or self-digestion, as suggested by some water fast proponents.

Mineral imbalance in the tissues is one of the main causes of diminished oxygenation, and consequent disease and premature aging. Generous amounts of minerals in the juices help to restore the biochemical and mineral balance in the tissues and cells.

Also, according to Dr. Ralph Bircher, raw juices contain an as yet unidentified factor which stimulates what he calls a micro-electric tension in the body and is responsible for the cells' ability to absorb nutrients from the blood stream and effectively excrete metabolic wastes.

In *PART ONE* of this book, we list specific juices which can be used in the treatment of various diseases. These juices, which possess specific medicinal properties, should be used both during the juice fasting, and/or when the patient is on a specific therapeutic diet, even if he does not fast.

How do you fast?

It is advisable to prepare yourself for fasting by a short cleansing diet. For 2 or 3 days, eat nothing but raw fruits and vegetables — one meal a day of any available fruits, the other of fresh vegetable salad.

Fasting usually begins with an effective bowel cleansing with the help of purgatives, such as Glauber's salts or castor oil. Dr. Buchinger uses an ounce and a half of Glauber's salts in one and a quarter pints of warm water on the morning of the first day of fasting. Since the Glauber's salt drink is not very tasty, it is usually followed by a glass of fruit juice. Glauber's salts will cause repeated and powerful evacuations and cleanse your bowels thoroughly. Some European clinics use castor oil for the same purpose. On the first day of fasting, one or two hours before an enema, 2 tbsp. of pure castor oil is taken in a glass of water to which the juice of half a lemon has been added. Of course, you can begin your fasting without a purgative, just by taking a double enema. First take 1 pint of plain water and let it out. Then repeat with a full quart of water, into which camomile tea or a few drops of lemon juice have been added.

The next day, and each following day of the fast, you follow this program:

UPON ARISING: Enema.

AFTER ENEMA: Dry brush massage, followed by hot and cold shower (see *Directions: 4*).

9:00 A.M.: Cup of herb tea — warm, not hot. Health food stores carry a large assortment of herb teas. When fasting therapeutically, use the herbs that are listed in *PART ONE* — specific herbs for specific conditions. See *Directions: 6* for instructions regarding preparation of herb teas.

11:00 A.M.: A glass of freshly-pressed fruit juice, diluted 50-50 with water.

11:00 A.M. to
1:00 P.M. Walk or mild exercise, or sunbathing, if the weather permits. Various therapeutic baths or other treatments can be given at this time.

1:00 P.M.: A glass of freshly made vegetable juice or a cup of vegetable broth (see *Recipes*).

1:30 to
4:00 P.M.: Rest in bed.

4:00 P.M.: Cup of herb tea.

4:15 to
7:00 P.M.: Walk, therapeutic baths, exercises and other treatments.

7:00 P.M.:   Glass of diluted vegetable or fruit juices.

9:00 P.M.:   Cup of vegetable broth.

Drink plain lukewarm water, or mineral water, when thirsty. The total juice and broth volume during the day should be between 1½ pints and 1½ quarts. Never dilute fresh juices with vegetable broth, only with pure water. The total liquid intake should be approximately 6 to 8 glasses — but don't hesitate to drink more, if thirsty.

I suggest that a therapeutic fast be supervised by a doctor or by someone who is well initiated in it. Under expert supervision, such a fast could be undertaken at home up to 30 days, if necessary. If you suffer from some illness and are under your doctor's care, you may wish to show him this book, or my fasting book and the fasting instructions, and ask him to supervise your fasting and examine your condition as the fast progresses. Without expert supervision I would not advise fasting longer than one week to 10 days at a time. After a few weeks on a Optimum health-building diet your fasting program may be repeated.

If you do decide to fast on your own, I strongly urge that you acquire my fasting book, which contains all the detailed instructions for do-it-yourself fasting. When you fast, you should be well informed on all the details and phases of fasting, and thoroughly convinced of its safety and superior healing potential.

How the fast is broken

Whether your fast will turn out to be a success or a failure will depend largely on how you break your fast. Breaking a fast is the most significant phase of it. The beneficial effect of fasting could be totally undone if the fast is broken incorrectly. As Dr. Otto H. F. Buchinger says: "Even a fool can fast, but only a wise man knows how to break the fast properly and to build up properly after the fast!"

The main rules for breaking the fast are:

1. Do not overeat!
2. Eat slowly and chew your food extremely well.
3. Take several days of gradual transition to the normal diet.

First day: Eat one half apple in the morning and a very *small* bowl of fresh vegetable soup at lunch, in addition to the usual juice and broth menu.

Second day: A few soaked prunes or figs (with soaking water) for breakfast. Small bowl of fresh vegetable salad for lunch. Vegetable soup made without salt at dinner.

	Two apples eaten between meals. All this in addition to the usual juices and broths.
Third day:	Same as second day, but add a glass of yogurt and 5-6 raw nuts (finely ground in a seed grinder) for breakfast. Increase the salad portion at lunch, and add a boiled or baked potato. A slice of whole grain bread with butter and a slice of cheese with soup at evening.
Fourth day:	You may start eating normally, adhering to a cleansing Airola Diet, as recommended in *Directions: 1.* If you fasted longer than 10 days, the break-in period should be extended one day for every 4 days of fasting.

In order to benefit from fasting to the greatest possible extent, it is of paramount importance that after fasting, a build-up diet of vital natural foods be maintained. Such a diet will supply the healing and regenerative forces of your body with all the needed elements, so that the cleansing, regenerative, rejuvenative and healing processes, initiated by the body during fasting, can be continued.

But first and foremost, always keep in mind the first rule of breaking the fast; *do not overeat!* This rule also happens to be the first rule of keeping healthy and staying younger longer.

Some important tips on fasting

1. *Enema.* During fasting a huge amount of morbid matter, dead cells and diseased tissues are burned; and the toxic wastes which have been accumulated in the tissues for years, causing disease and premature aging, are loosed and expelled from the system. These wastes are eliminated from the system by way of kidneys, bowels, skin and lungs. But the alimentary canal, the bowels, is the main road by which these toxins are thrown out of the body. Since, during fasting, the natural bowel movements cease to take place, the toxic wastes would have no way of leaving the system, except with the help of enemas. If you fast without enemas, these toxins remain in your colon and are re-absorbed into the system, poisoning your whole body. Your body will try to get them out through other eliminative organs, particularly through the kidneys, which, as a result, will often be overloaded and even damaged.

This is why enemas during fasting are an absolute must. Enemas during fasting will assist the body in its cleansing and detoxifying effort by washing out all the toxic wastes from the alimentary canal.

Enemas should be taken at least once, but preferably twice a day: the first thing in the morning and the last thing before going to bed. One pint to one quart of lukewarm water is sufficient. Enema bags are available in any drugstore.

2. *Drugs.* As a rule, a complete withdrawal of drugs is advised during fasting. Exceptions are: digitalis in heart disease, insulin in diabetes, and cortisone in arthritis — if these drugs have been taken previously for prolonged periods of time. Those who are on any kind of drugs would be wise to have their fast supervised by an experienced practitioner.

3. *Vitamins.* During fasting, the intake of vitamins and food supplements should be discontinued completely. Three exceptions: a) *In serious heart cases*, vitamin E should be taken while fasting; b) *Very sick persons* can be given extra vitamin C (up to 3,000 mg. a day) with fruit juices; c) *Very weak patients* can be given 1 or 2 tsp. of natural honey, possibly as a sweetener in herb teas.

4. *Smoking and drinking.* No smoking, no alcohol, and no coffee, of course. Incidentally, fasting is the best way to *quit* smoking and drinking. After about two weeks of fasting, all the desire for smoking or alcohol will be gone, as testified by hundreds of fasting patients. (See sections on *Smoking* and *Alcoholism* in *PART ONE*.)

5. *Contra-indications.* In advanced cases of diabetes, active tuberculosis, active malignancies, mental diseases and weak hearts in older patients, fasting is not recommended. Where there is any kind of disease, do not attempt fasting without consulting your doctor and abiding by his decision on the advisability of undertaking a fast in your situation.

6. *Juices.* All juices should be made fresh immediately before drinking. Do not use canned or frozen juices. This means that if you fast on your own, you have to have your own juicer (see *Directions: 2*). Canned or frozen juice can be used sparingly, only in an emergency situation when fresh juices are not available.

7. *Herb teas.* The best herb teas to drink during fasting are peppermint, rose hips and camomile; but you may drink any of your favorites. Your health food store has a good supply of these and many other herb teas (see *Directions: 6*). When fasting for the purpose of healing, use specific herbs for specific conditions as suggested in *PART ONE*.

8. *Work.* Must you discontinue your regular work and rest or stay in bed while fasting? Not at all! On the contrary, staying in bed while fasting is definitely harmful, except for sleeping at night and for an afternoon siesta. You may live your normal life and do your regular work while you fast. You will have plenty of strength to do it, too — unless you are a ditch digger, of course, in which case we advise you to take it easy.

9. *Exercise.* Your body needs lots of assistance in the form of fresh air, motion and exercise, in order to accomplish a thorough cleansing of the blood and tissues and effectively regenerate and revitalize all the

body functions. Therefore, you should do lots of walking and mild exercising in the fresh air — especially deep breathing exercises — in addition to sunbathing. Always sleep with windows open.

10. *Daily baths.* About one third of all body impurities and wastes are eliminated through your skin. Since the internal cleansing and speedy elimination of toxic wastes is a prime purpose of fasting, it is important to keep the skin pores wide open and the elimination through the skin as efficient as possible. Daily showers, especially in connection with dry brush massage (see *Directions: 4*) are recommended. If the heart and circulation are good (your doctor must determine this) then hot baths, sauna, and hot and cold showers should be taken frequently (see *Directions: 7*).

11. *Drinking water.* The fasting program, as suggested in this chapter, will give you 6 glasses of juices, broth and herb teas during 24 hours. If you still feel thirsty, you may drink additional regular water: pure, uncontaminated water, of course. Avoid chlorinated or fluoridated water. Natural, hard water is better than distilled water (see Section on water in *Directions: 1*).

12. *Hunger.* Will you feel hungry while fasting? Yes, naturally, but only during the first 3 or 4 days. After that, the unbelievable will happen: the longer you fast, the less hungry you will feel, until the time when the body has completed its cleansing work, at which time you will suddenly feel an excruciating hunger — a reliable signal that it is time to break the fast and start eating.

13. *Positive attitude.* Mental attitude during fasting is of paramount importance. Avoid negative influences or thoughts. Don't listen to the terrified relatives and "friends", and their "warnings". Have total confidence in what you are doing. Remember, hundreds of thousands of people have done it successfully before you. Perhaps thinking that you are on a juice *diet* instead of juice *fast* will make you feel safer!

14. *Diet after the fast.* The wonderful results achieved by fasting will be nullified in a very short time if fasting is followed by the improper diet that created the undesirable condition of ill health in the first place — a condition that fasting corrected so successfully. The regenerative, rejuvenative and healing processes initiated by your body during fasting must continue *after* the fast is broken.

Therefore, fasting should be followed by the Airola Diet — the health-building diet of optimum nutrition as described in *Directions: 1* of this book. Following the Airola Diet for optimum health after your fasting will insure that you are building upon — not tearing down — the good results the fasting has accomplished.

DRY BRUSH MASSAGE

A SIMPLE BUT MIRACULOUS HEALTH AND REJUVENATION TREATMENT

I am going to reveal to you a simple technique, which will cost you a total of fifty cents, which will take only 5 to 10 minutes a day to perform, but which will give a million dollars worth of benefits in terms of better health, better looks and longer life. I have tested it for 25 years on myself and thousands of patients and students. The technique is called *dry brush massage.* It is described in my books, *THERE IS A CURE FOR ARTHRITIS, HEALTH SECRETS FROM EUROPE* and *ARE YOU CONFUSED?.* I have received numerous glowing reports of great benefits derived by those who incorporate this simple method into their daily routine. It is of specific importance to those who are bed-ridden or convalescing after an illness.

How do you take dry brush massage.

First, you have to get a suitable brush. The best brush for a massage is a natural bristle brush about the size of your hand, or larger if you can get it. Unfortunately, it is more and more difficult to find a natural bristle brush, especially in the United States. The brush should have a long handle so you can reach all parts of your body. If you cannot find a natural bristle brush right away, but are anxious to start the dry brush program immediately, the following can be quite satisfactory:
- A regular, inexpensive natural plant-fiber vegetable brush which you can get at any drug store or hardware store.
- A coarse bath glove of twisted hogs' hair.
- A loofah mitt, a coarse natural sponge.

Warning: Do not use nylon or synthetic fiber brushes — they are too sharp and may damage the skin.

Another tip: It is advisable to start out with a less harsh brush, and brush gently at first, until your skin is "seasoned", then start using a coarser brush.

Starting with the soles of your feet, brush vigorously making rotary motions, and massage every part of your body. Press brush against your body as much as you can comfortably stand. Sensitivity of the skin varies, of course, with every individual. Some can stand much harder brushing than others. Also, the various parts of the body vary in sensitivity. The face, the inner part of the thighs, the abdomen and the chest are the most sensitive parts. Brush in this order: first feet and legs, then hands and arms, the back, abdomen, chest and neck.

Brush until your skin becomes rosy, warm and glowing. Five to ten minutes is the average time, although some people like to brush longer. But do not scrub all your skin off! Everything is best in moderation, including your dry brush massage.

The best time for dry brush massage is upon arising in the morning and again before going to bed.

Massage followed by shower

After dry brush massage it is advisable to take a shower or rub-down with a sponge or wet towel, to wash away dead skin particles. Brushing loosens up copious amounts of dead layers of skin that you can see as a dust on your body.

There are two ways to go about taking a shower. One, used mostly by the patients in European Clinics, is the alternating hot-and-cold shower, followed by dry brush massage. First, take a hot shower for 3 minutes or so, until you feel warmed up, then take a cold shower for about 10 to 20 seconds. Repeat this three times, always finishing with cold — as cold as you can stand. After this hot-and-cold shower, rub yourself dry with a coarse towel and then give yourself a brush massage that will warm you up thoroughly.

The other way, which is most suitable for relatively healthy people, is to take the dry brush massage first and finish with alternating hot-and-cold shower. Of course, if you can not tolerate the hot-and-cold shower, you can have a warm shower only. But the alternating hot-and-cold shower has an exceedingly beneficial and stimulating effect on all the vital functions of your body, particularly on the glandular system, and has a rejuvenating effect on your skin. The combination of the dry brush massage and a hot-and-cold shower is an excellent way to start and finish your day.

Why dry brush massage is so beneficial

The number one cause of all so-called degenerative diseases and premature aging is to be found in the derangement of cell metabolism and in slowed-down cell regeneration. This derangement is mainly caused by the accumulation of waste products in the tissues which interferes with the nourishment and oxygenation of the cells.

Normally, under ideal circumstances, your body cleanses itself automatically without any conscious effort on your part. It is an ingeniously designed self-cleansing, self-protecting and self-healing mechanism. Self-cleansing work is performed by a large group of specially designed organs, glands and transportation systems: alimentary canal, kidneys, liver, lungs, skin, lymphatic system, mucous membranes of various cavities, etc. But your largest eliminative organ is the *skin.*

It is estimated that one-third of all body impurities are excreted through the skin. Doctors often refer to the skin as "the third kidney" — and very appropriately so. Hundreds of thousands of tiny sweat glands act not only as the regulators of body temperature, but also as small kidneys, detoxifying organs, ready to cleanse the blood and free the system from health-threatening poisons. The chemical analysis of sweat shows that it has almost the same constituents as urine. Uric acid, the main metabolic waste product and a normal component of urine, is found in large amounts in perspiration. If the skin becomes inactive and its pores choked with millions of dead cells, uric acid and other impurities will remain in the body. The other eliminative organs, mainly the liver and kidneys, will have to increase their labor of detoxification because of the inactive skin, with the result that they will be overworked and eventually weakened or diseased. Toxins and wastes will then be deposited in the tissues. Thus, you must realize the great importance of always keeping your skin in perfect working condition.

The eliminative capacity of the skin is demonstrated by the fact that more than one pound of waste products is discharged through the skin every day. This explains why man discovered the healing effect of sweating very early in history. The Finnish sauna, and the Turkish, Russian and Roman baths have been used for healing purposes for thousands of years. The famous seventeenth-century Dutch physician, Sylvius, said, "One third of all diseases can be cured by sweating."

In addition to its eliminative work, skin has many other vital functions. The body actually breathes through the skin, absorbing oxygen and exhaling carbon dioxide which is formed in the tissues. Also, certain nutrients are absorbed into the body through the skin. Russian scientific studies show that minerals from the sea water and sea air are absorbed through the skin during seashore holidays. Other scientific studies have demonstrated that the skin is capable of assimilating various vitamins, minerals and even proteins applied directly to the skin. It has been long known, too, that by a mysterious chemical process, vitamin D is manufactured on the skin by the influence of the sun rays on the oils produced by the skin glands. Subsequently, vitamin D is absorbed into the system through the skin.

As you can see, your skin is a living, vital organ with a multiplicity of important functions. The tragedy is that the skin of modern man is the most neglected and mistreated organ. In our sheltered, air-conditioned existence skin is seldom exposed to life-giving fresh air or to stimulating temperature changes. How many times this week have you worked or exercised outdoors hard enough to cause profuse perspiration? Dry brush massage will give your skin stimulation, exercise and cleansing of which it is deprived by your sedentary way of life.

Here is an impressive list of benefits you derive from regular dry brush massage:

1. It will effectively remove the dead layers of skin and other impurities, and keep pores open.

2. It will stimulate and increase blood circulation in all underlying organs and tissues, and especially in the small blood capillaries of your skin.

3. It will revitalize and increase the eliminative capacity of your skin and help to throw toxins out of the system.

4. It will stimulate the hormone- and oil-producing glands.

5. It has a powerful rejuvenating influence on the nervous system by stimulating nerve endings in the skin.

6. It will help prevent colds, especially when used in combination with hot-and-cold showers.

7. It will contribute to a healthier muscle tone and a better distribution of fat deposits.

8. It will rejuvenate the complexion and make it look younger.

9. It will make you feel better all over.

10. It will improve your health generally, and help prevent premature aging.

Since the dry brush massage also happens to be one of the most *pleasant* and enjoyable do-it-yourself health measures, don't you think that the above list is impressive enough to convince you to give this million-dollar health and beauty secret an honest try? I am quite confident that once you try it, you will be "sold on it" for the rest of your life!

Some important tips on dry brush massage

1. Every two weeks or so wash your brush with soap and water and dry it in the sun or in a warm place. Your brush will be rapidly filled with impurities and should be washed regularly.

2. For hygienic reasons, use separate brushes for each member of the family.

3. Avoid brushing the parts of your skin that are irritated, damaged or infected.

4. The scalp should be brushed, too. For scalp brushing, a good natural bristle brush is a must — no other substitute will do. Scalp brushing will stimulate hair growth by increasing blood circulation, and keep scalp clean from dandruff, stale oils and other impurities.

5. The facial skin of most people is too sensitive for brushing; therefore, it is better to leave it alone.

6. If you don't have a brush with an extended handle, ask your husband or wife to help you with the brushing. Brush massage is doubly enjoyable when somebody else gives it to you. A mutual morning and evening brush massage session may even add a new dimension to your marriage!

7. If your skin is dry and shows the signs of premature aging, an excellent way to improve the quality of your skin and the looks of your complexion is to rub or massage your whole body with a nourishing oil immediately after dry brushing. I particularly recommend the following oils: sesame oil, avocado oil, almond oil. Or still better, use my *FORMULA F-PLUS* (see *Directions: 8*).

JUICES

HOW TO MAKE THEM AND HOW TO USE THEM

In *Part One* of this book, the therapeutic use of juices is suggested in the biological treatment of virtually every condition of ill health. Juice, as a medicine, is one of the major biological therapeutic modalities. Most biologically oriented doctors and biological clinics use juice therapy with remarkable results. In the famous Dr. Max Gerson's cancer clinic, fresh juice comprised a major part of the therapeutic program. All European biological clinics use raw juices in their programs of treatment, both in conjunction with fasting and in a therapeutic diet.

Juices, being extracts from plants and fruits, possess definite medicinal properties. Therefore, they should be used as suggested in various sections of *Part One* — specific juices for specific conditions.

In addition to specific medicinal properties, raw fruit and vegetable juices have an extraordinary revitalizing and rejuvenative effect on all the organs, glands and functions of the body. For this reason raw juices are universally used in all health and beauty spas.

Raw juices have a cleansing and detoxifying effect. They purify the blood and all the tissues of the body, neutralize the waste products of metabolism, and help in building new tissues. They are rightfully called "the internal baths of health and youth".

The favorable effect of raw juices in the treatment of disease, particularly in combination with juice fasting, is attributed to the following physiological facts:

- Raw juices are extremely rich in vitamins, minerals, trace elements, enzymes and natural sugars.
- Almost 100% of the vital nutritive elements in juices are assimilated directly from the stomach into the blood stream, without putting a strain on the digestive system.

- Raw juices speed the recovery from disease by supplying needed substances for the body's own healing activity and cell regeneration.
- Raw juices provide an alkaline surplus which is extremely important for normalizing the acid-alkaline ratio in the blood and tissues, since over-acidity is present in most conditions of ill health and is considered to be a contributing factor in disease development.
- Generous amounts of easily-assimilable organic minerals in juices, particularly calcium, potassium and silicon, help to restore biochemical and mineral balance in the tissues and cells. Mineral imbalance in the tissues is one of the main causes of diminished oxygenation which leads to premature aging of cells and disease.
- Raw juices contain nature's own medicines, vegetal hormones and antibiotics. String beans are known to contain insulin-like substances. Cucumber and onion juices contain hormones needed by the cells of the pancreas in order to produce insulin. Antibiotic substances are present in fresh juices of garlic, onions, radish and tomatoes.
- Studies show that raw juices contain an as yet unidentified factor which stimulates micro-electric tension in the tissues and is responsible for the cells' ability to absorb nutrients from the blood stream and effectively excrete metabolic wastes from the cell.
- Even coloring substances, yellow, red, green and blue, in all shades and intensities, which are present in large quantities in all raw vegetable and fruit juices, are vitally important from a therapeutic point of view. They increase production of red blood corpuscles, influence digestive and assimilative processes and take part in the metabolism of proteins and cholesterol.

It is easy to see from the above why raw vegetable and fruit juices have taken such a prominent place in the biological programs of treatment of virtually every known disease.

VITAL POINTS REGARDING JUICES

1. The only juices which should be used for therapeutic purposes are fresh, raw, natural juices, prepared on your own juicer immediately before drinking.

2. The best juicer for making fresh juices is a hydraulic press-type juicer. Although they are rather expensive for individual use, the juices made with them are superior in quality and have a greater mineral

content as compared with juices made with the more common, and less expensive, electric centrifugal juicers. Health food stores usually sell various types of juicers.

3. Only fresh, ripe fruits, plants, berries and vegetables, preferably organically grown, should be used for making juices.

4. If regular supermarket quality produce is used, they should be washed carefully. See washing instructions in *Part Two* ("*General Protective Measures Against Toxic Environment*").

5. Make only as much juice as needed for immediate use. In storage, even under refrigeration, raw juices oxidize rapidly and lose their medicinal value. Even after as short a time as 10 minutes of storage, raw juices lose much of their medicinal value.

6. If juices are very sweet, as is often the case with carrot, beet, grape, apple or pear juice, they should be diluted with water, 50-50, or mixed with other, less sweet juices. This is especially important in some specific conditions, such as diabetes, hypoglycemia, arthritis and high blood pressure.

7. Several fruits or vegetables are often combined to make blended juices. However, *never mix fruit and vegetable juices.* Fruit and vegetable juices should be made separately *and never drunk at the same time* — at least 1½ to 2 hours apart. Some writers advise making green juice by blending spinach, alfalfa, parsley or other greens with pineapple juice in the blender. This is definitely an incorrect way to make juice. When vegetables and fruit juices are mixed together, digestion and assimilation is impaired, resulting in gas and only partial assimilation of nutrients.

8. As a rule, vegetable or fruit juices should be drunk between meals or one hour *before* meals, but not *with* meals.

HOW TO MAKE GREEN JUICE

"Green Juice" is recommended often in *Part One* of this book for treatment of various diseases. It is extremely beneficial in most conditions of ill health, supplying valuable chlorophyll and an abundance of vitamins, minerals, trace elements, enzymes, coloring substances and nature's own medicinal and healing factors.

Here's how you make green juice:

Take any available greens: any green leafy vegetable from the garden, such as parsley, spinach, kale, swiss chard, turnip tops, radish tops, lettuce, wheat grass, comfrey — anything available at the time. Also wild plants, such as dandelion, common nettle, wild carrot tops, alfalfa, etc., can be used.

If you have hydraulic-type juicer, all these greens can be ground and pressed as any other vegetable. Then mix about 1/3 of green juice with

2/3 of carrot, celery, beet or other vegetable juice. If your juicer is a regular, electric centrifugal juicer, which is the most common type, then first make one glass of juice from carrot, beet and celery. Pour the juice into the electric *blender* and switch on low. Feed your available greens into blender slowly. Finally, switch on high and blend very well. Your green juice — the healing, rejuvenating and life-giving drink — is ready to drink!

Drink it, as well as all other juices, *slowly*; salivate well.

LACTIC ACID JUICES

There are several brands of fermented vegetable juices on the market, most of them imported. According to most European biological doctors, and particularly the foremost expert on the therapeutic value of lactic acid fermented foods, Dr. Johannes Kuhl, fermented juices possess extraordinary medicinal properties and should be used in the biological treatment of many diseases. Cancer, arthritis, digestive disorders and diseases of kidneys and liver are especially suited for treatment with fermented juices. In *Part One* of this book we specified such juices for several conditions.

Fermented lactic acid juices are sold in most health food stores.

HOW TO USE HERBS AND HERB TEAS THERAPEUTICALLY

Herbs have been used as healing agents since the beginning of time by every race upon the earth. Primitive people in every corner of this planet possessed remarkable knowledge of the medicinal value of certain roots, barks, seeds and plants that grew in their environment. This knowledge was handed down from one generation to the next.

Later, when the primitive medicine man was replaced by modern medical doctors, almost 90 percent of the medical pharmacopoeia that doctors used was made up of botanical medicines: herbs, roots, etc. The oldest medical literature, such as *Papyrus Ebers* (2nd century B.C.), *Atherva Veda*, and all the records of Persian, Roman, Hebrew, Chinese and Egyptian medicine, show that herbal medicine was in highest regard and used extensively to cure practically every ill known to man. As late as in the 1800's, fully 80 percent of medicines available to doctors were plant derivatives.

Although with the advance of chemical science doctors of today have all but forgotten the healing treasures of nature, in many parts of the world herbs are still used as remedial agents. In Mexico, botanical medicine was highly advanced during Mayan, Incan and Aztec cultures and has survived until present times. It is not an exaggeration to say that more herbs than chemical drugs are used in Mexico today for healing purposes, judging by the amount of herbs sold in numerous herbal shops and stands on every market in every town, village and city. In India, China, Central and South America, Africa and the Pacific Islands, herbs are still widely used — the art of botanical medicine having been carefully preserved by skillful herbalists.

Even modern 20th century medical science, after being contemptuous of herbal medicine for decades, is now turning "back to nature" and is engaged in world-wide research of old-time herbal remedies. Some of our largest pharmaceutical companies are testing thousands of herbs and plants in hopes of isolating the supposedly active medicinal ingredient and put it in tablet form. Some of today's most commonly used tranquilizers are made from a plant called snakeroot (Rauwolfia). A commonly used heart medicine, digitalis, is made from the leaves of the plant called foxglove. In Mexico, testosterone tablets (male sex hormone) are now manufactured by a leading drug company from sarsaparilla root. Chemists from all major drug companies are studying old books on herbs in hopes to find effective and harmless medicines to replace some of the harmful and ineffective chemicals in modern drugstores. Even the National Cancer Institute is now seriously investigating natural plant cures for cancer. Several universities, notably the University of Arizona, California College of Medical Evangelists, Utah University, and others, backed by government and private grants, are engaged in search of medicinal plants that can cure a mushrooming list of diseases that chemical drugs are powerless against: cancer, arthritis, multiple sclerosis, psoriasis, heart disease, etc.

Medical science is now confirming what the Bible has been telling from the beginning and what "primitive" people around the world knew all along, that man's best medicine is right close to him and all around him — in the plant kingdom. There is not a single disease in man that does not have a corresponding remedy or cure in some herb, root, bark or other botanical medicine. As it is said, "for every disease there is a cure," and this cure was given to man by a wise and loving Creator right in his close environment — in the plant kingdom. It behooves us to learn about and use these God-given herbal remedies to cure our ills.

In *Part One* of this book the most effective herbal remedies are listed for almost every condition. Most of the mentioned herbs are available in all better health food stores. They are also sold by mail by numerous herb houses. Look in the yellow pages of your telephone directory for one nearest you. They also usually advertise in health magazines.

Some of the herbs listed may grow in your own environment: dandelion, birch leaves, camomile, common nettle, alfalfa, peppermint, comfrey, rose hips, raspberry leaves, chaparral, eucalyptus leaves, juniper berries, parsley — to name a few. These herbs can be picked and dried for future use. They should be picked early in the summer, preferably when the plant is in full bloom. Herbs should then be dried outside in the shade, in a well ventilated area. When thoroughly dry, keep them in tightly closed glass jars, or in heavy brown paper bags. The same applies to barks and roots, although they require a much longer time for drying.

How to prepare herbs for use

The most common way to use herbs, especially leaves, blossoms and small plants, is in the form of *herb tea*, or what is professionally called *infusions*.

Here's how you make herb tea: Take 1 tsp. of dried herbs to a cup of water, or 1 ounce of the herb to 1 pint of water, if a larger quantity is desired. Boil the water. Place herbs in a cup or container and pour the boiling water over the herb. Cover and let it steep for 15 minutes. After that, stir, let settle, strain and let cool down to drinkable temperature — never drink the tea boiling hot! There is no wisdom in curing acne and dying of stomach cancer, which drinking boiling hot liquids surely can cause! Tea can be sweetened with a little natural honey. *NOTE: Infusions* or *herb teas* should never be boiled!

Another way to use herbs is in form of so-called *decoctions.* Decoctions are made by boiling herbs in water for a considerable length of time. Hard materials, such as roots, barks, seeds, etc., are normally prepared as decoctions, since it would require a longer time to extract the active ingredients from them.

Here's how to make decoctions: Place 1 ounce of roots, bark or seeds in 1½ pints of cold water. Cover and let boil for ½ hour. Let stand and steep for another ½ hour. Then strain, cool and drink, or store in glass jar in refrigerator for future use. While teas should be made fresh every day, decoctions can be stored for about one week.

Some herbs are used in the form of *tinctures.* Tinctures are herb extractions made with help of pure or diluted spirits of alcohol, or brandy, or vodka. The main reasons for making tinctures is that the medicinal property of some herbs is destroyed by the use of heat, and some herbs will not yield the active ingredient to water alone.

Tinctures are made in the following way: 1 ounce of *powdered* herb is mixed with 12 oz. of pure spirits diluted with 4 oz. of water. Vodka or brandy do not require water and can be used straight. The mixture is allowed to stand for 10 to 14 days; the bottle should be shaken every day. After that the contents are strained through a fine flannel, sediments discarded and the clear tincture is bottled for future use.

Poultices are another way to use herbs. There are two ways poultices are usually applied.

1. Fresh whole leaves − usually large leaves of such plants as comfrey, cabbage, raspberries or nettles − are placed directly on the affected part, such as the joints, abdomen, etc., in layers of several leaves over each other, then covered with a piece of cloth and finally wrapped with a large towel or blanket. Such a poultice "draws" the disease out of the affected part and soothes the pain.

2. Fresh leaves or plants are crushed and heated in a little water (sometimes in castor oil), then spread as hot as can be tolerated directly on the affected parts and covered with cloth. A plastic sheet is placed over, then a towel, and above all an electric heating pad. The poultice should be left on for 1/2 to 1 hour. The medicinal property of the herb in combination with heat has a powerful healing effect, especially in rheumatic and arthritic conditions. Dried herbs can be also used, if fresh are not available, for such a poultice. For example, a very effective stimulating and healing poultice for application on joints affected by arthritis is made from cayenne (red pepper powder) and a few other herbs (see section on *Arthritis* in *PART ONE*).

THERAPEUTIC BATHS

*How to use or administer overheating baths, sitz baths,
sauna, hot-and-cold shower, Kneipp baths, salt water baths, etc.*

Water has been used for remedial purposes since time immemorial. Natives in various parts of the earth, sought the healing effect of natural waters, mineral springs, sea water, rivers and springs. When medical science saw its birth, healing disease with water was recognized as one of the most important therapeutic modalities. Hippocrates, Celus, Galen and other ancient greats of medicine praised water for its many curative properties. In all major ancient civilizations, bathing was held in esteem not only for its remedial properties, but as an important health-building and disease-preventive measure.

In modern times, the therapeutic properties of water were popularized by Father Kneipp, Maria Schlenz, Priessnitz, and other European water-cure pioneers. There are hundreds of Spas and "Bads" in most European countries where therapeutic baths are used as a major healing measure, especially so-called Kneipp-baths. As Father Kneipp said, "Water contains great healing power" — and millions of yearly visitors to these "bads" can testify that water, indeed, does possess great therapeutic value.

Here are some therapeutic baths that can be employed in healing the sick and in preventing disease. Some of these, like overheating baths, should be supervised by a doctor or nurse, but most can be employed in a do-it-yourself manner in your own home.

HOT-AND-COLD SHOWER

Biological clinics attach great importance to alternating hot and cold baths. Such baths stimulate all the body functions, but particularly the adrenal and other endocrine glands, and reactivate their functions. They are excellent means of revitalizing skin activity and improving circulation.

The procedure is as follows. First, take a warm shower for about 3 to 5 minutes, to warm up the body. Then switch rapidly to cold water — as cold as it comes — for about 10-15 seconds. Switch back to warm water for 3 to 5 minutes. Make three changes, always finishing with cold. After the shower, warm yourself up by rubbing with a coarse bath towel and follow with dry brush massage (see *Directions: 4*).

KNEIPP SITZ BATH

There are three kinds of sitz baths: hot sitz bath, cold sitz bath and alternating hot-and-cold sitz bath.

The hot sitz bath is beneficial for relieving pain and inflammation in the reproductive organs and other organs of the pelvic region. The water should be as hot as can be borne comfortably and the duration of the bath should be 10 to 15 minutes.

The cold sitz bath has a stimulating and invigorating effect on the reproductive organs and the spine. It is popularly called a "youth bath," because of its rejuvenative effect as the result of increasing blood circulation to the vital centers. The temperature of the water should be 50-65 degrees F, and the duration of the bath from 3 to 5 minutes. After the bath, rub yourself warm with a coarse bath towel.

The alternate hot-and-cold sitz bath has great therapeutic value in most internal disorders. Not only organs and glands of the pelvic region are stimulated and revitalized, but practically all body functions are beneficially affected. This bath is especially beneficial for all who have lowered vitality.

For the alternate hot-and-cold sitz bath, two tubs are required: one containing hot and the other cold water. For a do-it-yourself sitz bath, some large metal or plastic household tubs (like a baby bath, for example) can be used. The temperature of the hot water is about 98-100 degrees, and the cold water is about 50-65 degrees. Sit in hot water first for 5 minutes, then switch to cold water for 5 to 10 seconds. Repeat twice.

For hot *or* cold sitz bath, you can use the regular bath tub in your home. Fill the bath tub with water about 8 inches high, or a little less than half-full. Sit in the tub with your knees drawn up (use a little box or stool) so that only the "sitz" is covered by the water. If a cold sitz bath is given to a patient in very weak condition, it is advisable to place his feet in a small tub or pan filled with warm water.

A sitz bath can be taken 2 or 3 times a week.

KNEIPP FOOT BATH

You need two small tubs for this bath. Fill one with hot water, 97 to 110 degrees; the other with cold water, 50 to 65 degrees. Water should be 8 to 12 inches deep.

Place feet in hot tub for 3 to 5 minutes. Switch to cold for 30 seconds. Repeat twice.

A foot bath is an excellent treatment for colds, chronic headaches, neuritis, catarrh, sinusitis, cold feet, poor circulation, nervous disorders and congestion in the abdomen and pelvic organs.

KNEIPP ARM BATH

Use two small tubs, or one large wash basin and an extra tub. Fill one with hot water, 97 to 105 degrees; the other with cold, 50 to 65 degrees.

Keep arms, preferably deeper than the elbows, in hot water for 5 minutes, then in cold for 15 seconds. Repeat 3 times.

An arm bath is very beneficial in heart conditions, rheumatic conditions in hands and arms, bursitis and neuritis.

COLD SHOWER

Famous nature-cure pioneer, Dr. Henry Lindlahr, said: "There is no such thing as a 'cure-all' — a remedy or panacea for all ailments — *but if there were* such a thing, it would be *cold water*, properly applied."

A cold shower treatment has a special tonic-like magic of exerting a rejuvenative and healing effect on the entire system. It stimulates circulation and increases muscle tone and nerve force. It stimulates the entire glandular system. It improves digestion and speeds up general metabolism. It will increase resistance to infections and colds, if used regularly. It has a powerful influence on the central nervous system, on the brain and on all the vital organs of the body. It increases the blood count, as shown in actual studies. It has an electro-magnetic effect on the body, stimulating the flow of life energies and increasing the intake of oxygen to a remarkable degree.

As you see, Dr. Lindlahr wasn't kidding!

If you can regulate the force of the water stream, set it on as forceful a flow as possible. The harder the stream, the greater the therapeutic value of the shower.

A cold shower can be taken twice a day — morning and evening. If you have a large enough shower room to place a cot, or at least a chair in it, you may take a *long* shower, keeping water at a comfortable temperature (even warm if necessary) and let the forceful stream pound the body, exposing every part of your body as you turn over on your cot. Showers like this have been taken for several hours, resulting in great health benefits.

SALT WATER BATH

Of all natural living waters, salt sea water has the greatest curative power. Sea water is extremely rich in all the beneficial minerals. It can be taken internally, 2 tbsp. a day, as a mineral supplement. Minerals are absorbed through the skin during ocean bathing and even by inhaling mineral-rich air by the seashore.

If you are not fortunate enough to live by the seashore, here is an easy do-it-yourself salt water bath which you can enjoy right in your own bathtub.

Three or four pounds of sea salt is dissolved in a tub half-full of cool water. Enjoy salt-water swimming by rubbing yourself briskly, then drying yourself warm with a coarse towel.

If sea salt is not available (health food stores are the most likely places to find it), the following ingredients can be substituted for it:

3½ lb. common salt
½ lb. magnesium chloride
½ lb. Epsom salts

SULPHUR BATH

A sulphur bath is used in rheumatic diseases, skin disorders, nervous conditions and neuritis. Drugstores usually carry ready-made fluid preparations for sulphur bath; use according to directions.

MINERAL BATHS

Mineral baths have been used for curative purposes as long as man has lived upon this earth. In many European countries, modern scientists have studied the therapeutic value of mineral baths and concluded that they "work." In Germany, in Russia, and in many East European countries, there are thousands of mineral spas where millions of people use mineral waters both for drinking and bathing, often under direction of licensed medical doctors.

If you can get to some mineral springs for a few weeks of "cure," consider yourself lucky. There are several mineral springs in the United States and Mexico. Hot mineral baths have a curative effect on virtually every disease in the medical book but particularly rheumatic and arthritic conditions, diseases of the heart and circulation, nervous disorders, skin conditions and diseases of old age and senility.

OVERHEATING THERAPY

"Give me a chance to create fever and I will cure any disease," said the great physician, Parmenides, 2,000 years ago.

Fever is one of the body's own defensive and healing forces, created and sustained for the deliberate purpose of restoring health. The high temperature speeds up metabolism, inhibits the growth of the invading virus or bacteria, and literally burns the enemy with heat. Fever is an effective protective and healing measure not only against colds and simple infections, but against such serious diseases as polio and cancer. In biological clinics, overheating therapies or artificially induced fever are used effectively in the treatment of acute infectious diseases, arthritis and rheumatic diseases, skin disorders, insomnia, muscular pain and cancer, to name a few conditions. Such giants of medical science as Nobel Prize Winner, Dr. A. Lwoff, Dr. Werner Zabel, and Dr. Josef Issels, recommend and use fever therapies extensively. Recently, a research team under the direction of Dr. David S. Muchles, from Oxford University, reported that the studies confirmed what ancient physicians and biological doctors knew all along — that fever is effective in combating many diseases, including cancer.

There are many ways to induce fever. Some doctors use certain vaccines (like BCG) or drugs to create artificial fever. Personally, I prefer a more natural approach. Although fever induced with BCG or drugs can have a beneficial effect by "waking up" and stimulating the body's natural defensive and immunological mechanism, there is less stress on the body if fever is induced with an overheating bath. Schlenz-bath has been used for this purpose for nearly a century.

SCHLENZ-BATH

Here's how the curative Schlenz-bath is administered. First, the patient should not eat for at least two hours before treatment. If possible, the bladder and the colon should be emptied. The bath tub should be as large and as deep as possible. If a regular American bath tub is used, you may need to plug the emergency outlet to raise the water to the top of the tub.

The patient must be *totally covered with water*, including his head; only his nose, eyes and mouth — and as little as possible of them — should be left uncovered. Start with a low temperature of about 95 degrees, or about the temperature of the skin. Let warm water run slowly from the faucet and stir constantly. In 15 to 20 minutes, bring the temperature in the tub to about 100 degrees; later to about 103 or even slightly higher, depending on the patient's reaction.

The length of the treatment is about one hour. Although the temperature of the water is not too high, when the patient is *totally* covered by the water there is no heat escaping from the body and its temperature will invariably rise to match the temperature of the water.

The Schlenz-bath, if given to sick patients, must be supervised. The pulse should not go over 130 or 140. The temperature of the water should be monitored at all times with a bath thermometer. If the patient feels any discomfort, he should be raised out of the water to a sitting position for a while. It is also recommended that the nurse massage the patient with a bristle brush during the bath. This brings the blood to the surface of the skin and relieves the heart from undue pressure.

SAUNA

A sauna, or Finnish steam bath, is another excellent way to benefit from overheating therapy. In addition to an artificially induced fever, which a prolonged steam bath always accomplishes, the sauna bath is specifically conducive to profuse therapeutic sweating.

The skin is our largest eliminative organ — "the third kidney." It is generally considered that the skin should eliminate 30 percent of the body wastes by way of perspiration. Due to lack of physical work and an overly sedentary life, the skin of most people today has degenerated as an eliminative organ, since it is hardly ever subjected to sweating. If health is to be restored, it is of vital importance that the eliminative activity of the skin is revitalized. Taking sauna or steam baths regularly, once or twice a week, will help to restore and revitalize the cleansing activity of the skin.

The therapeutic property of the sauna is attributed to the following facts:
- Overheating stimulates and speeds up the metabolic processes and inhibits the growth of virus and bacteria.
- All the vital organs and glands are stimulated to increased activity.
- The body's healing forces are aided and assisted, and healing is accelerated.
- The eliminative, detoxifying and cleansing capacity of the skin is dramatically increased by the profuse sweating.

DO-IT-YOURSELF SAUNA

If you do not have your own sauna, and have no easy access to a sauna, you can make a do-it-yourself sauna in your own bedroom, as follows:

First take a hot bath, as hot as you can stand. Then dry yourself and wrap in a heavy bath towel. Put a plastic or rubber sheet on your bed to protect it from damage by perspiration. Lie on the rubber sheet, take a couple of hotwater bottles and cover yourself with an electric blanket, turned on high, leaving just a crack for breathing. Use several heavy blankets, if necessary. Remain in bed while profuse sweating occurs — half an hour or more. Finish with a shower.

NOTE: Although fever is a natural, constructive, beneficial symptom, and fever therapy is one of the most effective means in the arsenal of biological modalities, I must stress the fact that fever therapy should always be supervised by an expert practitioner and undertaken on the advice of a doctor. The patient's heart condition, his ability to perspire and his general vitality should be checked and his reaction during the therapy closely supervised. Also, the length of the overheating therapy, and the dosage of fever-inducing drugs (if they are used), should be determined by the doctor.

The above warning is in regard to patients who are *ill*. There is, of course, no danger for *healthy* people to take sauna or other steam or hot baths, or even a Schlenz-bath, on a regular basis as a preventive, cleansing and health-building measure, as millions of people are doing both here and in Europe.

FORMULA F-PLUS

In *Part One* of this book, *Airola Formula F-Plus* is recommended as a part of the biological program in the treatment of many diseases, particularly skin conditions.

This is my own formula, which was first printed some years ago in my book, *Swedish Beauty Secrets*, which, by the way, contains many other excellent do-it-yourself natural internal and external cosmetics which can be made in your own kitchen.

Formula F-Plus contains only natural, easily obtained substances, and can be made by anyone in the home. The listed ingredients are sold in all better health food stores.

Here's how you make

AIROLA FORMULA F-PLUS

2 tbsp. sesame oil
1 tbsp. olive oil
2 tbsp. avocado oil
2 tbsp. almond oil
2,000 IU vitamin E, mixed tocopherols
100,000 USP Units vitamin A
A drop or two of your favorite perfume

Pour the oils into an empty bottle or small jar. Take 10 gelatin capsules of vitamin E, 200 IU each (or 5 capsules of 400 IU each) and 4 capsules of vitamin A, 25,000 units each (or 10 capsules 10,000 each). Puncture the capsules with a needle, or cut the ends off with scissors, and squeeze the contents into the bottle. Add a drop or two of your favorite perfume, close tightly and shake well. Keep in the refrigerator. Do not use Eau-de-Cologne, but pure essence of perfume. *Formula F-Plus* could be made, of course, without the perfume, if you don't mind an oily and slightly fishy aroma. By the way, to avoid the fishy aroma which natural vitamin A capsules sometime have, a synthetic form of vitamin A can be substituted.

I composed this *Formula* specifically for those who have badly deteriorated complexions and prematurely aged, dry, lifeless skin, covered with wrinkles and blemishes. The healing, nourishing and beautifying oils of *Airola Formula-F-Plus*, fortified with vitamins A and E, will feed your skin with nutrients it needs and help to revitalize and restore its normal activity. *Formula F-Plus* is also an excellent topical application in hemorrhoids and many skin disorders, particularly in acne, eczema and psoriasis.

The most effective way to use *Airola Formula F-Plus* is in the evenings, before going to bed. Wash your face, neck, hands and arms with mild natural soap and warm water (do not use soap in such conditions as psoriasis). Take a few drops of *Formula F-Plus* and massage gently into your face, neck, hands and arms (or all over the body, if you wish), and leave it on overnight. The oil will be totally absorbed into the skin by morning and your complexion will not only look and feel velvety soft, smooth and lusciously healthy, but its physiological functions and healthy activity will be restored by the action of the healing and rejuvenative property of the ingredients in the *Formula F-Plus*.

Use *Airola Formula F-Plus* regularly and you will be amazed at the rejuvenative and healing effect it will have on deteriorated, diseased, blemished, dry, lifeless, wrinkled and prematurely aged complexions.

PART FOUR:

RECIPES

For Special Foods and Dietary Supplements
Recommended in This Book

RECIPES

For Special Foods and Dietary Supplements
Recommended in This Book

MILLET CEREAL

1 cup hulled millet
3 cups water
½ tsp. honey
½ cup powdered skim milk

Rinse millet in warm water and drain. Place in a pan of water mixed with powdered skim milk and heat mixture to boiling point. Then simmer for ten minutes, stirring occasionally to prevent sticking and burning. Remove from heat and let stand for a half hour or more. Serve with milk, honey, oil or butter — or homemade applesauce. And treat yourself to the *most nutritious cereal in the world!*

Here's another, even better way to make millet cereal (or any other cereal, for that matter).

Place all ingredients in a pan with a tight cover. Use heatproof utensils: pyrex, earthenware or stainless steel, if possible. Put in an electric or gas oven turned to 200°, or less, and leave for 3-4 hours, or longer, if necessary; but the cereal will be ready to eat after about 3 hours. To speed the process, the cereal could be heated to a boiling point before putting into the oven.

This cooking method is superior because of the low temperature, which makes the nutrients — especially the proteins — of millet or other grains more easily assimilable.

Millet is a truly wonderful, complete food. It can rightfully be called the king of all cereals, possibly sharing this distinction with buckwheat. It is high in complete proteins and low in starches. It is very easily digested and never causes gas and fermentation in the stomach, as some other cooked cereals, high in starches, often do. Dr. Harvey Kellogg, famed nutritionist, said that millet is the only cereal that can sustain or support human life when used as the *sole item in the diet*. Besides complete proteins, millet is rich in vitamins, minerals and important trace elements, such as molybdenum and lecithin.

I consider millet and buckwheat to be two of the most important cereals in the Airola Diet.

KASHA
(Buckwheat cereal)

1 cup whole buckwheat grains
2 to 2½ cups water

Bring water to a boil. Stir the buckwheat into the boiling water and let boil for two to three minutes. Turn heat to low and simmer for 15 to 20 minutes, stirring occasionally. If seasoning is desired use a very little sea salt. When all the water is absorbed, take from the stove and let stand for another 15 minutes. Kasha must never be mushy. Serve hot with sunflower seed oil, olive oil, sesame seed oil or butter.

This is a favorite cereal in Russia and many other Eastern European countries. It has an unusual, mellow flavor and it is extremely nutritious. It contains complete proteins of high biological value, equal in quality to animal proteins, as shown in recent studies.

It is preferable to cook it the "oven-way", as described above in the section on millet cereal.

POTATO CEREAL

2 large raw potatoes
2 tbsp. whole wheat flour
1 tbsp. wheat bran
1 tbsp. wheat germ (make sure it is fresh, not rancid)
4 cups water

Heat water to boiling point. Mix flour and bran in pan and simmer for two to three minutes. Place a fine shredder over pan and quickly shred potatoes directly into pan. Stir vigorously and lift from the stove. Let stand for a few minutes and serve hot with milk, butter or cream; sprinkle wheat germ on top.

This is an alkaline and exceptionally nutritious cereal. It is used often in Swedish biological clinics, especially in diets for patients with rheumatic diseases, in which case wheat flour should be excluded, and only the bran and wheat germ used.

MOLINO CEREAL

1 tbsp. coarse whole wheat flour
2 tbsp. wheat bran
2 tbsp. whole flaxseed
2-3 chopped figs or soaked prunes
1 tbsp. unsulphured raisins

Place all the ingredients in a pan with one cup of water and boil for five minutes, stirring occasionally to prevent burning. Serve immediately with sweet milk, a little honey, or homemade applesauce.

This cereal is served in European clinics to patients with weak digestion, diverticulosis and a tendency toward constipation.

WAERLAND FIVE-GRAIN KRUSKA
(for four persons)

1 tbsp. whole wheat
1 tbsp. whole rye
1 tbsp. whole barley
1 tbsp. whole millet
1 tbsp. whole oats
2 tbsp. wheat bran
2 tbsp. unsulphured raisins

Take five grains and grind them coarsely on your grinder. Place in a pot with 1 to 1½ cups of water and add bran and raisins. Boil for 5 to 10 minutes, then wrap the pot in a blanket or newspapers and let it stand for few hours. Experiment with the amount of water used — kruska must not be mushy, but should have the consistency of a very thick porridge. Serve hot with sweet milk and homemade applesauce or stewed fruits.

Kruska is an extremely nutritious dish and should be eaten as a meal in itself.

UNCOOKED QUICK KRUSKA

Use the same ingredients as above. Pour boiling water over the freshly ground grains and other ingredients and let stand and steep for half an hour. This quick *kruska* is delicious and more easily digested because of the preserved enzymes. Serve warm and eat the same way as the cooked *Five-Grain Kruska*.

FRUIT SALAD Á LÁ AIROLA

1 bowl fresh fruits, organically grown if possible
1 handful raw nuts and/or sunflower seeds
3-4 soaked prunes or handful of raisins, unsulphured
3 tbsp. cottage cheese, preferably homemade, unsalted
1 tbsp. raw wheat germ, only if you can buy it fresh
3 tbsp. yogurt
1 tbsp. wheat germ oil
2 tsp. natural, unpasteurized honey
1 tsp. fresh lemon juice

Wash and dry all fruits carefully. Use any available fruits and berries, but try to get at least three or four different kinds. Peaches, grapes, pears, papaya, bananas, strawberries, and fresh pineapple are particularly good for producing a delightful bouquet of rich, penetrating flavors. A variety of colors will make the salad festive and attractive to the eye.

Chop or slice bigger fruits, but leave grapes and berries whole. Place them in a large bowl and add prunes and nuts (nuts and sunflower seeds could be crushed). Make a dressing with one teaspoon honey (or more if most of the fruits used are sour), one teaspoon of lemon juice, and two tablespoons of water. Pour over the fruit, add wheat germ, and toss well. Mix cottage cheese, yogurt, wheat germ oil, and one teaspoon of honey in a separate cup until it is fairly smooth in texture, and pour it on top of the salad. Sprinkle with nuts and sunflower seeds. Serve at once.

This is not only a most delicious dish but it is the most nutritious and perfectly balanced meal I know. It is a storehouse of high-grade proteins and all the essential vitamins, minerals, fatty acids and enzymes you need for optimum health.

HOW TO MAKE SPROUTS

First, make sure that the seeds or grains you buy for sprouting are packaged for food. Under no circumstances use seeds that are sold for planting; they more likely than not contain mercury compounds or other toxic chemicals. Play it safe and buy your seeds and sprouting grains at your health food store.

The seeds most commonly used for sprouting are: alfalfa, mung beans, soybeans and wheat.

There are many different methods of sprouting seeds. Slow germinating seeds, such as wheat or soybeans, can be soaked in water for two days (changing water twice a day) then spread thinly on a plate or paper towel for two or three days, rinsing them under running water three times a day to prevent molding.

Here's my own way of sprouting seeds: Place two tablespoons of alfalfa seeds in a quart size jar and fill with water. Let soak overnight. Rinse seeds well the following morning and place them back in the glass jar without water, covering the jar with a cheese cloth held on by a rubber band. Keep rinsing the seeds three or four times a day. In two or three days, alfalfa sprouts are ready for eating. When seeds are fully sprouted, that is, the sprouts are one to two inches long, place the top on the jar and keep them in the refrigerator if they are not eaten right away. Sprouts can be eaten as they are or mixed with salads or other foods. They can be also ground up in a drink, preferably with vegetable juices.

HOMEMADE YOGURT

Take a bottle of skim milk and heat it almost to boiling, then cool to room temperature. Add two to three tablespoons of yogurt, which can be bought in a grocery store or health shop. Stir well. Pour into a wide-mouthed thermos bottle. Cover and let it stand overnight. In five to eight hours it will be solid and ready to serve. If you do not have a thermos jar, use an ordinary glass jar, and place it in a pan of warm water over an electric burner switched on "warm" for four to five hours, then switch off until milk is solid.

Use two to three spoonfuls of your fresh, homemade yogurt as a culture for the next batch.

HOMEMADE KEFIR

To make your own kefir, you will need kefir grains. There is a mail order company, R. A. J. Biological Laboratory, 35 Park Ave., Blue Point, Long Island, New York, which sells kefir grains by mail directly to customers. The kefir grains will last indefinitely; there is never any need to reorder. Merely follow the instructions which will come with each order.

Place 1 tbsp. of kefir grains in a glass of milk, stir and allow to stand at room temperature overnight. When the milk coagulates, it is ready for eating. Strain and save the grains for the next batch. Kefir is a true "elixir of youth", used by centenarians in Bulgaria, Russia and Caucasus as an essential part of their daily diet.

HOMEMADE COTTAGE CHEESE (kvark)

Take homemade soured milk and warm it to about 110° F, by placing the container in warm water. When the milk has curdled, place a clean linen canvas or cheese cloth over a deep strainer and pour the curdled milk over it. Wait until all liquid whey has seeped through the strainer. What remains in the strainer is fresh, wholesome and delicious homemade cottage cheese. If the cheese is too hard, add a little sweet or sour cream, and stir. The higher the temperature, the harder the cheese, and vice versa. Raw homemade cottage cheese (kvark) can be made by straining soured milk through a fine cheese cloth, without warming it up first.

By the way, don't throw the whey away — it is an exceptionally nutritious and rejuvenating drink.

HOMEMADE SOURED MILK

Use only unpasteurized, raw milk. Place a bottle of milk in a pan filled with warm water, and warm it to about body temperature. Fill a cup or a deep plate, stir in a tablespoon of yogurt, cover with a paper towel (for dust) and keep in a warm place — for example, near the stove, radiator, or wherever there is a constant warm temperature. The milk will coagulate in approximately 24 hours.

Use one or two spoonfuls of soured milk as a culture for your next batch (use yogurt or commercial buttermilk only as a starting culture for the first batch).

HALVAH

> 1 cup sesame seeds
> 2 tsp. honey, preferably coagulated solid honey

Grind sesame seeds in a small electric seed grinder. Pour sesame meal into a larger cup and knead honey into the meal with a large spoon until honey is well mixed and the halvah acquires the consistency of a hard dough. Serve it as it is, or make small balls and roll them in whole sesame seeds, shredded coconut, or sunflower seeds. This is an excellent, nutritious and delicious candy, loved by children and grown-ups alike.

SOUR RYE BREAD
(Black Bread Russian Style)

> 8 cups freshly ground whole rye flour
> 3 cups warm water
> ½ cup sourdough culture

Mix seven cups of flour with water and sourdough culture. Cover and let stand in a warm place for 12 to 18 hours. Add remaining flour and mix well. Place in greased pans. Let rise for approximately a half-hour. Bake at 350° F, one hour or more, if needed. Always save ½ cup of dough as a culture for the next baking. Keep the culture in a tightly closed jar in your refrigerator. For the initial baking it will be necessary to obtain a sourdough culture from a commercial baker.

This recipe makes 2 two-pound loaves.

VEGETABLE BROTH

> 2 large potatoes, chopped or sliced
>   to approximately half-inch pieces
> 1 cup carrots, shredded or sliced
> 1 cup celery, chopped or shredded, leaves and all
> 1 cup any other available vegetable:
>   beet tops, turnip tops, parsley, or a little
>   of everything. However, broth can be made with
>   only potatoes, carrots and celery

Add some garlic, onions and/or any of the
natural herbal spices

Put all vegetables into a stainless steel utensil, add 1½ quarts of
water, cover and cook slowly for about a half-hour. Strain, cool until just
warm, and serve. If not used immediately, keep in refrigerator and warm
up before serving.

Vegetable broth is one of the standard beverages in all biological
clinics in Sweden. Fasting patients always start the day with a big mug of
vegetable broth — a cleansing, alkalizing and mineral-rich drink.

EXCELSIOR

1 cup of vegetable broth, as above
1 tbsp. whole flaxseed
1 tbsp. wheat bran

Soak flaxseed and wheat bran in vegetable broth overnight. In the
morning, warm up, stir well, and drink — seeds and all. Do not chew the
seeds, drink them whole. *Excelsior* is especially beneficial for patients
with constipation problems. It helps to restore normal peristaltic rhythm.
When used during fasting, *Excelsior* must be strained.

HOMEMADE SAUERKRAUT

Use a small wooden barrel, or a large earthenware pot. Possibly, a
large stainless steel pail or a glass jar could be used, but under no
circumstances use an aluminum utensil.

Cut white cabbage heads into narrow strips with a large knife or
grater, and place in a barrel. When the layer of cabbage is about four to
six inches deep, sprinkle a few juniper berries, cummin seeds and/or
black currant leaves on top — use your favorite or whatever you have
available. A few strips of carrots, green peppers and onions can also be
used. Add a little sea salt — not more than two ounces for each 25
pounds of cabbage. Then add another layer of grated cabbage and spices,
until the container is filled. Each layer should be pressed and stamped
very hard with your fists or a piece of wood so that there will be no air
left and the cabbage will be saturated with its own juice.

When the container is full, cover cabbage with a clean cheese cloth,
place a wooden or slate board over it, and on the top place a clean heavy
stone. Let stand for 10 days to two weeks; longer if temperature is below
70° F. Now and then remove the foam and the possible mildew from the
top, from the stone and from the barrel edges. The cheese cloth, board
and stone should occasionally be removed, washed well with warm water
and then cold water, and replaced. When the sauerkraut is ready for

eating, it can be left in the barrel, which now should be stored in a cool place, or put in glass jars and kept in the refrigerator.

Sauerkraut is best eaten *raw* — both from the point of taste and for its health-giving value. Drink sauerkraut juice, too. It is an extremely beneficial and wonderfully nutritious drink.

HOMEMADE PICKLED VEGETABLES

Use the same method as described above for homemade sauerkraut to make health-giving lactic acid vegetables. Beets, carrots, green and red peppers, beet tops, swiss chard and celery are particularly adapted for pickling.

HOMEMADE SOUR PICKLES

Use only small, fresh, hard cucumbers. Place them in cold water overnight, then dry them well.

Place cucumbers in a wooden barrel, or a large earthenware or glass jar. Place a few leaves of black currants, cherries, mustard seeds and dill branches in with the cucumbers.

Boil a sufficient amount of salt water, using about four ounces of sea salt for five quarts of water. Let water cool down, then pour it over the cucumbers. Cover with cheese cloth, place a wooden board over it, and on the top a clean heavy stone. There should be enough salt water to cover the board. Keep the container in a warm place for about one week, then move to a cooler place. Pickles are ready for eating in about 10 days to 2 weeks — longer if temperature is cold. Every week or so remove the stone and the covers, and wash them well, first in warm water then in cold water; then replace them. Keep the top of the water clean of foam and mildew. When pickles are ready for eating they can be placed in glass jars and kept in the refrigerator.

PART FIVE

CHARTS AND TABLES

VITAMIN GUIDE

Common vitamins, their functions, deficiency symptoms,
natural sources, Recommended Dietary Allowances (RDA)*
and usual therapeutic doses.

Vitamin A

Known as Anti-Ophthalmic Vitamin. Usually measured in retinol equivalents (RE) or International Units (IU).

FUNCTIONS

Builds resistance to all kinds of infections. It is a "membrane conditioner" — it keeps mucous linings and membranes of the body in healthy condition. Prevents eye diseases, counteracts night blindness and weak eyesight by helping in formation of visual purple in the eye. Plays vital role in nourishing skin and hair. Essential during pregnancy and lactation. Helps to maintain testicular tissue in a healthy state. Promotes growth and vitality. Aids in secretion of gastric juices and in digestion of proteins. By improving the stability of tissue in cell walls it helps to prevent premature aging and senility; increases life expectancy and extends youthfulness. Protects against the damaging effect of polluted air. Increases the permeability of blood capillaries contributing to better tissue oxygenation.

DEFICIENCY SYMPTOMS

Prolonged deficiency may result in eye inflammations, poor vision, nightblindness; increased susceptibility to infections, especially in the respiratory tract; frequent colds; retarded growth in children; lack of appetite and vigor; defective teeth and gums; rough, scaly and dry skin, and such skin disorders as acne, pimples, boils, premature wrinkles and psoriasis; dry, dull hair, dandruff and excessive hair loss; nails which peel or are ridged; poor senses of taste and smell.

---

*RDA, Recommended Dietary Allowances, only indicates the officially established need of healthy individuals sufficient to prevent deficiency diseases. Persons who are ill, or those who suffer from nutritional deficiencies, should obtain several times this amount. Information about common therapeutic doses is based on our study of what most American nutritionists and nutritionally oriented doctors recommend to their patients. Unless otherwise specified, RDA indicated in this section is for adults.

NATURAL SOURCES

Colored fruits and vegetables, particularly carrots, green leafy vegetables (such as kale, turnip greens, and spinach), melon, squash, yams, tomatoes, eggs, summer butter, fertile eggs and whole milk. The richest natural source is fish liver oils.

RDA

800 mcg. RE (2,700 IU) – 1,000 mcg. RE (3,300 IU), Usual therapeutic doses 25,000 to 50,000 units a day. Can be given up to 125,000 a day for a limited period of not more than four weeks, under doctor's supervision.

VITAMIN B₁

Thiamine. Thiamine Chloride. Thiamine HCl. Measured in milligrams (mg.).

FUNCTIONS

Known as anti-beriberi, anti-neuritic and anti-aging vitamin. Essential for effective protein metabolism. Promotes growth, protects heart muscle, stimulates brain action. Indispensable for the health of the entire nervous system. Aids in digestion and metabolism of carbohydrates. Improves peristaltis and helps prevent constipation. Helps maintain normal red blood count. Protects against the damaging effect of lead poisoning. Prevents edema, or fluid retention, in connection with heart condition. Improves circulation. Prevents fatigue and increases stamina. Helps prevent premature aging.

DEFICIENCY SYMPTOMS

Deficiency may lead to loss of appetite; muscular weakness; slow heart beat; irritability; defective hydrochloric acid production in the stomach with accompanied digestive disorders; chronic constipation; loss of weight; diabetes; mental depression and nervous exhaustion. Prolonged, gross deficiency can cause beriberi, neuritis, edema. Deficiency can be induced by excess of alcohol and dietary sugar, and the excess of processed and refined foods.

NATURAL SOURCES

Brewer's yeast; wheat germ and wheat bran; rice polishings; most whole-grain cereals, especially wheat, oats and rice; all seeds and nuts, and nut butters; beans, especially soybeans; milk and milk products; and such vegetables as beets, potatoes and leafy green vegetables.

RDA

1.0 mg. Therapeutically, up to 100 mg. for limited periods.*

---

*For best result, all other vitamins of B-complex should be administered simultaneously. Prolonged ingestion of large doses of any one of the isolated B-complex vitamins may result in high urinary losses of other B-vitamins and lead to deficiencies of these vitamins.

VITAMIN B₂

Riboflavin. Vitamin G. Measured in milligrams (mg.).

FUNCTIONS

Essential for growth and general health. Essential for healthy eyes, skin, nails and hair. May help in prevention of some types of cataracts.

DEFICIENCY SYMPTOMS

Deficiency may result in bloodshot eyes; abnormal sensitivity to light; itching and burning of the eyes; inflammations in the mouth; sore, burning tongue (magenta-colored tongue); cracks on the lips and in the corners of the mouth; dull hair or oily hair; oily skin; premature wrinkles on face and arms; eczema; split nails; and such aging symptoms as "disappearing" upper lip. Can be a contributing cause to such disorders as seborrhea, anemia, vaginal itching, cataracts and ulcers.

NATURAL SOURCES

Milk, cheese, whole grains, brewer's yeast, torula yeast, wheat germ, almonds, sunflower seeds, liver, cooked leafy vegetables.

RDA

1.2 mg. – 1.7 mg. Usual therapeutic doses 25 to 50 mg.

VITAMIN B₃

Niacin. Nicotinic Acid. Niacinamide. Niacin Amide. Nicotinamide. Measured in milligrams (mg.). Niacinamide is similar in effect and therapeutic value to niacin, but does not cause burning, flushing and itching of the skin that usually occurs when the isolated form of niacin is taken.

FUNCTIONS

Anti-pellagra vitamin. Important for proper circulation and for healthy functioning of the nervous system. Maintains normal functions of gastro-intestinal tract. Essential for proper protein and carbohydrate metabolism. Helps maintain healthy skin. May prevent migraine headaches. Dilates blood vessels and increases the flow of blood to the peripheral capillary system. Often prescribed in cases of cold feet and hands. In mega-doses (massive doses), niacin has been successfully used in the treatment of schizophrenia.

DEFICIENCY SYMPTOMS

Mild deficiency may cause coated tongue, canker sores, irritability, nervousness, skin lesions, diarrhea, forgetfulness, insomnia, chronic headaches, digestive disorders, anemia. Severe, prolonged deficiency may cause pellagra, neurasthenia, mental disturbances, depression, mental dullness, disorientation and mental disease.

NATURAL SOURCES

Brewer's yeast, torula yeast, wheat germ, rice bran and rice polishings, nuts, sunflower seeds, peanuts, whole wheat products, brown rice, green vegetables, liver.

RDA

13-19 mg. Therapeutically, 100 mg. or more with each meal (preferably together with other B-complex vitamins).

NOTE: Although niacin is currently used in massive doses (up to 25,000 mg.) in treatment of such conditions as schizophrenia, high cholesterol and arteriosclerosis, some authorities warn that prolonged ingestion of massive doses of B_3 can be dangerous and may cause stomach ulcers, liver damage, jaundice, colitis and male impotence.

VITAMIN B_6
Pyridoxine. Pyridoxine HCl. Measured in milligrams (mg.).

FUNCTIONS

Aids in food assimilation and in protein and fat metabolism, particularly in metabolism of essential fatty acids. Activates many enzymes and enzyme systems. Involved in the production of antibodies which protect against bacterial invasions. Essential for synthesis and proper action of DNA and RNA. Helps in the healthy function of the nervous system and brain. Important for normal reproductive processes and healthy pregnancies. Prevents nervous and skin disorders, such as acne. Protects against degenerative diseases, such as elevated cholesterol, some types of heart disease and diabetes. Prevents tooth decay. Has been used as natural diuretic. Some studies show that it can prevent or lessen epileptic seizures. Helps prevent and relieve premenstrual edema; also effective in overweight problems caused by water retention. Vitamin B_6 regulates the balance between the minerals sodium and potassium in the body, which is of tremendous importance for vital body functions. Cases of Parkinson's Disease have responded to B_6 injections (in combination with magnesium). B_6 is required for the absorption of vitamin B_{12} and for the production of hydrochloric acid.

DEFICIENCY SYMPTOMS

Deficiency of B_6 may cause anemia, edema, mental depression, skin disorders, sore mouth and lips, halitosis, nervousness, eczema, kidney sto1es, inflammation of the colon, insomnia, tooth decay, irritability, los; of muscular control, migraine headaches, diseases of old age and premature senility.

NATURAL SOURCES

Brewer's yeast, bananas, avocados, wheat germ, wheat bran, soybeans, walnuts, blackstrap molasses, cantaloupe, cabbage, milk, egg yolks, liver, green leafy vegetables, green peppers, carrots and peanuts. Pecans are an especially rich source. Raw foods contain more B_6 than cooked foods. Cooking and food processing destroys vitamin B_6.

1.8-2.2 mg. (0.3-1.6 mg. for infants and children, 2.5 mg. for pregnant and lactating women). Therapeutically, up to 200 mg. have been used daily for several months, preferably combined with other B-complex vitamins.

BIOTIN

Vitamin H. Measured in micrograms (mcg.).

FUNCTIONS

Involved in metabolism of proteins and fats. Related to hair growth and healthy hair. Prevents hair loss. Antiseptic. It has been used in treatment of malaria.

DEFICIENCY SYMPTOMS

Deficiency may cause eczema, dandruff, hair loss, seborrhea, skin disorders, such as pallor, heart abnormalities, lung infections, anemia, loss of appetite, extreme fatigue, confusion, mental depression, drowsiness and hallucinations.

NATURAL SOURCES

Best and richest natural source is brewer's yeast. Also: unpolished rice, soybeans, liver, kidneys. Biotin is also normally produced in the intestines if there is sufficient amount of healthy intestinal flora.

RDA

100-200 mcg. (Estimated safe and adequate intake.)

FOLIC ACID

Vitamin B_9. Pteroylglutamic acid. Folate. Measured in micrograms (mcg.).

FUNCTIONS

As a co-worker with vitamin B_{12}, folic acid is essential for the formation of red blood cells. Necessary for the growth and division of all body cells and for the production of RNA and DNA, the nucleic acids that carry the hereditary patterns. Aids in protein metabolism and contributes to normal growth. Essential for healing processes. Helps build antibodies to prevent and heal infections. Essential for the health of skin and hair. Helps prevent premature graying of the hair. Its need is indicated in diarrhea, dropsy, stomach ulcers and menstrual problems. It has been used in treatment of atherosclerosis, circulation problems, anemia, radiation injuries and burns, and in treatment of sprue, a tropical nutritional deficiency disease, whose symptoms are anemia and acute diarrhea.

DEFICIENCY SYMPTOMS

Deficiency of folic acid may cause nutritional megaloblastic anemia of pregnancy, serious skin disorders, loss of hair, impaired circulation, a grayish-brown skin pigmentation, fatigue, mental depression, reproductive disorders, such as spontaneous abortions, difficult labor, high infant death rate. Also, loss of libido in males.

NATURAL SOURCES

Deep green leafy vegetables, broccoli, asparagus, lima beans, Irish potatoes, spinach, lettuce, brewer's yeast, wheat germ, mushrooms, nuts, peanuts, liver.

RDA

400 mcg. To correct anemia and deficiencies, 5 mg. or more are needed daily. Potencies higher than 0.1 mg. (100 mcg.) in one tablet are available only by prescription. Usual dose prescribed by doctors is 5 to 10 milligrams daily. It has been proven safe in large doses if taken together with B-complex (brewer's yeast) and B_{12}. *NOTE*: Some authorities believe that folic acid is contraindicated in leukemia and cancer.

PABA

Para-amino-benzoic acid. Vitamin B_x. Measured in milligrams (mg.).

FUNCTIONS

A growth promoting factor. Stimulates metabolism and all vital life processes, possibly in conjunction with folic acid. Prevents skin changes due to aging. Prevents graying of the hair. Has been used, in combination with pantothenic acid, choline and folic acid, in treatment of gray hair, with some success. Essential for healthy skin. Soothes the pain of burns and sunburns. When added to a salve and applied to the skin, may protect against sunburn, and even prevent skin cancer. Helpful in a variety of skin disorders, including eczemas and lupus erythematosus.

DEFICIENCY SYMPTOMS

Deficiency may cause extreme fatigue, eczema, anemia, gray hair, reproductive disorders, infertility, vitiligo and loss of libido.

NATURAL SOURCES

Brewer's yeast, whole grain products, milk, eggs, yogurt, wheat germ, molasses and liver. PABA is also synthesized by friendly bacteria in the healthy intestines.

RDA

Not established. Potencies of PABA higher than 30 milligrams per tablet are available only by prescription. Much higher potencies are used therapeutically, up to several hundred milligrams. *NOTE:* According to some researchers, continuous ingestion of high doses of PABA is not recommended, as it can be toxic to the heart, kidneys and liver.

PANTOTHENIC ACID

Vitamin B$_5$. Calcium Pantothenate. Measured in milligrams (mg.).

FUNCTIONS

Involved in all vital functions of the body. Stimulates adrenal glands and increases production of cortisone and other adrenal hormones. Primarily used as an anti-stress factor. Protects against most physical and mental stresses and toxins. Increases vitality. Wards off infections and speeds recovery from ill health. Helps in maintaining normal growth and development of the central nervous system. Can help prevent premature aging, especially wrinkles and other signs of aging. Can help protect against damage caused by excessive radiation.

DEFICIENCY SYMPTOMS

Deficiency can cause chronic fatigue, increased tendency for infections, graying and loss of hair, mental depression, irritability, dizziness, muscular weakness, stomach distress and constipation. May lead to skin disorders, retarded growth, painful and burning feet, insomnia, muscle cramps, adrenal exhaustion, low blood sugar (hypoglycemia) and low blood pressure. Considered to be one of the causes of allergies and asthma.

NATURAL SOURCES

Brewer's yeast, wheat germ, wheat bran, royal jelly, whole-grain breads and cereals, green vegetables, peas and beans, peanuts, crude molasses, liver and egg yolk.

RDA

Not established, but estimated to be between 4-7 mg. a day. In some studies, 1,000 mg. and more were given daily for six months without side effects. Usual therapeutic doses 50 to 200 mg. *NOTE:* It is considered that folic acid helps in the assimilation of pantothenic acid.

CHOLINE

A member of the vitamin B-complex. One of the "Lipotropic Factors." Measured in milligrams (mg.).

FUNCTIONS

The most important function of choline is in its teamwork with inositol as a part of lecithin. Essential for proper fat metabolism. Lecithin helps to digest, absorb and carry in the blood fats and fat-soluble vitamins: A, D, E and K. Necessary for the synthesis of nucleic acids, DNA and RNA. Minimizes excessive deposits of fat and cholesterol in the liver and arteries. Essential for the health of myelin sheaths of the nerves. Regulates and improves liver and gallbladder function. Necessary for the manufacture of a substance in the blood called phospholipid. Choline is useful in treatment of nephritis. Can prevent formation of gallstones. Useful in reducing high blood pressure. Has been used to treat atherosclerosis, kidney damage, glaucoma and myasthenia gravis.

DEFICIENCY SYMPTOMS

Prolonged deficiency may cause high blood pressure, cirrhosis and the fatty degeneration of the liver, atherosclerosis and hardening of arteries.

NATURAL SOURCES

Granular or liquid lecithin (made from soybeans), brewer's yeast, wheat germ, egg yolk, liver, green leafy vegetables and legumes.

RDA

Not established, but many authorities estimate it to be 1,000 mg., or more. Usual therapeutic dose 500 to 1,000 mg. Not toxic in doses under 6,000 mg. *NOTE*: Prolonged ingestion of massive doses of isolated choline may induce a deficiency of vitamin B_6. Therefore it should always be taken with other vitamins of B-complex.

Choline can also be manufactured in the body of healthy individuals receiving optimum nutrition, particularly adequate amounts of vitamins B_6 and B_{12}, magnesium, folic acid and methionine (an amino acid).

INOSITOL

A member of B-complex vitamin family.

FUNCTIONS

Vital for hair growth and can prevent thinning hair and baldness. As a part of lecithin, participates in all of its activity. Important for healthy heart muscle. Can help reduce blood cholesterol. Has been used in the treatment of obesity and schizophrenia (as part of brain cell nutrition).

DEFICIENCY SYMPTOMS

Deficiency may contribute to hair loss, constipation, eczema (dermatitis) eye abnormalities and high blood cholesterol.

NATURAL SOURCES

Brewer's yeast, wheat germ, lecithin, unprocessed whole grains, especially oatmeal and corn, nuts, milk, crude unrefined molasses, citrus fruits and liver.

RDA

Not established, but most authorities recommend the same amounts of inositol as choline. More inositol is found in the human body than any other vitamin except niacin. One tablespoon of yeast provides approximately 40 milligrams each of choline and inositol. Therapeutic doses 500 to 1,000 mg. a day, if taken in tablet form.

VITAMIN B$_{12}$

Cobalamin. Cyanocobalamin. Also known as the "Red-Vitamin." Usually measured in micrograms (mcg.).

FUNCTIONS

Essential for the production and regeneration of red blood cells. Prevents anemia. Promotes growth in children. Involved in many vital metabolic and enzymatic processes.

DEFICIENCY SYMPTOMS

Deficiency may cause nutritional and particularly pernicious anemia, poor appetite and growth in children, chronic fatigue, sore mouth, feelings of numbness or stiffness, loss of mental energy, difficulty in concentrating.

NATURAL SOURCES

Milk, eggs, aged cheese such as roquefort, liver, fortified brewer's yeast, sunflower seeds, comfrey leaves, kelp, bananas, peanuts, concord grapes, sunflower seeds, raw wheat germ, pollen.

RDA

3.0 mcg. Therapeutic doses up to 50 and 100 mcg. Because vitamin B$_{12}$ is difficult to assimilate when taken by mouth, most doctors give it in the form of injection when used for therapeutic purpose. Since B$_{12}$ is present in vegetable foods only in small amounts, vegetarians are advised to use milk and/or fortified brewer's yeast, or take vitamin B$_{12}$ in a tablet form as a supplement.

VITAMIN B$_{13}$

Orotic Acid.

FUNCTIONS

Essential for the biosynthesis of nucleic acid. Vital for the regenerative processes in cells. Considered to be of special value in the treatment of multiple sclerosis.

DEFICIENCY SYMPTOMS

Deficiencies are not known, but it is believed that they may lead to liver disorders and cell degeneration and premature aging; also overall degeneration as in multiple sclerosis.

NATURAL SOURCES

Present in whey portion of milk, particularly in soured milk.

RDA

Not known.

VITAMIN B$_{15}$

Pangamic acid. Calcium Pangamate, Measured in milligrams (mg.).

FUNCTIONS

Increases the body's tolerance to hypoxia, or insufficient oxygen supply to the tissues and cells. Helps to regulate fat metabolism, stimulates the glandular and nervous systems and is helpful in the treatment of heart disease, angina, elevated blood cholesterol, impaired circulation and premature aging. Can help protect against the damaging effect of carbon monoxide poisoning. B$_{15}$ is also a good detoxicant.

DEFICIENCY SYMPTOMS

May cause diminished oxygenation of cells, hypoxia, heart disease, glandular and nervous disorders.

NATURAL SOURCES

Whole grains, seeds and nuts; whole brown rice.

RDA

Not known. Usual therapeutic dose: 100 mg. a day, 50 mg. in the morning before breakfast, and 50 mg. at night. Used extensively in medical practice in Russia and some other countries, but not in the United States.

VITAMIN B$_{17}$

Nitrilosides. Amygdalin. Known as Laetrile when used in medical dosage form. Measured in milligrams (mg.).

FUNCTIONS

Specific preventive and controlling anti-cancer effect, as proposed by its discoverer, Ernst T. Krebs, Jr.

DEFICIENCY SYMPTOMS

Prolonged deficiencies may lead to diminshed resistance to malignancies.

NATURAL SOURCES

Most whole seeds of fruits and many grains and vegetables, such as apricot, peach and plum pits; apple seeds; raspberries, cranberries, blackberries and blueberries; mung beans, lima beans, garbanzas; millet, buckwheat and flaxseed.

RDA

Vitamin B$_{17}$ is not accepted officially as a vitamin, and, thus, no need in human nutrition has been established. Therapeutic doses are determined by doctors who use it in cancer treatment. If apricot and other fruit pits are included in the diet for preventive purposes they should be used only in small amounts, only a few pits a day. It is considered that if the diet contains an abundance of whole seeds, grains, nuts, beans and other foods mentioned above, deficiency of this factor will be unlikely. (See section on *CANCER* in *PART ONE* of this book.)

VITAMIN C

Ascorbic acid. Cevitamin acid. Usually measured in milligrams (mg.). In Europe, occasionally in Units: 1 mg. equals 20 Units.

FUNCTIONS

Essential for the healthy condition of collagen, "intercellular cement". Involved in all the vital functions of all glands and organs. Necessary for healthy teeth, gums and bones. Strengthens all connective tissues. Essential for proper functioning of adrenal and thyroid glands. *Promotes healing in every condition of ill health.* Helps prevent and cure the common cold. Protects against all forms of stress: physical and mental. Protects against harmful effects of toxic chemicals in environment, food, water and air. Counteracts the toxic effect of drugs. Has been used successfully in rattlesnake bite, and as a general natural antibiotic. Specific against fever, all sorts of infections and gastrointestinal disorders. General detoxicant. Specific protector against toxic effects of cadmium.

DEFICIENCY SYMPTOMS

Deficiency may lead to tooth decay, soft gums (pyorrhea), skin hemorrhages, capillary weakness, deterioration in collagen, anemia, slow healing of sores and wounds, premature aging, thyroid insufficiency, lowered resistance to all infections and toxic effect of drugs and environmental poisons. Prolonged efficiency may cause scurvy.

NATURAL SOURCES

All fresh fruits and vegetables. Particularly rich sources: rose hips, citrus fruits, black currants, strawberries, apples, persimmons, guavas, acerola cherries, potatoes, cabbage, broccoli, tomatoes, turnip greens and green bell peppers.

RDA

Official recommendation: 60 mg. Therapeutically used in large doses, from 100 to 10,000 mg. a day. In acute poisonings or infections, 1,000 to 2,000 mg., preferably in injection form, can be given each 1½ or 2 hours. Vitamin C is non-toxic, even in massive doses.

VITAMIN D

Ergosterol, Viosterol, Calciferol. Known as the "Sunshine Vitamin." Measured in micrograms (mcg.) or International Units (IU).

FUNCTION

Assists in assimilation of calcium, phosphorus and other minerals from the digestive tract. Necessary for the healthy function of parathyroid glands, which regulate the calcium level in the blood. Essential for the health of thyroid gland. Very important in infancy and adolescence for the proper formation of teeth and bones. Prevents rickets. Helps prevent tooth decay and pyorrhea. Some scientists feel that vitamin D is a hormone rather than a vitamin, as its functions parallel those of hormones.

DEFICIENCY SYMPTOMS

Prolonged deficiency may lead to rickets, tooth decay, pyorrhea, osteomalacia, osteoporosis, retarded growth and poor bone formation in children, muscular weakness, lack of vigor, deficient assimilation of minerals and premature aging.

NATURAL SOURCES

Fish liver oils, egg yolks, milk, butter, sprouted seeds, mushrooms, sunflower seeds. Vitamin D is produced by sunlight on the oily skin and absorbed by the body through the skin.

RDA

5-10 mcg. (200-400 IU). Therapeutically, up to 4,000 to 5,000 units a day *for adults,* or half of this for children, is a safe dose, if taken for not longer than one month. Can be toxic if taken in excessive doses, especially by infants.

VITAMIN E

Tocopherol. D-alpha tocopherol, or tocopheryl; di-tocopherol. Mixed tocopherols. For most therapeutic purposes, only *d-alpha tocopherol* is used. Usually measured in International Units (IU) or alpha tocopherol equivalents.

FUNCTIONS

Oxygenates the tissues and markedly reduces the need for oxygen intake. Prevents unsaturated fatty acids, sex hormones and fat soluble vitamins from being destroyed in the body by oxygen. Prevents rancidity when added to other substances. An effective vasodilator — dilates blood vessels and improves circulation. Prevents scar tissue formation in burns and sores. An effective anti-thrombin and natural anti-coagulant — prevents death through thrombosis or blood clot. Can improve circulation in tiniest capillaries. Protects lungs and other tissues from damage by polluted air. Retards the aging processes. Essential for healthy function of reproductive organs. Indispensable for the prevention and treatment of heart disease, asthma, phlebitis, arthritis, burns (speeds healing and prevents scar-building), angina pectoris, emphysema, leg ulcers, "restless" legs, varicose veins, hypoglycemia, and many other conditions. Improves glycogen storage in the muscles. Has been used successfully in the prevention and treatment of reproductive disorders, miscarriages, male and female infertility, stillbirths, and menopausal and menstrual disorders.

DEFICIENCY SYMPTOMS

Deficiency may lead to degenerative developments in coronary system, pulmonary embolism, strokes and heart disease. May cause degeneration of the epithelial and germinal cells of the testicles and lead to loss of sexual potency. Prolonged deficiency may cause reproductive disorders, abortions, miscarriages, male or female sterility, muscular disorders and increased fragility of red blood cells.

NATURAL SOURCES

Unrefined, cold-pressed, crude vegetable oils, particularly wheat germ oil and soybean oil. All whole raw or sprouted seeds, nuts and grains – especially whole wheat. Fresh wheat germ (must be absolutely fresh, less than a week old; rancid wheat germ does *not* contain vitamin E). Green leafy vegetables and eggs.

RDA

8-10 mg. tocopherol equivalents (12-15 IU). Expert nutritionists estimate the actual requirement at 100 to 200 IU a day. Therapeutic doses: From 200 to 2,400 IU daily, depending on condition. Persons with high blood pressure, heart conditions or rheumatic heart disease, or those taking more than 600 IU a day, should ask their doctor to determine the best dosage for them, *Known antagonists* (which interfere with or destroy vitamin E in the body): inorganic iron, estrogen (synthetic estrogen taken as drugs), chlorine, or chlorinated water.

BIOFLAVONOIDS

Vitamin P. Bioflavonoid complex: citrin, hesperidin, quercitin. Rutin. Considered to be a part of the vitamin C-complex. Measured in milligrams (mg.).

FUNCTIONS

Strengthens capillary walls and prevents or corrects capillary fragility. Prevents capillary hemorrhaging and acts as an anti-coagulant. May prevent strokes. Protects vitamin C from destruction in the body by oxidation. Vitamin C synergist – enhances its property. Beneficial in hypertension, respiratory infections, hemorrhoids, varicose veins, hemorrhaging, bleeding gums, eczema, psoriasis, cirrhosis of the liver, retinal hemorrhages, radiation sickness, coronary thrombosis, arteriosclerosis.

DEFICIENCY SYMPTOMS

Causes capillary fragility. Appearance of purplish or blue spots on the skin. Diminished vitamin C activity. Susceptibility to above-mentioned conditions.

NATURAL SOURCES

Fresh fruits and vegetables; buckwheat; citrus fruits, especially the pulp; green peppers; grapes, apricots, strawberries, black currants, cherries, prunes. Cooking largely destroys bioflavonoids.

RDA

Not established. Usual therapeutic doses 50 to 200 mg. or more. The FDA has determined that bioflavonoids do not have any nutritional, therapeutic, or preventive value. Therefore, the above information regarding the function, deficiency symptoms and sources of bioflavonoids is offered for educational and experimental purposes only, not as an endorsement or recommendation.

VITAMIN F

Essential fatty acids, linoleic and linolenic being considered the most important fatty acids. Measured in grams or milligrams (mg.).

FUNCTIONS

Considered to be important in lowering blood cholesterol in atherosclerosis and, thus, preventing heart disease. Essential for normal glandular activity — especially the adrenal glands. Necessary to healthy skin and all mucous membranes. A growth-promoting factor. Needed for many metabolic processes. Promotes the availability of calcium and phosphorus to the cells. Can protect from damage by excessive radiation.

DEFICIENCY SYMPTOMS

Deficiency may lead to skin disorders, such as eczema, acne and dry skin, gallstones, falling hair, retarded growth, impairment in reproductive functions, kidney disorders, prostate disorders, menstrual disturbances.

NATURAL SOURCES

Unprocessed and unrefined vegetable oils, especially soybean oil, corn oil, flaxseed oil, safflower oil and sunflower oil. Also available in capsule form.

RDA

Not established. National Research Council says that "fat intake (should) include essential unsaturated fatty acids to extent of at least 1 percent of the total calories."

VITAMIN K

Menadione. Measured in milligrams (mg.).

FUNCTION

Essential for the production of prothrombin, a substance which aids in blood clotting. Important for normal liver function. An "anti-hemorrhaging" vitamin. An important vitality and longevity factor. Involved in energy-producing activities of the tissues, particularly the nervous system.

DEFICIENCY SYMPTOMS

May cause hemorrhages anywhere in the body due to prolonged blood-clotting time, such as nosebleeds, bleeding ulcers, etc. Lowered vitality. Premature aging.

NATURAL SOURCES

Kelp, alfalfa and other green plants, soybean oil, egg yolks, cow's milk, liver. Also manufactured by the normal bacteria in the healthy intestines.

RDA

Not established. Estimated safe and adequate intake: 70-140 mcg.

VITAMIN T

Sesame seed factor, known to be present, but unidentified, often referred to as vitamin T.

FUNCTION

Re-establishes platelet integrity in the blood. Useful in correcting nutritional anemia. Promotes the formation of blood platelets and combats anemia and hemophilia. Useful in improving fading memory.

NATURAL SOURCES

Sesame seeds, "Tahini," raw sesame butter, egg yolks and some vegetable oils.

VITAMIN U

Vitamin-like factor found in some vegetables, notably cabbage.

FUNCTION

Promotes healing activity in peptic ulcers, particularly in duodenal ulcers.

NATURAL SOURCES

Raw cabbage juice, fresh cabbage, homemade sauerkraut.

IMPORTANT NOTE ON VITAMINS

The deficiency symptoms listed in this *Vitamin Guide* could occur only after a prolonged inadequate dietary intake or the body's chronic inability to assimilate dietary vitamins. The symptoms listed do not alone prove an existing nutritional deficiency, as similar symptoms may be caused by a great number of conditions or functional disorders. If, after an adequate vitamin supplementation, these symptoms persist, they may indicate a condition other than a vitamin or nutritional deficiency.

When suffering from serious diseases, it is unwise to attempt self-treatment, with vitamins, minerals or any other way, but it is advisable to consult a doctor, preferably one who is nutritionally oriented, and to abide by his expert advice on the choice of suitable therapy.

MINERAL GUIDE

Common minerals and trace elements, their functions,
deficiency symptoms, natural sources and
Recommended Daily Allowances (RDA)

CALCIUM (Ca)

FUNCTIONS

Essential for all vital functions of the body. Needed to build bones and teeth, and for normal growth. Essential for heart action and all muscle activity. High calcium dietary intake can protect against radioactive strontium 90. Needed for normal clotting of the blood, and in many enzyme functions. Is of extreme importance in pregnancy and lactation. Speeds all healing processes. Helps to maintain balance between Na, K and Mg. Essential for proper utilization of phosphorus and vitamins D, A and C.

DEFICIENCY SYMPTOMS

Deficiency may cause osteomalacia and osteoporosis (porous and fragile bones), retarded growth, tooth decay, rickets, nervousness, mental depression, heart palpitations, muscle cramps and spasms, insomnia and irritability.

NATURAL SOURCES

Milk and cheese; most raw vegetables, especially dark leafy vegetables such as endive, lettuce, watercress, kale, cabbage, dandelion greens, brussels sprouts and broccoli. Sesame seeds are excellent source. Other good sources are oats, navy beans, almonds, walnuts, millet, sunflower seeds, tortillas. Bone meal or calcium lactate are rich natural supplements.

RDA

Adults: 800-1200 mg. Children, or women during pregnancy or lactation: 1,000-1,400 mg.

PHOSPHORUS (P)

FUNCTION

Phosphorus is a mineral colleague of calcium. They work together and must be present in proper balance to be effective. Needed for building bones and teeth. It is an important factor in carbohydrate metabolism and in maintaining an acid-alkaline balance in the blood and tissues. Needed for healthy nerves and for efficient mental activity.

DEFICIENCY SYMPTOMS
May result in poor mineralization of bones, in retarded growth, rickets, deficient nerve and brain function, reduced sexual power, general weakness.

NATURAL SOURCES
Whole grains, seeds and nuts, legumes, dairy products, egg yolks, fish, dried fruits, corn.

RDA
Adults: 800-1,200 mg. Children, or women during pregnancy or lactation: 1,000 to 1,400 mg. Deficiencies of phosphorus are rare, as it is one of the most plentiful elements in diet.

MAGNESIUM (Mg)

FUNCTIONS
Important catalyst in many enzyme reactions, especially those involved in energy production. Helps in utilization of vitamins B and E, fats, calcium and other minerals. Needed for healthy muscle tone, healthy bones and for efficient synthesis of proteins. Essential for heart health. Regulates acid-alkaline balance in the system. Involved in lecithin production. A natural tranquilizer. Prevents building up of cholesterol and consequent atherosclerosis.

DEFICIENCY SYMPTOMS
Continuous deficiency will cause a loss of calcium and potassium from the body, with consequent deficiencies of those minerals. Deficiency can lead to kidney damage and kidney stones, muscle cramps, atherosclerosis, heart attack, epileptic seizures, nervous irritability, marked depression and confusion, impaired protein metabolism and premature wrinkles.

NATURAL SOURCES
Nuts, soybeans, raw and cooked green leafy vegetables, particularly kale, endive, chard, celery, beettops, alfalfa, figs, apples, lemons, peaches, almonds, whole grains, sunflower seeds, brown rice and sesame seeds.

RDA
350-400 mg. Therapeutic doses up to 700 mg. a day. Magnesium chloride is the best form of supplementary magnesium, although other forms can be used also.

POTASSIUM (K)

FUNCTIONS

Important as an alkalizing agent in keeping proper acid-alkaline balance in the blood and tissues. Prevents over-acidity. Essential for muscle contraction, therefore it is important for proper heart function, especially for normal heart beat. Promotes the secretion of hormones. Helps the kidneys in detoxification of blood. Prevents female disorders by stimulating the endocrine hormone production. Involved in proper function of the nervous system.

DEFICIENCY SYMPTOMS

Severe deficiency may cause excessive accumulation of sodium (salt) in the tissues, with severe consequences of sodium poisoning, edema, high blood pressure and heart failure. May damage the heart muscle and lead to heart attacks. Prolonged deficiency causes constipation, nervous disorders, extreme fatigue, muscular weakness and low blood sugar (hypoglycemia).

NATURAL SOURCES

All vegetables, especially green leafy vegetables, oranges, whole grains, sunflower seeds, nuts and milk. Potatoes, especially potato peelings, and bananas are especially good sources.

RDA

1,875-5,625 mg. (Estimated safe and adequate intake.)

SODIUM (Na)

FUNCTIONS

Sodium is closely associated with potassium and chlorine in many vital functions in the body. These three minerals are known to maintain proper electrolyte balance by changing into electrically charged ions which carry nerve impulse conduction and transportation. They control and maintain osmotic pressure, which is responsible for the transportation of nutrients from the intestines into the blood. They are involved in keeping the body fluid at normal levels. Sodium is necessary for hydrochloric acid production in the stomach, and plays a part in many other glandular secretions.

DEFICIENCY SYMPTOMS

Deficiencies are rare, and may be caused by excessive sweating, prolonged use of diuretics or chronic diarrhea. Deficiency may cause nausea, muscular weakness, heat exhaustion, mental apathy, respiratory failure. Oversupply of sodium is a more common problem because of overuse of dietary sodium chloride (common salt). Too much sodium may lead to water retention, high blood pressure, stomach ulcers, stomach cancer, hardening of arteries and heart disease.

NATURAL SOURCES

Kelp, celery, romaine lettuce, watermelon, asparagus, sea water supplement, sea salt.

RDA

1,100-3,300 mg. (estimated safe and adequate intake). 200 mg. to 600 mg. a day, according to Dr. Ragnar Berg. Some authorities list as 2 to 4 grams. More than sufficient in normal diet of natural foods without added salt.

CHLORINE (Cl)

FUNCTIONS

Essential for the production of hydrochloric acid in the stomach, which is needed for proper protein digestion and for mineral assimilation. Helps liver in its detoxifying activity. Involved in the maintenance of proper fluid and electrolyte balance in the system.

DEFICIENCY SYMPTOMS

Impaired digestion of foods. Derangement of fluid levels in the body.

NATURAL SOURCES

Seaweed (kelp), watercress, avocado, chard, tomatoes, cabbage, endive, kale, turnip, celery, cucumber, asparagus, pineapple, oats, salt water fish.

RDA

500 mg.

SULFUR (S)

FUNCTIONS

"The beauty mineral." Vital for healthy hair, skin and nails. Involved in oxidation-reduction processes.

DEFICIENCY SYMPTOMS

Brittle nails and hair. Skin disorders: eczema, rashes, blemishes.

NATURAL SOURCES

Radish, turnip, onions, celery, horseradish, string beans, watercress, kale, soybeans, fish, meat.

RDA

Not established. Considered to be sufficient in an adequate diet.

IRON (Fe)

FUNCTIONS

Essential for the formation of hemoglobin, which carries the oxygen from the lungs to every cell of the body. Builds up the quality of the blood and increases resistance to stress and disease.

DEFICIENCY SYMPTOMS

Deficiency of dietary iron may cause nutritional anemia, lowered resistance to disease, a general run-down feeling, shortness of breath during exercise, headaches, pale complexion and low interest in sex. Deficiencies are common among young girls and pregnant women.

NATURAL SOURCES

Apricots, peaches, bananas, black molasses, prunes, raisins, brewer's yeast, whole grain cereals, turnip greens, spinach, beettops, alfalfa, beets, sunflower seeds, walnuts, sesame seeds, whole rye, dry beans, lentils, kelp, dulse, liver, egg yolks.

A sufficient amount of gastric enzymes, especially of hydrochloric acid, is needed for proper assimilation of iron. Older people are often anemic in spite of plentiful iron in the diet, because they lack sufficient hydrochloric acid in their stomachs. For these reasons, the iron-containing fruits, which contain their own enzymes and acids needed for iron digestion and assimilation, are the most reliable sources of dietary iron. Vitamin C (up to 500 mg. daily) also aids in the absorption of dietary and supplementary iron. *NOTE*: Coffee and tea interfere with iron absorption.

RDA

10 mg. for males, 18 mg. for females.

COPPER (Cu)

FUNCTIONS

Similar to those of iron. Iron cannot be absorbed without copper. Necessary for production of RNA. Involved in protein metabolism, in healing processes and in keeping the natural color of the hair. Aids development of bones, brain, nerves and connective tissues.

DEFICIENCY SYMPTOMS

Deficiency of copper may cause anemia, loss of hair, impaired respiration, digestive disturbances, graying of hair, heart damage.

NATURAL SOURCES

Foods rich in copper are generally those rich in iron. Especially good sources: almonds, beans, peas, green leafy vegetables, whole grain products, prunes, raisins, pomegranates, liver.

RDA

2-3 mg. (Estimated safe and adequate intake.)

IODINE (I)

FUNCTIONS

Essential for formation of *thyroxin* — the thyroid hormone which regulates much of physical and mental activity. Regulates the rate of metabolism, energy production, and body weight. Helps to prevent rough and wrinkled skin. Plentiful dietary iodine can prevent poisoning by radioactive iodine 131. Essential for the health of thyroid gland.

DEFICIENCY SYMPTOMS

Deficiency may cause goiter and enlargement of the thyroid gland, or exophthalmic goiter. Prolonged deficiency may result in cretinism. Dietary lack may lead to anemia, fatigue, lethargy, loss of interest in sex, slowed pulse, low blood pressure and a tendency toward obesity. A serious deficiency may result in thyroid cancer, high blood cholesterol and heart disease.

NATURAL SOURCES

The best dietary sources of iodine are kelp, dulse and other seaweed (available in tablet form). Other good sources are: swiss chard, turnip greens, garlic, watercress, pineapples, pears, artichokes, citrus fruits, egg yolks, and, of course, seafoods and fish liver oils.

RDA

150 mcg. (0.15 mg.)

MANGANESE (Mn)

FUNCTIONS

Important component of several enzymes which are involved in the metabolism of carbohydrates, fats and proteins. Combined with choline, helps in fat digestion and utilization. Helps to nourish the nerves and brain and assists in the proper coordinative action between brain, nerves and muscles in every part of the body. Involved in normal reproduction and the function of mammary glands.

DEFICIENCY SYMPTOMS

Deficiency may cause retarded growth, digestive disturbances, abnormal bone development and deformities, male and female sterility, impotence in men, poor equilibrium, asthma and myasthenia gravis.

NATURAL SOURCES

Green leafy vegetables, spinach, beets, Brussels sprouts, blueberries, oranges, grapefruit, apricots, the outer coating of nuts and grains (bran), peas, kelp, raw egg yolk and fresh wheat germ.

RDA

Not known. Estimated safe and adequate intake: 2.5-5.0 mg.

ZINC (Zn)

FUNCTIONS

Essential for the formation of RNA and DNA and for the synthesis of body protein. Involved in many enzymatic processes and hormone activities, especially in reproductive hormones. Affects tissue respiration and normal growth processes. Needed in the construction of insulin molecule. As a constituent of insulin, involved in carbohydrate and energy metabolism. Essential for normal growth and development of sex organs and for the normal function of prostate gland. Helps the body to get rid of toxic carbon dioxide. Increases the rate of healing of burns and wounds. Needed for proper metabolism of vitamin a. Essential for bone formation.

DEFICIENCY SYMPTOMS

Retarded growth, birth defects, hypogonadism or underdeveloped gonads (sex organs), enlargement of prostate gland and impaired sexual functions, loss of fertility, lowered resistance to infections, slow healing of wounds and skin diseases, white spots on finger and toe nails, poor sense of taste and smell. Deficiency may cause lethargy, apathy, hair loss, dandruff and loss of interest in learning. Zinc deficiency is also associated with atherosclerosis, epilepsy and osteoporosis.

NATURAL SOURCES

Wheat bran and fresh wheat germ, pumpkin seeds, sunflower seeds, brewer's yeast, milk, eggs, onions, oysters, herring, nuts, green leafy vegetables. Zinc in grains and seeds is not easily available for assimilation because it is "locked" by phytin, but becomes "unlocked" by the fermentation process (as in sour bread) and by sprouting.

RDA

15 mg. (estimated safe and adequate intake). Supplementary doses up to 30 mg. Therapeutic doses under doctor's supervision up to 600 mg. a day.

SILICON (Si)

FUNCTIONS

Essential for building strong bones and for normal growth of hair, nails and teeth. Beneficial in all healing processes and protects body against many diseases, such as tuberculosis, irritations in mucous membranes and skin disorders.

DEFICIENCY SYMPTOMS

Soft brittle nails, aging symptoms of skin such as wrinkles, thinning or loss of hair, poor bone development, insomnia, osteoporosis.

NATURAL SOURCES

Young green plants, such as horsetail, common nettle and alfalfa; kelp, flaxseed, steel-cut oats, apples, strawberries, grapes, beets, onions, parsnips, almonds, peanuts, sunflower seeds.

RDA

Not known.

FLUORINE (F)

FUNCTIONS

Essential for bone and tooth building. Protects against infections. Acts as an internal antiseptic. Excessive fluorine, especially in form of sodium fluoride (as in fluoridated water) causes mottled teeth and can be toxic.

DEFICIENCY SYMPTOMS

Unknown.

NATURAL SOURCES

Organic fluorine is found in steel-cut oats, sunflower seeds, milk and cheese, carrots, garlic, beettops, green vegetables and almonds. Also, normally present in sea water and naturally hard water.

RDA

Not known. May be needed in minute quantities.

CHROMIUM (Cr)

FUNCTIONS

Integral part of many enzymes and hormones. Co-factor with insulin to remove glucose from the blood into cells. Important in cholesterol metabolism. Essential for proper utilization of sugar. Involved in the synthesis of heart protein. Contains so-called Glucose Tolerance Factor.

DEFICIENCY SYMPTOMS

Severe deficiency may be a contributing cause of diabetes, high or low blood sugar, hardening of arteries and heart disease.

NATURAL SOURCES

Normally present in natural waters, particularly in hard (highly mineralized) water. The natural complex of the chromium, the Glucose Tolerance Factor, is present in whole grain bread, mushrooms, liver, brewer's yeast, raw sugar and cane juice.

RDA

Not known. Estimated safe and adequate intake: 0.05-2.0 mg. Needed in minute quantities. White sugar in the diet contributes to the loss of chromium from the body and consequent deficiency.

MOLYBDENUM (Mo)

FUNCTIONS

Integral part of certain enzymes, particularly those involved in oxidation processes. Considered to be an antagonist to copper, thus may have protective action in copper poisoning. Involved with proper carbohydrate metabolism.

DEFICIENCY SYMPTOMS

Unknown.

NATURAL SOURCES

Whole cereals, especially brown rice, millet and buckwheat, brewer's yeast, legumes, naturally hard water.

RDA

Not known. Estimated safe and adequate intake: 0.15-0.5 mg. Needed in minute quantities.

COBALT (Co)

FUNCTIONS

Integral component of vitamin B_{12} and necessary for the synthesis of this vitamin. If cobalt is present in the system in needed amounts, vitamin B_{12} can be synthesized in the system. Aids in hemoglobin formation.

DEFICIENCY SYMPTOMS

May lead to development of pernicious anemia.

NATURAL SOURCES

Liver. All green, leafy vegetables.

RDA

Not known. Needed in minute quantities.

LITHIUM (Li)

FUNCTIONS

Involved in sodium metabolism and its transportation in nerves and muscles. Associated with function of the autonomic or involuntary nervous systems.

DEFICIENCY SYMPTOMS

May lead to nervous and mental disorders, particularly paranoid schizophrenia.

NATURAL SOURCES

Kelp, sea water, natural lithium-rich mineral springs.

Not known. For therapeutic uses, lithium is available in tablet form, as lithium carbonate, on prescription. Can be highly toxic in overdoses.

SELENIUM (Se)

FUNCTIONS
Antioxidant; its biological activity closely related to vitamin E. Has a "sparing" effect on the body's uses of vitamin E. Prevents the hemoglobin in red blood cells from being damaged by oxidation. Can help in regeneration of the liver after damage, especially by cirrhosis. May slow down the aging processes by an inhibiting action on formation of free radicals. Protects body from toxic damage by mercury poisoning. Is essential for the function of the enzyme glutathione peroxidase.

DEFICIENCY SYMPTOMS
Liver damage, muscle degeneration, premature aging. Prolonged, severe deficiency may lead to development of cancer, especially in digestive and eliminative tract.

NATURAL SOURCES
Brewer's yeast (not primary grown yeast), sea water, kelp, garlic, mushrooms, organically grown foods, seafoods, milk, eggs, cereals and most vegetables.

RDA
Not established. Estimated safe and adequate intake: 0.05-0.2 mg. Toxic in overdoses.

IMPORTANT NOTES ON TRACE MINERALS
There are a few other trace minerals, or micronutrients, which are considered to be important in human nutrition, such as *boron, strontium, nickel, bromine,* and *vanadium,* to name a few. They have been found in the human body in minute quantities (traces), but whether they are important for the body processes or not, has not been determined, as deficiency symptoms have not been observed.

We wish to caution those who attempt to supplement their diets with the trace elements discussed in this section that although microscopic amounts of these substances are required for nutritional welfare, these micronutrients can be extremely toxic if taken in too large amounts. Therefore, great care should be exercised when considering supplementation of the diet with any isolated minerals, but particularly with trace minerals, so that the body's delicate chemistry will not be upset and possible harmful effects will be avoided. The best way to avoid toxicity and imbalances, is to use multi-mineral-trace element supplementation, especially in such natural forms as sea water, mined minerals, mineral waters, bone meal, kelp, raw vegetable and fruit juices, and natural foods mentioned in this *Mineral Guide.*

ACID-ALKALINE FOOD CHART

Balanced body chemistry is of utmost importance for the maintenance of health and correction of disease. Acidosis, or over-acidity in the body tissues, is one of the basic causes of many diseases, especially the arthritic and rheumatic diseases.

All foods are "burned" in the body — more commonly called "digested" — leaving an ash as the result of the "burning", or the digestion. This food ash can be neutral, acid or alkaline, depending largely on the mineral composition of the foods. Some foods leave an acid residue or ash, some alkaline. The acid ash (acidosis) results when there is a depletion of the alkali reserve or the diminution in the reserve supply of fixed bases in the blood and the tissues of the body.

It is, therefore, vitally important that there is a proper ratio between acid and alkaline foods in the diet. The natural ratio in a normal healthy body is approximately 4 to 1 — four parts alkaline to one part acid, or 80% to 20%. When such an ideal ratio is maintained, the body has a strong resistance against disease. In the healing of disease, when the patient usually has acidosis, the higher the ratio of alkaline elements in the diet, the faster will be the recovery. Alkalis neutralize the acids. Therefore in the treatment of most diseases it is important that the patient's diet includes plenty of alkaline-ash foods to offset the effect of acid-forming foods and leave a safe margin of alkalinity.

A healthy body usually keeps large alkaline reserves which are used to meet the emergency demands if too many acid-producing foods are consumed. But these normal reserves can be depleted. When the alkaline-acid ratio drops to 3 to 1, health can be seriously menaced. Your body can function normally and sustain health only in the presence of adequate alkaline reserves and the proper acid-alkaline ratio in all the body tissues and the blood.

The Airola Diet, as described in *Directions: 1*, will assure a balanced body chemistry and a proper alkaline-acid ratio, as the acid-forming foods from the first food group (seeds, nuts and grains) are well balanced by the alkali-forming foods from the second and third food groups (vegetables and fruits). For optimum health and maximum resistance to disease, it is imperative that your diet is slightly over-alkaline. The ideal ratio, according to the world's foremost authority on the relationship between the acid-alkaline ratio in the diet in health and disease, Dr. Ragnar Berg, is about 80% alkali-producing foods and 20% acid-producing foods.

Here are tables of common foods with an approximate potential acidity or alkalinity, as present in one ounce of food.

ALKALI-FORMING FOODS

Figs	30.0	Potatoes	2.0
Soybeans	12.0	Pineapple	2.0
Lima beans	12.0	Cabbage	1.8
Apricots	9.5	Grapefruit	1.7
Spinach	8.0	Tomatoes	1.7
Turnip or beettops	8.0	Peaches	1.5
Raisins	7.0	Apples	1.0
Almonds	3.6	Grapes	1.0
Carrots	3.5	Bananas	1.0
Dates	3.0	Watermelon	1.0
Celery	2.5	Millet	0.5
Cucumber	2.5	Brazil nuts	0.5
Cantaloupe	2.5	Coconuts	0.5
Lettuce	2.2	Buckwheat	0.5
Watercress	2.0		

NEUTRAL (OR NEAR-NEUTRAL) ASH FOODS

Milk	Vegetable oils
Butter	White sugar

ACID-FORMING FOODS

Oysters	5.0	Rice	2.5
Veal	3.5	Whole wheat or	
Most fish	3.5	rye bread	2.5
Organ meats	3.0	Most nuts, except almonds	
Liver	3.0	and Brazil nuts	2.0
Chicken	3.0	Natural cheese	1.5
Most meats and fowl	3.0	Lentils	1.5
Eggs	3.0	Peanuts	1.0
Most grains	3.0		

Most grains are acid-forming, except millet and buckwheat, which are considered to be alkaline. Sprouted seeds and grains become more alkaline in the process of sprouting.

All vegetable and fruit juices are highly alkaline. The most alkali-forming juices are: fig juice, green juices of all green vegetables and tops, carrot, beet, celery, pineapple and citrus juices. Vegetable broth (see *Recipes*) is an extremely alkalizing drink.

(Designed for the maintenance of good nutrition

BASED ON TABLES PUBLISHED BY FOOD AND NUTRITION
RESEARCH COUNCIL.

| | AGE | WEIGHT | | HEIGHT | | PROTEIN | FAT-SOLUBLE VITAMINS | | |
| | | | | | | | VITAMIN A ACTIVITY | VITAMIN D | VITAMIN E ACTIVITY |
	From up to years :	kg.	lb.	cm.	in.	Gm	mcg. RE[a]	mcg.[b]	mg. ∝ TE[c]
INFANTS	0.0-0.5	6	13	60	24	kg. x 2.2	420	10	3
	0.5-1.0	9	20	71	28	kg. x 2.0	400	10	4
CHILDREN	1-3	13	29	90	35	23	400	10	5
	4-6	20	44	112	44	30	500	10	6
	7-10	28	62	132	52	34	700	10	7
MALES	11-14	45	99	157	62	45	1000	10	8
	15-18	66	145	176	69	56	1000	10	10
	19-22	70	154	177	70	56	1000	7.5	10
	23-50	70	154	178	70	56	1000	5	10
	51 +	70	154	178	70	56	1000	5	10
FEMALES	11-14	46	101	157	62	46	800	10	8
	15-18	55	120	163	64	46	800	10	8
	19-22	55	120	163	64	44	800	7.5	8
	23-50	55	120	163	64	44	800	5	8
	51 +	55	120	163	64	44	800	5	8
	Pregnant					+ 30	+ 200	+ 5	+ 2
	Lactating					+ 20	+ 400	+ 5	+ 3

[a]Retinol equivalents. 1 retinol equivalent = 1 mcg retinol or 6 mcg beta carotene.

[b]As cholecalciferol. 10 mcg. cholecalciferol = 400 IU of vitamin D.

[c]alpha-tocopherol equivalents. 1 mg. d-alpha tocopherol = 1 alpha (∝) TE.

[d]1 NE (niacin equivalent) is equal to 1 mg. of niacin or 60 mg. of dietary tryptophan.

DIETARY ALLOWANCES

of practically all healthy people in the U.S.A.)

BOARD, NATIONAL ACADEMY OF SCIENCE, NATIONAL

Revised 1980.

WATER-SOLUBLE VITAMINS							MINERALS					
VITAMIN C	B₁ (Thiamine)	B₂ (Riboflavin)	B₃ (Niacin)	B₆ (Pyridoxine)	FOLIC ACID (Folacin)	B₁₂	CALCIUM	PHOSPHORUS	MAGNESIUM	IRON	ZINC	IODINE
mg	mg.	mg.	mg^d NE	mg.	mcg.	mcg.	mg.	mg.	mg.	mg.	mg.	mcg
35	0.3	0.4	6	0.3	30	0.5	360	240	50	10	3	40
35	0.5	0.6	8	0.6	45	1.5	540	360	70	15	5	50
45	0.7	0.8	9	0.9	100	2.0	800	800	150	15	10	70
45	0.9	1.0	11	1.3	200	2.5	800	800	200	10	10	90
45	1.2	1.4	16	1.6	300	3.0	800	800	250	10	10	120
50	1.4	1.6	18	1.8	400	3.0	1,200	1,200	350	18	15	150
60	1.4	1.7	18	2.0	400	3.0	1,200	1,200	400	18	15	150
60	1.5	1.7	19	2.2	400	3.0	800	800	350	10	15	150
60	1.4	1.6	18	2.2	400	3.0	800	800	350	10	15	150
60	1.2	1.4	16	2.2	400	3.0	800	800	350	10	15	150
50	1.1	1.3	15	1.8	400	3.0	1,200	1,200	300	18	15	150
60	1.1	1.3	14	2.0	400	3.0	1,200	1,200	300	18	15	150
60	1.1	1.3	14	2.0	400	3.0	800	800	300	18	15	150
60	1.0	1.2	13	2.0	400	3.0	800	800	300	18	15	150
60	1.0	1.2	13	2.0	400	3.0	800	800	300	10	15	150
+20	+0.4	+0.3	+2	+0.6	+400	+1.0	+400	+400	+150	e	+5	+25
+40	+0.5	+0.5	+5	+0.5	+100	+1.0	+400	+400	+150	e	+10	+25

[e]The increased requirement during pregnancy cannot be met by the iron content of habitual American diets nor by the existing iron stores of many women; therefore the use of 30-60 mg. of supplemental iron is recommended. Iron needs during lactation are not substantially different from those of nonpregnant women, but continued supplementation of the mother for 2-3 months after parturition is advisable in order to replenish stores depleted by pregnancy.

COMPOSITION OF FOODS
100 grams, edible portion

(dash (—) denotes lack of reliable data for a constituent believed to be present in measurable amount)

FOOD	CALORIES	PROTEINS grams	FATS grams	CARBOHYDRATES grams	CALCIUM mg.	PHOSPHORUS mg.	MAGNESIUM mg.	IRON mg.	SODIUM mg.	POTASSIUM mg.	VITAMIN A VALUE IU	B₁ mg.	B₂ mg.	NIACIN mg.	VITAMIN C mg.
ACEROLA cherry, raw	28	.4	.3	6.8	12	11	—	.2	8	83	—	.02	.06	0.4	1,300
ACEROLA JUICE, raw	23	.4	.3	4.8	10	9	—	.5	3	—	—	.02	.06	.4	1,600
ALMONDS, dried	598	18.6	54.2	19.5	234	504	270	4.7	4	773	0	.24	.92	3.5	trace
APPLES, freshly harvested	58	.2	.6	14.5	7	10	8	.3	1	110	90	.03	.02	.4	7-20
APPLE JUICE, canned or bottled	47	.1	trace	11.9	6	9	4	.6	1	101	—	.01	.02	.1	1
APRICOTS, raw	51	1.0	.2	12.8	17	23	12	.5	1	281	2,700	0.3	.04	.6	10
APRICOTS, dried, uncooked	260	5.0	.5	66.5	67	108	62	5.5	26	979	10,900	.01	.16	3.3	12
ARTICHOKES, globe or French, raw	9-47	2.9	.2	10.6	51	88	—	1.3	43	430	160	.08	.05	1.0	12
cooked	8-44	2.8	.2	9.6	51	68	—	1.1	30	301	150	.07	.04	.7	8
ARTICHOKES, Jerusalem, raw	7-75	2.3	.1	16.7	14	78	11	3.4	—	—	20	.2	.06	1.3	4
ASPARAGUS, raw spears	26	2.5	.2	5.0	22	62	20	1.0	2	278	900	.18	.20	1.5	33
cooked spears	20	2.2	.2	3.6	21	50	14	.6	1	183	900	.16	.18	1.4	26
AVOCADOS, raw	167	2.1	16.4	6.3	10	42	45	.6	4	604	290	.11	.20	1.6	14
BANANAS, common, raw	85	1.1	.2	22.2	8	26	33	.7	1	370	190	.05	.06	.7	10
BARLEY, pearled, light	349	8.2	1.0	78.8	16	189	37	2.0	3	160	0	.12	.05	3.1	0

Food															
BEANS, common white, cooked	118	7.8	.6	21.2	50	148	37	2.7	7	416	0	.14	.07	.7	0
red, cooked	347	7.8	.5	21.4	38	140	–	2.7	3	340	trace	.11	.06	.7	–
pinto, raw	349	22.9	1.2	63.7	135	457	–	6.4	10	984	–	.84	.21	2.2	–
lima, immature cooked	123	8.4	.5	22.1	52	142	46	2.8	2	650	290	.24	.12	1.4	29
lima, mature, cooked	138	8.2	.6	25.6	29	154	48	3.1	2	612	20	.13	.06	.7	–
mung, sprouted, raw	38	3.8	.2	6.6	19	64	–	1.3	5	223	600	.8	.13	.8	19
green, raw	32	1.9	.2	7.1	56	44	32	.8	7	243	540	.07	.11	.5	19
green, cooked	25	1.6	.2	5.4	50	37	21	.6	4	151	20	.03	.09	.5	12
BEETS, red, raw	43	1.6	.1	9.9	16	33	25	.7	60	335	20	.03	.05	.4	10
red, cooked	32	1.1	.1	7.2	14	23	15	.5	43	208	20	.03	.04	.3	6
BEET GREENS, raw	24	2.2	.3	4.6	119	40	106	3.3	130	570	6,100	.10	.22	.4	30
cooked	18	1.7	.2	3.3	99	25	–	1.9	76	332	5,000	.07	.15	.3	15
BLACKBERRIES, raw	58	1.2	.9	12.9	32	19	30	.9	1	170	200	.03	.04	.4	21
BLUEBERRIES, raw	62	.7	.5	15.3	15	13	6	1.0	1	81	100	.03	.06	.5	14
BRAZIL NUTS, raw	654	14.3	66.9	10.9	186	693	225	3.4	1	715	trace	.96	.12	1.6	–
BROCCOLI, raw spears	32	3.6	.3	5.9	103	78	24	1.1	15	382	2,500	.10	.23	.9	113
cooked	26	3.1	.3	4.5	88	62	21	.8	10	267	2,500	.09	.20	.8	90
BRUSSELS SPROUTS, raw	45	4.9	.4	8.3	36	80	29	1.5	14	390	550	.10	.16	.9	102
cooked	36	4.2	.4	6.4	32	72	21	1.1	10	273	520	.08	.14	.8	87
BUCKWHEAT, whole grain	335	11.7	2.4	72.9	114	282	229	3.1	–	448	0	.60	–	4.4	0
BUTTER, salted	716	.6	81.	.4	20	16	2	0	987	23	3,300	–	–	–	0
unsalted	720	.6	82.	.4	20	16	–	0	8	9	3,35–	–	–	0	–
BUTTERMILK, cultured, from skim milk	36	3.6	.1	5.1	121	95	14	trace	130	140	trace	0.4	.18	.1	1
CABBAGE, white, raw	24	1.3	.2	5.4	49	29	13	.4	20	233	130	.05	.05	.3	47
red, raw	31	2.0	.2	6.9	42	35	–	.8	26	268	40	.09	.06	.4	61
savoy, raw	24	2.4	.2	4.6	67	54	–	.9	22	269	200	.05	.08	.3	55
CAROB FLOUR	180	4.5	1.4	80.7	352	81	–	.7	–	–	–	–	–	–	–
CARROTS, raw	42	1.1	.2	9.7	37	36	23	3.8	47	341	11,000	.06	.05	.6	8
CASHEW NUTS	561	17.2	45.7	29.3	38	373	267	1.1	15	464	100	.43	.25	1.8	–
CAULIFLOWER, raw	27	2.7	.2	5.2	25	56	24	.7	13	295	60	.11	.10	.7	78
cooked	22	2.3	.2	4.1	21	42	–	.7	9	206	60	.09	.08	.6	55
CELERY, raw	17	.9	.1	3.9	39	28	22	3.2	126	341	240	.03	.03	.3	9
CHARD, Swiss, raw	25	2.4	0.3	4.6	88	39	65	1.8	147	550	6,500	.06	.17	.5	32
cooked	18	1.8	.2	3.3	73	24	–	–	86	321	5,400	.04	.11	.4	16

FOOD	CALORIES	PROTEINS grams	FATS grams	CARBOHYDRATES grams	CALCIUM mg.	PHOSPHORUS mg.	MAGNESIUM mg.	IRON mg.	SODIUM mg.	POTASSIUM mg.	VITAMIN A VALUE IU	B1 mg.	B2 mg.	NIACIN mg.	VITAMIN C mg.
CHEESE, Blue or Roquefort	368	21.5	30.5	2.0	315	339	48	.5	700	82	1,240	.03	.61	1.2	
Cheddar	398	25.0	32.2	2.1	750	478	45	1.0	229	85	1,310	.03	.46	.1	
Cottage, creamed	106	13.6	4.2	2.9	94	152	—	.3	229	72	170	.03	.25	.1	
Cottage, uncreamed	86	17.0	.3	2.7	90	175	—	.4	290	104	10	.03	.28	.1	
Swiss	370	27.5	28.0	1.7	925	563	—	.9	710	—	1,140	.01	.40	.1	
Brick	370	22.2	30.5	1.9	730	455	—	.9	—	—	1,240	—	.45	.1	
CHERRIES, sour, red, raw	58	1.2	.3	14.3	29	19	14	.4	2	191	1,000	.05	.06	.4	10
sweet, raw	70	1.3	.3	17.4	22	19	9	.4	2	191	110	.05	.06	.4	10
frozen, sour, red	55	1.0	.4	13.4	13	22	10	.7	2	188	1,000	.04	.07	.3	5
CHESTNUTS, fresh	194	2.9	1.5	42.1	27	88	41	1.7	6	454	—	.22	.22	.6	—
COCONUT MEAT, fresh	346	3.5	35.3	9.4	13	95	46	1.7	23	256	0	.05	.02	.5	3
dried	662	7.2	64.9	23.0	26	187	90	3.3	—	588	0	.06	.04	.6	0
COCONUT WATER, from green coconuts	22	.3	.2	4.7	20	13	28	.3	25	147	0	trace	trace	.1	2
COLLARDS, raw, leaves	45	4.8	0.8	7.5	250	82	57	1.5	—	450	9,300	0.16	.31	1.7	152
cooked	33	3.6	.7	5.1	188	52	38	.8	—	262	7,800	.11	.20	1.2	76
CORN, whole-grain, dried, raw	348	8.9	3.9	72.0	22	268	147	2.1	1	284	490	.37	.12	2.2	—
SWEET, on-the-cob, raw	96	3.5	1.0	22.0	3	111	48	.7	trace	280	400	.15	.12	1.7	12
cooked on the cob	91	3.3	1.0	21.0	3	89	19	.6	trace	196	400	.12	.10	1.4	9
flour	368	7.8	2.6	76.8	6	164	106	1.8	1	—	340	.20	.06	1.4	—
bread, whole-grain	207	7.4	7.2	29.1	120	211	—	1.1	628	157	150	.13	.19	.6	1
CRANBERRIES, raw	46	.4	.7	10.8	14	10	8	.5	2	82	40	.03	.02	.1	11
CUCUMBERS, raw	15	.9	.1	3.4	25	27	11	1.1	6	160	250	.03	.04	.2	11

CURRANTS, black, raw	54	1.7	.1	13.1	60	40	15	1.1	3	372	230	.05	.05	.3	200
DANDELION GREENS, raw	45	2.7	.7	9.2	187	66	36	3.1	76	397	14,000	.19	.26	—	35
DATES	274	2.2	.5	72.9	59	63	58	3.0	1	648	50	.09	.10	2.2	0
EGGS, whole, raw	163	12.9	11.5	.9	54	205	11	2.3	122	129	1,180	.11	.30	.1	0
yolks, raw	348	16.0	30.6	.6	141	569	16	5.5	52	98	3,400	.22	.44	.1	0
cooked, whole	163	12.9	11.5	.9	54	205	—	2.3	122	129	1,180	.09	.28	.1	0
EGGPLANT, cooked	19	1.0	.2	4.1	11	21	—	.6	1	150	10	.05	.04	.5	3
ELDERBERRIES, raw	72	2.6	.5	16.4	38	28	10	1.6	—	300	600	.07	.06	.5	36
ENDIVE, raw	20	1.7	.1	4.1	181	54	20	1.7	14	294	3,300	.07	.14	.5	10
FIGS, raw	80	1.2	.3	20.3	35	22	—	.6	2	194	80	.06	.05	.4	2
dried	274	4.3	1.3	69.1	126	77	71	3.0	34	640	80	.10	.10	.7	0
FILBERTS (hazelnuts)	634	12.6	62.4	16.7	209	337	184	3.4	2	704	—	.46	—	.9	trace
GARLIC, raw	137	6.2	.2	30.8	29	202	36	1.5	19	529	trace	.25	.08	.5	15
GOOSEBERRIES, raw	39	0.8	.2	9.7	18	15	9	0.5	1	155	290	—	—	—	33
GRAPEFRUIT, raw	41	.5	.1	10.6	16	16	12	.4	1	135	80	.04	.02	.2	38
juice	39	.5	.1	9.2	9	15	12	.2	1	162	80	.04	.02	.2	38
GRAPES, raw	69	1.3	1.0	15.7	16	12	13	.4	3	158	100	.05	.03	.3	4
juice, bottled	66	.2	trace	16.6	11	12	13	.3	2	116	—	.04	.02	.2	trace
GUAVAS, whole, raw	62	.8	.6	15.	23	42	13	.9	4	289	280	.05	.05	1.2	242
HONEY	304	.3	0	82.3	5	6	3	.5	5	51	0	trace	.04	.3	1
HORSERADISH, raw	87	3.2	.3	19.7	140	64	34	1.4	8	564	—	.07	—	—	81
KALE, leaves, raw	53	6.0	.8	9.0	249	93	37	2.7	75	378	10,000	.17	.26	2.1	186
cooked	39	4.5	.7	6.1	187	58	—	1.6	43	221	8,300	.10	.18	1.6	93
KELP, raw		5.0	1.1		1,093	240	740	3.7	3,007	5,273	—	—	—	—	5-140
KOHLRABI, raw	29	2.0	.1	6.6	41	51	37	.5	8	372	20	.06	.04	.3	66
KUMQUATS, raw	65	.9	.1	17.1	63	23	10	.4	7	236	600	.08	.10	—	36
LEMONS, peeled, raw	27	1.1	.3	8.2	26	16	8	.6	2	138	20	.04	.02	.1	53
LEMON JUICE, raw	25	.5	.2	8.0	7	10	—	.2	1	141	20	.03	.01	.1	46
LENTILS, dry, cooked	106	7.8	trace	19.3	25	119	80	2.1	—	249	20	.07	.06	.6	0
LETTUCE, raw, romaine	18	1.3	.3	3.5	68	25	11	1.4	9	264	1,900	.05	.08	.4	18
iceberg, New York	13	.9	.1	2.9	20	22	—	.5	9	175	330	.06	.06	.3	6
MANGOS, raw	66	.7	.4	16.8	10	13	18	.4	7	189	4,800	.05	.05	1.1	35

FOOD	CALORIES	PROTEINS grams	FATS grams	CARBOHYDRATES grams	CALCIUM mg.	PHOSPHORUS mg.	MAGNESIUM mg.	IRON mg.	SODIUM mg.	POTASSIUM mg.	VITAMIN A VALUE IU	B1 mg.	B2 mg.	NIACIN mg.	VITAMIN C mg.
MILK, cow's, whole	65	3.5	3.5	4.9	118	93	13	trace	50	144	140	.03	.17	.1	1
skim	36	3.6	.1	5.1	121	95	14	trace	52	145	trace	.04	.18	.1	1
dry, whole	502	26.4	27.5	38.2	909	708	98	.5	405	1,330	1,130	.29	1.46	.7	6
dry, skim non-instant	363	35.9	.8	52.3	1,308	1,016	143	.6	532	1,745	30	.35	1.80	.9	7
MILK, goat's, raw	67	3.2	4.0	4.6	129	106	17	.1	34	180	160	.04	.11	.3	1
MILLET, whole-grain	327	9.9	2.9	72.9	20	311	162	6.8	–	430	0	.73	.38	2.3	0
MOLASSES, blackstrap	213	–	–	55	684	84	258	16.1	96	2,927	–	.11	.19	2.0	–
MUSHROOMS, cultivated, raw	28	2.7	.3	4.4	6	116	13	.8	15	414	trace	.10	.46	4.2	3
MUSKMELONS, raw, cantaloupe	30	.7	.1	7.5	14	16	16	.4	12	251	3,400	.04	.03	.6	33
honeydew	33	.8	.3	7.7	14	16		.4	12	251	40	.04	.03	.6	23
MUSTARD GREENS, raw	31	3.0	.5	5.6	183	50	27	3.0	32	377	7,000	.11	.22	.8	97
NECTARINES, raw	64	.6	trace	17.1	4	24	13	.5	6	294	1,650	–	–	–	13
OATMEAL or rolled oats, dry	390	14.2	7.2	68.2	53	405	144	4.5	2	352	0	.60	.14	1.0	0
cooked	55	2.0	1.0	9.7	9	57	21	.6	–	61	0	.08	.02	.1	0
OKRA, raw	36	2.4	.3	7.6	92	51	41	.6	3	249	520	.17	.21	1.0	31
ONIONS, mature, raw	38	1.5	.1	8.7	27	36	12	.5	10	157	40	.03	.04	.2	10
green, bulb & top	36	1.5	.2	8.2	51	39		1.0	5	237	2,000	.05	.05	.4	32
ORANGES, peeled, raw	49	1.0	.2	12.2	41	20	11	.4	1	200	200	.10	.04	.4	50
ORANGE JUICE, raw	45	.7	.2	10.2	11	17	11	.2	1	200	200	.09	.03	.4	50
PAPAYA, raw	39	.6	.1	10.0	20	16		.3	3	234	1,750	.04	.04	.3	56
PARSLEY, raw	44	3.6	.6	8.5	203	63	41	6.2	45	727	8,500	.12	.26	1.2	172
PARSNIPS, raw	76	1.7	.5	17.5	50	77	32	.7	12	541	30	.07	.08	.1	10
PEACHES, raw	38	.6	.1	9.7	9	19	10	.5	1	202	1,330	.02	.05	1.0	7
PEANUTS, raw, with skins	564	26.0	47.5	18.6	69	401	206	2.1	5	674	–	1.14	.13	17.2	0

PEARS, raw	61	.7	.4	15.3	8	11	7	.3	2	130	20	.02	.04	.1	4
PEAS, raw, from pods	53	3.4	.2	12.0	62	90	35	.7	1	170	680	.28	.12	—	21
green, cooked	71	5.4	.4	12.1	23	99	—	1.8	1	196	540	.28	.11	2.3	20
split, cooked	115	8.0	.3	20.8	11	89	—	1.7	13	296	40	.15	.09	.9	—
PECANS	687	9.2	71.2	14.6	73	289	142	2.4	trace	603	130	.86	.13	.9	2
PEPPERS, raw, sweet, green	22	1.2	.2	4.8	9	22	18	.7	13	213	420	.08	.08	.5	128
raw, red	31	1.4	.3	7.1	13	30	—	.6	trace	—	4,450	.08	.08	.5	204
PERSIMMONS, raw	127	.8	.4	33.5	27	26	8	2.5	1	310	—	—	—	—	66
PINEAPPLE, raw	52	0.4	0.2	13.7	17	8	13	0.5	1	146	70	.09	.03	.2	17
juice, canned, unsweetened	55	.4	.1	13.5	15	9	12	.3	1	149	50	.05	.02	.2	9
PLUMS, prune-type, raw	75	.8	.2	19.7	12	18	9	.5	1	170	300	.03	.03	.5	4
POTATOES, raw	76	2.1	.1	17.1	7	53	34	.6	3	407	trace	.10	.04	1.5	20
baked in skin	93	2.6	.1	21.1	9	65	—	.7	4	503	trace	.10	.04	1.7	20
boiled in skin	76	2.1	.1	17.1	7	53	—	.6	3	407	trace	.09	.04	1.5	16
PUMPKIN, raw	26	1.0	.1	6.5	21	44	12	.8	1	340	1,600	.05	.11	.6	9
PUMPKIN SEEDS, dry	553	29.0	46.7	15.0	51	1,144	—	11.2	—	—	70	.24	.19	2.4	—
RADISHES, raw	17	1.0	.1	3.6	30	31	15	1.0	18	322	10	.03	.03	.3	26
RAISINS, natural, uncooked	289	2.5	.2	77.4	62	101	35	3.5	27	763	20	.11	.08	.5	1
RASPBERRIES, raw, black	73	1.5	1.4	15.7	30	22	30	0.9	1	199	trace	.03	.09	0.9	18
red	57	1.2	.5	13.6	22	22	20	0.9	1	168	130	.03	.09	0.9	25
RICE, brown, cooked	119	2.5	.6	25.5	12	73	29	.5	3	70	0	.09	.02	1.4	0
RICE BRAN	276	13.3	15.8	50.8	76	1,386	—	19.4	trace	1,495	0	2.26	.25	29.8	0
RICE POLISHINGS	265	12.1	12.8	57.7	69	1,106	—	16.1	trace	714	0	1.84	.18	28.2	0
RUTABAGAS, raw	46	1.1	.1	11.0	66	39	15	.4	5	239	580	.07	.07	1.1	43
cooked	35	.9	.1	8.2	59	31	—	.3	4	167	550	.06	.06	.8	26
RYE, whole-grain	334	12.1	1.7	73.4	38	376	115	3.7	1	467	0	.43	.22	1.6	0
flour, dark	327	16.3	2.6	68.1	54	536	73	4.5	1	860	0	.61	.22	2.7	0
SAUERKRAUT, solids and liquid	18	1.0	.2	4.0	36	18	—	.5	—	140	50	.03	.04	.2	14
SESAME SEEDS, dry, whole	563	18.6	49.1	21.6	1,160	616	181	10.5	60	725	30	.98	.24	5.4	0
SOYBEANS, dry, raw	403	34.1	17.7	33.5	226	554	265	8.4	5	1,677	80	1.10	.31	2.2	—
cooked	130	11.0	5.7	10.8	73	179	—	2.7	2	540	80	.21	.09	.6	0
sprouted, raw	46	6.2	1.4	5.3	48	67	—	1.0	—	—	80	.23	.20	.8	13
sprouted, cooked	38	5.3	1.4	3.7	43	50	—	.7	—	—	80	.16	.15	.7	4

SOYBEAN CURD (TOFU)	72	7.8	4.2	2.4	128	126	111	1.9	7	42	0	.06	.03	.1	—
SOYBEAN FLOUR, full-fat	421	36.7	20.3	30.4	199	558	247	8.4	1	1,660	110	.85	.31	2.1	0
SOYBEAN MILK, powder	429	41.8	20.3	28.0	278	—	300	—	—	—	—	—	—	—	—
SPINACH, raw	26	3.2	.3	4.3	93	51	88	3.1	71	470	8,100	.10	.20	.6	51
cooked	23	3.0	.3	3.6	93	38	65	2.2	50	324	8,000	.07	.14	.5	28
SQUASH, summer, all varieties, raw	19	1.1	1.1	4.2	28	29	16	0.4	1	202	410	.05	.09	1.0	22
cooked	14	.9	.1	3.1	25	25	16	0.4	1	141	370	.05	.08	.8	22
winter, raw	50	1.4	.3	12.4	22	38	17	.6	1	369	3,700	.05	.11	.6	10
cooked (baked)	63	1.8	.4	15.4	28	48	17	.8	1	461	4,200	.05	.13	.7	13
STRAWBERRIES, raw	37	.7	.5	8.4	21	21	12	1.0	1	164	60	.03	.07	.6	59
SUNFLOWER SEED KERNELS, dry	560	24.0	47.3	19.9	120	837	38	7.1	30	920	50	1.96	.23	5.4	—
TOMATOES, ripe, raw	22	1.1	.2	4.7	13	27	14	.5	3	244	900	.06	.04	.7	23
TOMATO JUICE, canned	19	.9	.1	4.3	7	18	10	.9	200	227	800	.05	.03	.8	16
TURNIPS, raw	30	1.0	.2	6.6	39	30	20	.5	49	268	trace	.04	.07	.6	36
cooked	23	.8	.2	4.9	35	24	—	.4	34	188	trace	.04	.05	.3	22
TURNIP GREENS, raw	28	3.0	.3	5.0	246	58	58	1.8	—	—	7,600	.21	.39	.8	139
WALNUTS, black	628	20.5	59.3	14.8	trace	570	190	6.0	3	460	300	.22	.11	.7	—
English	651	14.8	64.0	15.8	99	380	131	3.1	2	450	30	.33	.13	.9	2
WATERCRESS, raw	19	2.2	.3	3.0	151	54	20	1.7	52	282	4,900	.08	.16	.9	79
WATERMELON, raw	26	.5	.2	6.4	7	10	8	.5	1	100	590	.03	.03	.2	7
WHEAT, whole-grain, spring	330	14.0	2.2	69.1	36	383	160	3.1	3	370	—	.57	.12	4.3	0
winter	330	12.3	1.8	71.7	46	354	160	3.4	3	370	—	.52	.12	4.3	0
WHEAT BRAN	213	16.0	4.6	61.9	119	1,276	490	14.9	9	1,121	0	.72	.35	21.0	0
WHEAT GERM, raw	363	26.6	10.9	46.7	72	1,118	336	9.4	3	827	0	2.01	.68	4.2	0
WHEY, powder	349	12.9	1.1	73.5	646	589	130	1.4	—	—	—	.50	2.51	.8	—
YAM, tuber, raw	101	2.1	.2	23.2	20	69	31	.6	—	600	50	.10	.04	.5	9
YEAST, brewer's debittered	283	38.8	1.0	38.4	210	1,753	231	17.3	121	1,894	trace	15.61	4.28	37.9	trace
torula	277	38.6	1.0	37.0	424	1,713	165	19.3	15	2,046	trace	14.01	5.06	44.4	trace
YOGURT, from whole milk	62	3.0	3.4	4.9	111	87	12	trace	47	132	140	.03	.16	.1	1
from skimmed milk	50	3.4	1.7	5.2	120	94	13	trace	51	143	70	.04	.18	.1	1

SOURCES: Agriculture Handbook No. 8., U.S. Dept. Agric. Washington, D.C.; Home and Garden Bulletin No. 72.

INDEX

Fredricks, Dr. Carlton, 124,
129, 131
Fruit salad á lá Airola,
recipe, 251

G

Gallbladder problems,
treatment, 92
Gallstones, 92
Garten, Dr. M. O., 45, 119
Gas, flatulence, 77, 162
Gastric ulcers, 154
Gerovital, or KH-3, 147
Gerson, Dr. Max, 59
Glaucoma, treatment, 95
Glutamine,
in treatment of alcoholism, 32
Gout, treatment, 97, 162
IQ and, 98
Gray hair, 162
to restore natural color to,
162
Gum problems, 68

H

Hair loss, treatment, 49
Halitosis, cause and treatment, 99
Halvah, how to make, 254
Hayfever, 162
Health, 200
emotional stress and, 200
exercise and, 200
nutrition and, 184
relaxation and, 200-201
Health menu, 201
Heart disease, 101
Hemorrhoids, causes,
treatment, 107
Hegsted, Dr. D. M., 140
Herbs
how to prepare, 235
how to use therapeutically,
234, 236
High blood pressure, treatment,
109
emotional causes, 111
low blood pressure, 111

High-protein diet
arteriosclerosis and, 194
danger of in reducing, 137
danger of overindulgence in,
137, 192, 194
mineral deficiencies caused
by, 193
premature aging and, 194
pyorrhea and, 193
schizophrenia and, 193
Hirschfelt, M., 34
Hoffer, Dr. A., 151, 152
Honey, 191
Hornet stings, 162
Hyperkinetic children, 162
Hypoglycemia, treatment, 112
diet for, 113
peptic ulcers and, 156
Hypothalamus, 31
Hypothyroidism, 164

I

Impetigo, 162
Indigestion, 77
Infections, 162, 164
Inflammations, 164
Insomnia, 162
Intestinal worms, 160
Iron deficiency anemia, 36
Issels, Dr. Josef, 56, 241
Itchy skin, 162

J

Jaundice, treatment, 115
Juices, 230
green juice, 232
how to make, 231
lactic acid juices, 233
therapeutic use of, 230, 233

K

Kefir, how to make, 253
Keith, H. M., 91
Kelp, 191, 207
Kenyon, Dr. Herbert, 144

ABOUT THIS BOOK

"HOW TO GET WELL is extremely well organized, practical and helpful for the reader, and a giant example of research and work. I am sure that I will refer to it many times, giving you credit all the way . . . Many thanks, and congratulations!"

**Linda Clark, M.A., Author, Contributing
Editor, LET'S LIVE Magazine**

"Please send me a copy of Paavo Airola's HOW TO GET WELL. I am considering one or two of his books emphasizing biological medicine as text books in my Honors Class on nutrition-health relationship. I know of no better author on such matters."

**Dr. Louis Junker, Professor of Economics
Western Michigan University**

"Dr. Paavo Airola has done it again. This time it's HOW TO GET WELL — the crowning glory of his 30 years of the most discriminating world-wide research. With this book he firmly established the fact which we, a few of his long-time followers, knew all along — that he is THE MOST OUTSTANDING NUTRITIONIST in the world today."

**Richard Barmakian, Nutrition Consultant,
Pasadena, California**

"Your book is sensational! I am impressed with the way in which you conceived and constructed it, with your fabulous and expert presentation of the philosophy of biological medicine, and with common and academic sense that it makes . . . There are but few informed and courageous leaders concerned with the well-being of the public; leaders who have not only dedicated their lives to helping their fellow men, but who have the sufficient knowledge and qualifications to accomplish this. I am proud to tell you that I feel you to be one of those few. By writing this book, you rendered a great service to a disease-ridden mankind."

Dr. H. Rudolph Alsleben, M.D., Anaheim, California

"Your book is better than well written, IT IS EXCELLENT. Plus, it is precise and easy to understand for those who wish to renew their aspirations in the quest for Ideal Health."

Elmo Pinta, Glen Ellyn, Illinois

"Dr. Airola is not only the most knowledgeable, but also the most honest writer of them all."

Dr. Kathlene M. Fricia, D.C., Pasadena, California

"I stayed up all night reading your book . . . It's terrific."

Rev. Robert Strecker, Los Angeles, California

"Truly an amazing book. A health book to end all the other 'so-called' health books."

Ethel Adler, Nutrition Consultant, Los Angeles, California

"Paavo Airola's book, HOW TO GET WELL, is interesting, informative, and helpful. $8.95 worth of information on every page!"

I. M. Marynak, Skokie, Illinois

"I received HOW TO GET WELL yesterday and have spent several hours reading it. It's a book that should be in every home and I'm going to see that it is in quite a few! I now have nine of your books, and wouldn't part with any of them."

Martha Cutkomp, Lake Elmo, Minnesota

"Your book is wonderful . . . Congratulations that the first edition sold out so soon! This do-it-yourself sort of book is what the public is hungry for. No one deserves more than yourself the success you are having — you have worked hard many years and HAVE LIVED BY YOUR PHOSOPHY as a dynamic example of what you teach."

Betty Lee Morales, Nutrition Consultant, President, Cancer Control Society, Secretary, National Health Federation

"Congratulations on your fabulous new book. HOW TO GET WELL is doubtlessly the book of the century! At our store, it is selling better than even our paperbacks!"

Scott S. Smith, Vegetarian World.

"Thank you so much for the recent book order. Airola's book, HOW TO GET WELL, is a superior book to all that I have read on the subject of getting well."

John Mastel, Health Food Store Owner, St. Paul, Minnesota

"You are the best of the best . . . This is the most useful and practical book on natural therapies I've seen. It will help millions of people. This remarkable volume is worth its weight in gold."

David Troutman, Nutritionist, Los Angeles, California

"No doubt in my mind about it — you are the Number One nutritionist and the most knowledgeable health writer."

Audry Smith, Reg. Therapist. Escondido, California

"Your book, HOW TO GET WELL, arrived today. It is a good book — very well done."

Dr. Alan H. Nittler, M.D. Santa Cruz, California

"I wish to compliment you on your brilliant and dynamic presentation of contemporary health problems and how they can be overcome in a most logical and convincing sequence. I have received great pleasure and stimulation from reading your books, and feel you have given to the Western world some priceless teachings which they are so pathetically in need of."

Dr. M.O. Garten, N.D., D.C., San Jose, California

"HOW TO GET WELL is a tremendous book and it sells itself. Our customers agree that it is the most popular and informative book we have stocked at any time. We feel that it is 1974's best seller in the health book field."

Carl P. Pearson, Health Food Store Owner, Mount Vernon, Washington

"HOW TO GET WELL has so much information, it is a real GEM.

Helen P. Ahlbrecht, New York, N.Y.

"I have recently purchased your book, HOW TO GET WELL. I want to commend you for a very excellent book which will be a valuable guide in any physician's office."

Dr. David R. Anderson, M.A., N.D. Wheeling, Illinois

(There are hundreds of similar unsolicited comments in publishers' files.)